W9-AER-614

Praise for *Science Under Siege*

"Fumento's new book is a spiky attempt to introduce more intellect into the overemotional popular debate on environmental hazards. A must-read for journalists, *Science Under Siege* offers any reader with a large capacity for detail a lively, well-documented, pro-technology perspective on the risks of modern life."

John Wilkes
The Los Angeles Times

"Michael Fumento proved to be an accurate forecaster when he argued in his 1990 book, *The Myth of Heterosexual AIDS*, that the disease would not make apocalyptic inroads into America's general population. In *Science Under Siege* he debunks such popular scare threats as Alar, dioxin, pesticides, electromagnetic fields, food irradiation and video display terminals, as well as the air-cleansing claims made on behalf of gasoline additives."

Fred Singer
The Wall Street Journal

"This cranky, carefully documented and frequently funny book should be required reading for concerned citizens and community organizations. . . . It provides an invaluable rational antidote to the incessant squeal of hype and alarm issuing from our TV sets and news magazines."

Curt Suplee
The Washington Post

"Loudmouth technophobes are far more interested in grabbing a headline, bashing a technology, scaring up a rabble and selling a show than in drawing a line between good science and bad. An excellent new primer on the subject is Michael Fumento's *Science Under Siege* . . . ."

Peter Huber
Forbes

"Michael Fumento, with his new book, *Science Under Siege*, scathingly criticizes perpetrators of . . . environmental cancer scares."

Candace Crandall
The San Diego Union-Tribune

"Michael Fumento's book shows in detail how the environmental movement has used a caricature to frighten people into believing that modern life is carcinogenic."

Angelo M. Codevilla
National Review

THE MYTH OF
HETEROSEXUAL
AIDS

THE MYTH OF
HETEROSEXUAL
AIDS

MICHAEL FUMENTO

Regnery Gateway

WASHINGTON, D.C.

Due to lack of space, permissions appear on page 452.

Library of Congress Cataloging-in-Publication Data

Fumento, Michael.
    The myth of heterosexual AIDS / Michael Fumento.
        p.   cm.
    Previously published: New York: Basic Books, 1990.
    Includes bibliographical references and index.
    ISBN 0-89526-729-2
        1. AIDS (Disease)—Political aspects—United States. 2. AIDS
(Disease)—Social aspects—United States. 3. AIDS (Disease)—
Transmission. 4. AIDS (Disease)—Epidemiology. I. Title.
    RA644.A25F86 1993   93-26358
    362.1′969792—dc20   CIP

Published in the United States by Regnery Gateway, Inc. 1130 17th Street, NW
Washington, DC 20036

Distributed to the trade by National Book Network 4720-A Boston Way
Lanham, MD 20706

Printed on acid-free paper.

Manufactured in the United States of America.

10 9 8 7 6 5 4 3 2 1

To My Parents

CONTENTS

ACKNOWLEDGMENTS

I must state first that all the opinions expressed in this book are my own. Acknowledging that some individuals provided assistance in some areas in no way indicates that they necessarily endorse each and every idea, conclusion, and more importantly, criticism. I wish to thank Thomas (Burke) Balch for stretching his work weeks, already often 100 hours long, that much further to help me in almost all areas of this project, especially in editing the first draft. While I began the book before meeting him, the thought of having had to complete it without his help is terrifying. Thanks also to Matthew Kaufman for his editing and skills as a sounding board. The fortuity of his having been a time zone behind mine meant that poor Mr. Kaufman was the victim of many an excited late-night phone call. Mary Oliver's dogged efforts as research assistant for the paperback edition allowed me full insulation from the monstrosity known as the Los Angeles library system. Dr. Joel Hay now at the University of Southern California, Los Angeles has my appreciation for reviewing the entire manuscript and providing a constant flow of advice and new information. Chuck Fallis, public affairs specialist at the federal Centers for Disease Control (CDC) in Atlanta, is as efficient a public affairs official as one could ever hope to meet, and I note also the help I received from Sam Friedman of the New York Department of Health and the health department public affairs officials in San Francisco, Los Angeles, Houston, and elsewhere.

James Boulet, formerly of The Moral Majority, graciously opened up to me that organization's Washington office AIDS files. Allan Ryskind did likewise at *Human Events*, even though he was convinced that I was going to find material to use against his own publication. (I didn't.)

Thanks to Paul Noël for his ideas and Susan Adair for help in pulling articles and checking citations. Homer Giles, my publisher at the American Economic Foundation, and Leon Stevens, came through with some badly needed Nexis research.

Editors at *Commentary, The New Republic, The American Spectator*, and elsewhere have provided me with space to get some of this material across before it became of mere historical interest.

Robert Whelan provided valuable material from the United Kingdom and has been a tremendous help in promoting my own material in his country.

This project would not have been but for the faith of my editor Bill Newlin and that of my agents Glen Hartley and Lynn Chu. I have found, sadly, that our nation is not nearly so enamored of new ideas as it prides itself on being, and those few who are willing to support iconoclasm deserve our greatest respect.

Finally, I must acknowledge the epidemiologists. Dr. Alexander Langmuir is the former chief epidemiologist at CDC. Even though he is called "the grandfather of epidemiology" and his efforts at CDC laid the groundwork for tracking the AIDS virus decades before the epidemic hit, he is now scorned by colleagues many years his junior for daring to declare that the epidemic has been overstated. Both Langmuir and Dr. Rand Stoneburner, formerly Director of AIDS Research at the New York City Department of Health and now with the World Health Organization in Geneva, provided special assistance with the epidemiology sections and made sure I was never at a loss for the very latest data. Dr. Harold Jaffe, formerly chief AIDS epidemiologist at CDC, also lent far more time in answering my questions than I had any right to expect. Further, his bravery in challenging AIDS alarmism has been truly inspirational. Thanks finally to all the other epidemiologists, federal and local, AIDS and otherwise, whose names are far too numerous to mention but without whose work this book would not exist. Ignored though they have been by the politicians and reporters, the epidemiologists are truly the heroes of the AIDS epidemic.

INTRODUCTION TO THE PAPERBACK EDITION

"Until now, most experts have held that everyone is at risk of acquiring AIDS, so messages promoting less risky behavior, they say, should be broadcast scattershot . . . . But other experts are now arguing otherwise." So read the first paragraph of a front-page *New York Times* story, in March 1993, entitled "Targeting Urged in Attack on AIDS."[1] Six years have elapsed since my first article suggesting that AIDS be treated like other diseases by identifying and then reducing risk factors, and the time that suggestion appeared in America's newspaper of record. What happened during that time to me and to the first edition of this book shows how pervasively the AIDS debate has been dominated by politics, to the detriment of science and public health.

To begin with, this book came very close not to being published. It was rejected by publisher after publisher, not because of basic disagreement with the facts or because of skepticism as to its salability but because, as one house put it, "I'm not convinced that his argument—or the cause of curing AIDS for those who have it or are prone to it—is best served by publishing it in book form." Another stated, disingenuously, "I'm afraid I feel the book community is terribly overloaded on this subject, and also on Michael Fumento's point of view on this subject." Of course, there was no other book asserting "my point of view"; indeed, there were no anti-alarmist books available at all. There were, however, over two hundred AIDS books in print, most of which to varying extents put forth opposite positions.

I finally did acquire a publisher, but my tribulations were just beginning. In August of 1988, while employed as an AIDS analyst for the U.S. Commission on Civil Rights in the Office of the General Counsel, I published an article, a cover story in *The New Republic* (see chapter thirteen of this book), that criticized some conservatives' reaction to AIDS.[2] I was called onto the carpet and told that I had criticized people who were friends of the commission. Whether these criticisms were valid was not at issue, nor, I was told, was the First Amendment's guarantee of free speech. I was dropped from the AIDS project and relegated to checking other people's citations, and even then I was harassed. I had no choice but to resign.[3]

In the meantime, for a period of nine months I had been negotiating with a conservative think tank concerning a fellowship to complete the book. Everything had been confirmed and I was told that a letter would be sent in a matter of days with the official invitation. Then the article appeared. Several weeks went by without my receiving any letter. When I finally called I was told the fellowship had been denied and that was the end of it. There was never any written notification nor reason given. The infamous article, incidentally, was entitled "The Political Uses of an Epidemic."

Little did I know that what came before publication would be just a taste of what would come after. One paragraph in a letter I received from a Houston reader sums it up:

> Reality hit home when I tried to purchase *The Myth of Heterosexual AIDS* last November. Not only was I unable to locate a single book store in Houston carrying the book, but your publisher removed *Myth* from print. I then began researching the subject matter and soon realized that there is widespread collusion and conspiracy to discredit you and your book. The news media are playing a major part in what I now feel is deliberate and intended deceit, distortion, and misrepresentation on the entire subject of AIDS.[4]

Sound like right-wing paranoia? Yet it was all too true. Eventually, even the liberal *Washington Monthly* would agree, in an article by Leslie Kaufman that appeared in its March 1992 issue.

THE BANNING OF A BOOK

Months before the book was complete, letters were already circulating to book distributors asking that *Myth* be kept off store shelves. My editor and I originally thought that only a few stores would go along

with this boycott and none of the chains. We were wrong. Indeed, one of the largest chains in the country refused to buy a single copy until I announced their boycott on national TV. An ABC reporter called them about it, and then and there, it seems, they decided to begin stocking it, albeit too late for the book to take advantage of the publicity. A short while later, the president and CEO of this chain signed his name to a full-page advertise-ment in numerous newspapers condemning "diverse special interest groups" for, among other things, trying to keep certain titles out of stores. This threat to the Republic, of which the ad warned, was the effort of a Christian group to get the chain to stop selling girlie magazines. Perhaps if *Myth* had included some dirty pictures, the chain would have felt obligated to carry it.

Granted, not every store can carry every book, but that was not the problem here. For example, when one acquaintance asked the manager of a store in New York City why he didn't carry the book, he was told "for editorial reasons." Had he even seen the book? "No." A San Diego doctor reported to me that when he requested the book in that city, a store clerk said they wouldn't carry the book because it was "politically incorrect." In Cincinnati, when another acquaintance went to pick up the book from the store where he'd ordered it, the clerk tried to talk him out of buying it.

I use these anecdotes to illustrate motives behind a problem that occurs on a national scale with many so-called "conservative" books. Early in 1990, a group of thirty physicians in the Pacific Northwest (the states of Washington and Oregon) discovered they hadn't found a single store in either state that carried *Myth*. They reported this to a Seattle, Washington, TV station, KING, which in a televised report noted that it had contacted eighty different stores without finding a single copy of the book. Indeed, only one store had *ever* carried the book; it sold out quickly and didn't reorder until after KING contacted them. One university book store in Seattle claimed to have over 350,000 titles, including every single AIDS title in print. Except one.[5]

You might think that the San Francisco area, with the highest rate of AIDS of any metropolitan area, would have a high interest in *Myth* and that the book would be readily available there. Think again. Arthur Hu, writing in *Asian Week*, said, "The best book on AIDS hysteria today is *The Myth of Heterosexual AIDS*, by Michael Fumento, but it

has been so widely discredited by the AIDS political machine that it's practically a banned book in Bay Area bookstores."[6]

In metropolitan Denver, my home at the time, the Tattered Cover, one of the largest, best-known book stores in the nation, had told *Westword*, a local weekly for whom I had written on this subject, that "[B. Dalton and Waldenbooks] usually keep *The Myth of Heterosexual AIDS* in stock, but are currently sold out."[7] In an area with a population of about 2.5 million people, the book was therefore unavailable at the distributor level, and all the stores just happened to have sold out.

Both the Tattered Cover and a B. Dalton store advised me they had no intention of reordering the book, at least until the paperback version came out. At the Tattered Cover I was told they weren't carrying the book because "it is over six months old." I personally surveyed their massive collection of AIDS books and found that of the eighty books they carried on AIDS, sixty-eight were published in 1989 or earlier, making them at least nine months old (the time of the search was October of 1990). The store carried books that said AIDS is really syphilis, that the disease is the result of biological warfare, that AIDS can be cured through a positive mental attitude. It had Gene Antonio's book, the *AIDS Coverup*, which said that as much as a fifth of the U.S. population would be dead or dying of AIDS by 1990. It had AIDS books from publishing houses so tiny that some didn't even use typeset. But it did not have *The Myth of Heterosexual AIDS*, published by Basic Books, a subsidiary of one of the nation's largest publishers, HarperCollins.

Ironically, at the same time, the Tattered Cover, in celebration of Banned Books Week, had just organized a seminar on censorship,[8] mounting a large store display. Needless to say, *Myth* was not featured.

Interestingly, the owner of the Tattered Cover later wrote to *Westword* saying she couldn't imagine what I was talking about since *Myth* had sold quite well at the store and had been continuously stocked. Indeed, it had sold quite well until it was suddenly no longer available. At many stores, as at the Tattered Cover, the problem was not the distributor, or the failure of the store to order copies, but store clerks who would fail to put the book on the shelf or falsely claim to be out of copies.

This reveals the extent of the problem in getting *Myth* to would-be purchasers. Any one person in a chain connecting the publisher to the customer can keep a book from being available. If not the owner, it might be the manager. If not the manager, it might be the clerks, or any one given clerk. At any step of the way, a politically correct thinker could have kept the book away from customers—and usually someone did.

If *Myth* was difficult to find in the U.S., it was impossible to find in the UK, because not a single British publisher would print it. This despite articles in the *Sunday Times* and the *Daily Telegraph* virtually taunting the publishing industry for not doing so.[9] One publisher told the *Sunday Times* he rejected it because "it was addressed to a set of American concerns."[10] But the British media, like the American, had made a tremendous fuss over the book. Another publisher's comment was even more transparent: he "felt the author did not have enough research to base his conclusions on." No, and *no* amount of research would have been enough. In the end, the nation that provided safe harbor to *Satanic Verses* author Salman Rushdie effectively banned the book. You could read all about it in the British papers, hear about it on the radio, see its author on British TV, but you could not buy the book. In Australia and Germany, it was the same story, despite major publicity in both countries. The German-language representative for Basic Books informed me that one German publisher said he couldn't publish *Myth* because it went against what the government was saying. Yes, I thought. No doubt that was the reason for turning away books in the 1930s as well.

A FOUNDATION OF LIES

Having been so successful at keeping the book out of stores, activists then began removing it from library shelves and reporting it lost. You don't have to take anyone's word for this. Go to a couple of local libraries and try to find it. Most likely you will find that it was checked out and never returned.

Having denied the public the right to see the book, AIDS activists concentrated on telling them what they would have read had they been able to obtain a copy. Donna Minkowitz at the *Village Voice* said it was "bilge" built on "a foundation of lies."[11] Common epithets included labeling it cruel, uncompassionate, racist, sexist, and homophobic. AIDS activists routinely turned my conclusions on their heads in order to pronounce me a bigot or worse. For example, one reviewer, writing in the *Orange County Register,* stated:

> . . . he refers to the possibility that minorities are genetically predisposed to AIDS, and says that is one of the reasons AIDS in the minority community is growing rapidly. This kind of journalistic bigotry is unacceptable to me and needs to be called what it is—pure and simple racism.[12]

In fact, *Myth* states (page 33), that although one study pointed to a genetic predisposition to AIDS, its results had not been duplicated by other laboratories and the study was later retracted by the scientists citing laboratory error. Still, if the evidence had been that blacks were genetically predisposed to AIDS, as they are, for instance, to sickle cell anemia, how would reporting such a result make me a bigot?

Aside from finding myself branded the worst hate-monger since Adolf took the easy way out, what stunned me most about such reviewers was their willingness to contort what was clearly stated in the book. The same Donna Minkowitz who claimed that *Myth* was built on a "foundation of lies" wasn't beyond telling a few of her own, writing, "Heterosexual intercourse, he claims, is so intrinsically gentle that vaginal tissues are never broken."[13] Actually the book states: "While the vaginal wall is far more rugged than the anus, the science writer John Langone notes that the former is far from impervious to the sort of damage that might allow transmission of HIV . . ." (*Myth*, pages 49 and 50). While not doubting for a moment that the average *Village Voice* reader wanted to see *Myth* slammed, the reader still deserved an accurate description of what was in it.

Maybe the average *Village Voice* reader expects dishonest reviews. I would guess, however, that the average reader of science magazines does not. Thus, what happened with two of them was the most shocking of all.

Probably the most prestigious science journal in the world is the

British magazine *Nature*. *Nature*'s review of *Myth* ran quite early, just as the book was coming out, something journals will do when they are making a conscious effort to affect how a book will be received. The reviewer for *Nature* was Duncan Campbell who, among many other things, asserted:

> Only a writer whose prejudices deny humanity could write in such bad taste as this: "Although AIDS is no joke, there is good news and bad news about the length of HIV infectiousness . . . the 'good news' [is] that the great majority and perhaps almost all, of HIV-infected persons will develop debilitating symptoms or die."[14]

In fact, what the book says, on page 25, is:

> The "good news" here is actually terrible news for anyone infected. Originally, it was thought that only a small percentage of those infected with the virus would go on to develop the disease. While this was reassuring to infected persons, it made the long-term outlook for the spread of the disease look bad because it meant that large numbers of healthy persons would be spreading the virus to others indefinitely. But a consensus of opinion has now formed that the great majority, and perhaps almost all, of HIV-infected persons will develop debilitating symptoms or die.

How different, I wonder, is this from taking a statement like, "Judaism is not a gutter religion" and presenting it as "Judaism is . . . a gutter religion"?

There is no nice term for what Campbell did in his review. He lied. He lied blatantly, and he lied often. It was some consolation to know that some of these lies were self-evident even without reading my book. For example, he stated, "The true myth of this book—the proposition that heterosexual transmission of the 'pure' sort (which he labels tertiary transmission), cannot occur—is an invention by Fumento."[15] But then, just two paragraphs later, he wrote, "Fumento goes on to admit that tertiary transmission has been observed . . ."[16]

Campbell also engaged in such niceties as putting into quotation marks things I had not said. In order to back up his initial claim that *Myth* stated there was no tertiary transmission, he quoted the book as saying heterosexuals get HIV infection "only from shared needles, from transfusions, from clotting factor . . . from their mothers at or before birth, and sometimes through sexual intercourse with persons in these categories and bisexuals," to which he adds, as if it were a paraphrase, "but never from another heterosexual, infected hetero-sexually."[17] In fact, the quote, which appears on pages 15–16 and on the back of the first edition, does not contain that key word "only." But for Campbell to make his point it *had to* contain it, so he simply inserted it.

What's really remarkable, however, is that an esteemed scientific journal such as *Nature* should assign a nonscientist such as Duncan Campbell to review the book at all. The frankly left-wing *Village Voice* might be expected to employ a radical lesbian to review a work of science journalism. But *Nature*? Campbell's only AIDS background is as a homosexual AIDS activist. Further, when I offered a reply, *Nature* refused to run it. Acting Book Review Editor Maxine Clarke wrote back: "My own view is that Mr. Campbell is surely at least as qualified as you to comment on the AIDS epidemic." As to Campbell's misrep-resentations of fact and his bad science, she said only, "I am sure you appreciate that a reviewer is free to express his or her own opinions whether or not they concur with the author's view and so it would not, therefore, be appropriate to publish your letter."[18]

Chalk up another point for those who believe that everything concerning the AIDS epidemic is a matter of opinion. After all, it makes sense in its own perverse way. If one can take a statistic indicating that 85 percent of the nation's AIDS cases come from 5 percent of the population and say this means AIDS does not discrimi-nate, why not take a book that says one thing and quote it as saying something else? What counts is not what the epidemic is doing or what the book is saying but what the epidemic *should* do and what the book *should* say.

Fortunately, another respected British journal, the *Spectator*, did allow me to run an article in response, one which detailed the troubles I had had both in Britain and the U.S.

Back in the United States, *Science* is probably the most prestigious science magazine. But *Myth* fared no better there. Like *Nature*, *Science* skipped over any number of scientists, doctors, and science writers and turned *Myth* over to a professor of post-structuralist linguistics, Paula Treichler.

Treichler is best known for coediting *A Feminist Dictionary*, which enlightens readers on such topics as: "testosterone poisoning," "lesbian consciousness," "egotistical world view" (defined as "men's point of view on all issues"), "heterosexually impaired" (defined as "large group often ignorant of their condition"), "compulsory heterosexuality," and "de-dyking the apartment"—that's when the folks come over and you have to make it look like your lover isn't. She also introduces such colorful acronyms as SCUM, the "Society for Cutting Up Men"; LUNA, "Lesbians United in Non-Nuclear Action"; and DARE, "Dykes Against Racism Everywhere."[19]

Treichler is decidedly *not* known for her expertise in AIDS. Her major contribution on the subject was for a Marxist quarterly, *October* (the name refers to the Soviet October Revolution), where it was accompanied by such essays as "How to Have Promiscuity in an Epidemic," featuring drawings of men having anal and oral sex with each other (with a condom, of course).[20] Treichler's *October* essay railed against the assertion that the anus is more susceptible to penetration by the AIDS virus than the vagina, not on any scientific grounds but because it makes AIDS appear to be a "gay disease" which in turn "protects not only the sexual practices of heterosexuality but also its ideological superiority."[21]

Given her ideological disdain for discomfiting facts, unsurprisingly Treichler's review in *Science* was no less dishonest than Campbell's. For example, she wrote, "Incredibly, he [I] calls Africa a 'country'. . . ."[22] That certainly made me look foolish. Problem is, it wasn't true. Indeed, on four occasions, *Myth* refers to African nations as individual nations or to the continent of Africa as a continent (*Myth*, pages 111, 112, 113, and 115).

Wrote Treichler, "Fumento's own political agenda is never, after all, very far from his science. He calls, among other things, for AIDS estimates to be revised downward (for all groups, not only heterosexuals). . . ."[23] In fact, even as my book was appearing on store shelves in January, four months before Treichler's review appeared (in April), the federal Centers for Disease Control *did* revise downward the projections for all groups (this is discussed further in the new appendix). *Science*, too, refused to run a response to the Treichler review, although at least it refrained from sending me an abusive letter.

But it must be asked, who is more dishonest, Treichler or the book editor at *Science*? Treichler is a purely political animal. She assigns political motives to viruses. She only did what *Science* must have predicted she would do.

OF MICE AND MEN

Activists also pressured television shows and publications to lock me out. Four national television shows, including "Good Morning America" and "McLaughlin" on CNBC, "Eleventh Hour" on PBS, and "A Current Affair," scheduled me for appearances, then pulled out without giving a reason.

"A Current Affair" had already gone through considerable expense to send a reporter and crew to tape me. When the air date for the show came and went, my publicist called the producer, Whitney Trilling, who earlier had enthusiastically thanked me for writing the book. She said that reporter Rafael Abromowitz was still editing the piece, even though such editing jobs are usually done within a couple of days of the shooting. Several weeks later my publicist called again. This time the producer said, "It looks like it is just disappearing beneath our feet." We did not hear from "A Current Affair" again.

There were other such incidents. A reporter for the New York *Daily News* called my publicist, eager to interview me the next time I was in town. But when my publicist returned the call, the reporter said his editor had refused to allow him to do the story. Just one month before this introduction was written another writer expressed interest in a freelance article on the troubles surrounding *Myth*. When he tried to sell the article, a major newspaper magazine advised him that while it sympathized, it "was afraid of ACT-UP" (the "AIDS Coalition to Unleash Power"). At about the same time a reporter for the *New Yorker*, Peter Boyer, told me he had heard from *Newsday*'s Jack Schwartz of *Myth*'s troubles and expressed horror that such a thing could happen in this country. He asked to see a copy of the Kaufman article, and I faxed it. But he never called, nor did he return my repeated calls.

But of all the acts of cowardice surrounding *Myth*, the most painful concerned my job at the *Rocky Mountain News*. In October 1989, I moved out to the Denver area to take a job as editorial writer with the *News*, edited by Jay Ambrose. About four weeks after *Myth* started being shipped to stores and two days after *USA Today* photographed me in the newsroom for its upcoming profile, the *News* fired me without warning. The reason: I had "made too many phone calls." I've been at newspapers where reporters were criticized for not making *enough* phone calls ("I want to see you burning up those phone lines!" was a favorite of my editor at my previous newspaper), but this was something quite new. The man responsible for this indefensible charge, Managing Editor Michael Finney, had just weeks earlier responded to pressure from a feminist group by announcing an affirmative action plan, scheduling sensitivity sessions for white males, and publicly expressing his sorrow at being a white male. It wasn't too difficult to figure out what happened. After this, but for the occasional freelance piece, I was unemployed for a year-and-a-half.

The Forbes Incident—The Rest of the Story

In the introduction to the hardcover edition, I recounted how in June 1989 *Forbes* senior editor Joe Queenan wrote a profile article about me and my views for that magazine. The tone of the piece was dispassionate, much as if I had been a collector of interesting World War II memorabilia. It talked about my aforementioned trials and tribulations as much as it did about my views, with the blurb above the title stating, "Is the AIDS epidemic spreading? The answers to the question are as much political as medical, as Michael Fumento has been learning—at some cost."[24]

Little did Queenan know that I—and he—were about to suffer more of that cost. Eight days after the issue appeared, ACT-UP picketers gathered outside the building. ACT-UP a few weeks earlier had disrupted the international AIDS conference in Montreal (*Myth*, page 335) and the year before had picketed *Cosmopolitan* magazine after it ran a piece saying the risk of AIDS to heterosexuals had been overstated. Queenan's phone line started to buzz with denunciations, and even threats.[25]

The demonstrators, thirty to forty in number, soon barged into the building and demanded to speak to the magazine's editor-in-chief, multimillionaire Malcolm Forbes, Sr., who granted them an audience. Rather than stand up for his magazine's right to print mild-mannered articles about people with diverse opinions, Forbes printed an unprecedented retraction of the Queenan article in the next issue. He put in block letters "I AGREE" above an ACT-UP-supplied diatribe that included such statements as *"everyone is vulnerable to AIDS"* (emphasis in original).[26] In an introduction to the ACT-UP statement, he wrote that, "In the case of Michael Fumento's speculations in a forthcoming book, *The Myth of Heterosexual AIDS*, I find his views asinine."[27] Since the book wasn't even in galleys, and he could not possibly have seen it, he would be the first in a long line of critics who would blast the text they hadn't even seen. The "asinine" remark was gleefully picked up by the *New York Daily News*'s gossip columnist[28] and by *USA Today*.[29] But for columnist Pat Buchanan, not one journalistic soul publicly defended Queenan's or my right to free expression, though one writer for a homosexual New York paper said he did try, only to have it killed by his editors.[30] Queenan told me that among his journalism colleagues, it was pretty much the same case. He found the tenets of free speech didn't extend to this subject.

What I didn't say in that first introduction, for no longer applicable legal reasons, was that Forbes's shameful action was almost certainly due to an implied or explicit threat of being "outed" by ACT-UP. After Forbes's death in February 1991, the month after *Myth* came out, that closet door burst wide open. Several tabloids and a radical homosexual magazine, *Outweek*, documented Forbes's homosexuality.[31] Further details were sketched in Christopher Winan's biography, *Malcolm Forbes: The Man Who Had Everything*.[32] Winans wrote about the incident at great length.[33] Asked directly by journalist Cliff Kincaid if Forbes was blackmailed by ACT-UP, Winans responded, "It looks that way." He added that there was no evidence that a direct threat was made, but maybe Forbes saw it coming.[34]

THE AIDS TERRORISTS

The Forbes incident would not be the only case of direct terrorist action against me. After *Newsday* dared allow me to review two AIDS books,[35] the features editor of the now-defunct unofficial ACT-UP magazine *Outweek*, Michelangelo Signorile, became enraged, called the newspaper, and threatened to punish it for having allowed me to appear in their pages.[36] He then blasted the paper in his magazine and its book review editor, Jack Schwartz, with language that would make a child pornographer blush. Signorile said what he thought of me ("baboon, racist, homophobic") and demanded, in upper-case letters, "WHY THE FUCK WOULD *NEWSDAY* HAVE SUCH A HATE-FILLED, UNTALENTED, LYING LOSER RE-VIEW IMPORTANT BOOKS?"[37] He also called for a telephone bar-rage against Schwartz.

As Leslie Kaufman would later relate:

[Schwartz] began receiving anonymous phone calls late at night. Nasty calls. "They made a lot of threats," Schwartz recalls, "not the least of which was death." It was clear very few of the callers had actually read the review, says Schwartz. "What outraged these people was not the content of the review, which was very even-handed," he says, "but that we allowed this guy to write anything at all." The issue was Michael Fumento himself.[38]

On the second page of this raving, running alongside Signorile's article, was an advertisement for male prostitutes. There has never been much evidence that the hard-core AIDS activists of the ACT-UP variety care about preventing new HIV infections. They want money for AIDS research and treatment, they want more public and legal acceptance of homosexuality, and they want someone to hate.

Despite such aberrant antics as this, negative articles about ACT-UP in the mainstream media have been almost nonexistent. The media have plenty of space to condemn the hateful actions of a handful of pathetic, deranged "skinhead" neo-Nazis in Europe, but no stomach for criticizing similar tactics employed by ACT-UP members and other AIDS activists right here.

As Kaufman wrote, "Fumento is not the only AIDS writer who has been harassed for having an unpalatable point of view. Others, such as

Gina Kolata of the *New York Times* and Daniel Lynch of the *Albany Times Union*, have also been singled out for harassment by AIDS activists."[39] My colleague Joel Hay, a professor at the University of Southern California and an outspoken academic critic of the AIDS establishment, has had the unpleasant experience of having a man call his wife and tell her to tell him to stop writing about AIDS, adding simply, "I know where you live."[40]

AMERICAN NUREMBERG

The bottom line was that a book which received tremendous national and international publicity, was reviewed in virtually every major publication, was the subject of such TV shows as "Donahue," "Crossfire," the "Today Show," and "CBS This Morning"—"the kind of controversy publicists dream of,"[41] as Kaufman put it—quickly sold only twelve thousand copies and then no more.

That's where the figure has stopped because Basic, which usually stocks books for years, decided not to reprint the book. I found out about this only after I began receiving letters from people who said that not only could they not find the book in stores, they couldn't even get it from the publisher. "The decision was uncharacteristic for Basic," wrote Kaufman, "which has a reputation for keeping books in print even when back orders for them are low. Moreover, there was every reason to believe that *Myth* would continue to have an audience." The explanation, according to Martin Kessler, the chief editor at Basic, was that "the reps [representatives who sell the books to buyers] refuse to carry it."[42]

Continued Kaufman,

> Asked why the book didn't sell well, Clinton Morris, the Basic representative who sold to Waldenbooks in New York, says, "Look, it was going against everything we know about AIDS, against anything anybody who was reputable was telling us. Why buy a book like that?"[43]

This of a book that the *Journal of the American Medical Association* had termed "thoroughly researched, poignantly written, and a must read for anyone interested in learning the dynamics of the HIV epidemic or health care planning."[44] This of an author who, the *New England Journal of Medicine* said, "marshals a substantial amount of epidemiological data and interprets it in a credible fashion to support his contention. He demonstrates successfully that the 'heterosexual breakout' widely predicted in the mid-1980s has failed to materialize and does not seem likely to. The book is well worth reading for this critical reinterpretation of the available data."[45] This of a book that carried an endorsement by the former chief epidemiologist for the federal Centers for Disease Control and Prevention.

DEFENDERS OF FREE SPEECH? OUT TO LUNCH

François Marie Arouet Voltaire wrote in a letter, "Monsieur l'abbé, I detest what you write, but I would give my life to make it possible for you to continue to write." I've heard versions of that sentiment expressed many times in my life, but I no longer believe any but a very tiny handful of people actually mean it.

In his 1993 book *Ambition, Discrimination, and Censorship in the Libraries*, Jefferson Selth wrote:

> A colleague who helped me found the Southern California Coalition for Intellectual Freedom in 1979 later became a Unitarian Universalist minister. Writing her recently, I mentioned the latest example of suppression à la Ibsen or Capra: Michael Fumento's *The Myth of Heterosexual AIDS*, which had been withdrawn from most bookstores in the country because of a nationally planned program of theft, defacement, and threats against the store owners.

He continued:

> My friend's reply astounded me. She said she'd changed her position somewhat on intellectual freedom; some printed falsehoods can be so harmful that they should not be permitted to be sold freely. At the least, she said, if Fumento's work is sold in any store, it ought to be accompanied by a sign reading, THIS BOOK IS WRONG.[46]

Concluding on this point, Selth noted that, "not one intellectual freedom group has to my knowledge denounced [the book's] suppression." Indeed, none did. Virtually no one who disagreed with *Myth* would defend the public's right to see it.

During the time of the controversies surrounding my writings on AIDS, other controversies erupted in which the media rose as one in defense of the right of free expression. When Islamic extremists threatened Salman Rushdie and even stores that carried *Satanic Verses*, the temporary measures taken by some booksellers either not to sell or not to display the book were fiercely attacked by the media and by authors' groups.[47] When Cincinnati prosecuted a museum for displaying homoerotic photos by the late Robert Mapplethorpe, which included photos of whips dangling from anuses and depictions of the sex organs of children, they were denounced vociferously by some of the same papers—such as *USA Today*—that refused to come to my aid.[48] It is safe to asssume that many of the same AIDS activists who most bitterly denounced the museums that balked at displaying Mapplethorpe were in the forefront of those seeking to ban *Myth*.

No issue more strikingly illustrates the lock-step uniformity of the mainstream American media than its coverage of AIDS. Overseas, despite—and to some extent *because*—of the publishers' refusal to carry my book, I have been the subject of profiles and lengthy interviews or major excerpts in Germany, Belgium, France,[49] the UK, and Brazil.[50] The German magazine, *Esquire*, flew me to Munich for a lengthy interview and photo session, which were incorporated in a cover story that received tremendous play.[51] In the States, *Myth* was excerpted once, by the *Chicago Sun-Times*,[52] in addition to a pre-release section in *The New Republic*.[53]

Overseas, the book was divided up like a cow by piranha. Australia's largest weekly, the *Bulletin*, took a huge excerpt and borrowed the cover of the book for its cover.[54] In Britain, the nation's most prestigious newspaper, the *Sunday Times*, excerpted such large chunks that it had to run it over a space of two weeks.[55] Indeed, the editors maintained they felt *obligated* to do so because of the blacklisting, saying, "Michael Fumento has been pilloried, big British publishers have refused to handle the book."[56] Spain's biggest daily, *El Pais*, also excerpted it, as did the Greek magazine *Pontiki*.

IF AT FIRST . . .

"Ultimately," wrote Kaufman, "the fate of *Myth* is best explained by the very orthodoxies that it sought to expose."[57] In the original introduction I wrote that, in essence, this book isn't really about AIDS. What happened to it makes the point all the clearer. What is at stake is the concept of the public's right to know versus the desire of a special interest group with an enormous financial, emotional, and political stake that the public not know. The AIDS crisis and the way our government, our leaders, and the media have manipulated it have provided perhaps the single best example of the politically correct intellectual dark ages into which our country has fallen. If these forces can take a grim disease that has utterly devastated minority sectors of the population while leaving the majority essentially unscathed, and if they can declare through proclamations, hundreds of millions of dollars of advertising, and vast media publicity that it does "not discriminate," then truly the Newspeak dictionary is well on its way to completion. It is *1984* arrived just about on schedule, a world in which "Ignorance is Strength," to use the slogan of The Party which dominated George Orwell's nightmare world.

And yet, because of the courage of one publisher and the bull-headedness of one author, *The Myth of Heterosexual AIDS* rises like the proverbial phoenix from the ashes. Its fate I cannot guess. But what can be said with certainty is that during the six years that I have labored to get our nation and others to treat AIDS like a disease instead of a political weapon, hundreds of millions of dollars of AIDS-designated dollars have been squandered and tens of thousands of Americans have been needlessly infected and will die horribly. No matter how successful the second edition of this book, it will never bring them back.

Michael Fumento
July 1993

THE MYTH OF HETEROSEXUAL AIDS

1

The Reign of Terror

Hello everybody. AIDS has both sexes running scared. Research studies now project that one in five—listen to me, hard to believe—one in five heterosexuals could be dead from AIDS at the end of the next three years. That's by 1990. One in five. It is no longer just a gay disease. Believe me.[1]

Thus, early in 1987, began a segment of the most popular daytime show in America. The speaker, one of the most beloved women in the country: Oprah Winfrey. The message was clear and simple: far from threatening just the old risk groups, the homosexuals and the drug abusers, AIDS was now rival to the greatest epidemics in history, including those of the bubonic plague.

If Winfrey's statement was not authoritative enough, there was that of the nation's highest health official, then-Health and Human Services Secretary Otis Bowen: "If we can't make progress," we face a pandemic that will make others, including the Black Death, seem "pale by comparison."[2]* Then-Surgeon General C. Everett Koop declared the disease to be "the biggest threat to health this nation has ever faced."[4] The media were quick to jump on the bandwagon: The cover of *Life* told us, "Now No One Is Safe from AIDS."[5] *U.S. News & World Report* declared, "The disease of them suddenly is the disease of *us*. The slow death presumed just a few years ago to be confined to homosexuals, Haitians, and hemophiliacs is now a plague of the mainstream, finding fertile growth among heterosexuals."[6]

We were warned. We were told that AIDS "is not just a gay disease," that it could "break out into the heterosexual community," that it "just

---

*A year later an HHS spokesman tried to excuse this remark, saying "Nobody actually predicted another Black Death, but Secretary Bowen did say about two years ago that if it were to become rampant heterosexually, it could rival the Black Death. The point was more about the fatality of the disease than the number of deaths it would cause."[3]

happened to hit gays first." Then, suddenly, it was here. The apocalypse at last, the days of wine and roses come to an end. The covers of *Time, Newsweek, U.S. News & World Report, The Atlantic,* and other magazines all shrieked about the coming heterosexual holocaust. There had been some debate over whether this would happen, but the debate was settled now. Now it was all a matter of size—a large body count or an utterly incalculable one.

Reporters scrambled in search of reactions to the new plague. They announced the demise of the sexual revolution, pumping out articles with such titles as "Spread of AIDS May Send Sex Mores Back to the '50s,"[7] "For Many Singles, the Party Is Over,"[8] "Looking for Love in the Era of AIDS,"[9] "The Love or Life Choice,"[10] and "The New Dating Game."[11] They usually began something like this:

> As AIDS and the fear of it increasingly infect the nation, a new movement toward safer sexual practices is starting to gather momentum among heterosexuals. It promises to work a major change in male-female relationships and bedroom behavior if, as some health officials warn, the fatal disease reaches epidemic proportions in the general population.[12]

Like perpetual motion machines, the articles fed upon fear, and used it to breed still more fear. Heterosexuals were reported not only giving up casual sex but indeed marrying out of fear. Said one to a news magazine, "It's a matter of settle down or die."[13]

There was "panic in the sheets" as an epidemic of AIDS hysteria swept across the country, reaching the level of national obsession. A minister wrote a letter to the editor of a newspaper saying that AIDS is "a national disaster as great as a thermonuclear war,"[14] and declaring, with no intended irony, that more education is needed to alleviate panic.

Congress declared October 1987 as AIDS Awareness/Prevention Month. Some states (such as New York) sponsored "AIDS Doesn't Discriminate" campaigns, and $4.6 million of federal money was pumped into the giant firm of Ogilvy & Mather for an AIDS advertising blitz. The Ogilvy & Mather advertisements made virtually no mention of homosexual transmission of the AIDS virus, but concentrated instead on heterosexuals.

Clearly the articles and the ad campaign were taking their toll in terror. AIDS information hotlines, initially established for homosexuals and drug abusers, found themselves swamped by non–drug-using heterosexuals. Reported the *New York Times:*

Almost across the board, the upsurge of concern among heterosexuals is reflected in telephone calls received by AIDS hot lines and other health-crisis services. Since last November [1986], for instance, 58 percent of the calls received at a center in Miami were from heterosexuals. Previously, only 23 percent were. And of the 6,000 to 7,000 calls received each month by the AIDS Foundation Hot Line of Northern California, in the San Francisco area, nearly half are now from heterosexual women.[15]

Another surge hit the nation's hot lines in 1988 after the surgeon general sent out 107 million four-page AIDS brochures to households throughout the country. An Illinois spokesman said, "The majority of our questions are about transmission." The calls, he said, included "husbands and wives who have questions about each other's activities before marriage and if that could lead to AIDS."[16]

Heterosexuals also swamped AIDS testing sites. From July 1986 to July 1987, about 2,500 persons in New York sought free anonymous testing. Within three months after this period, that number doubled, forcing the city to allocate an extra $2.5 million that year for the service.[17] One exasperated doctor at a Long Beach, California, clinic expressed hope that the media would "burn itself out" on the topic of heterosexual AIDS, thus slowing the stampede of people seeking to know if they were infected.[18] AWARE, a San Francisco-based AIDS education and testing program for women, had two counselors whose primary job was to reassure women who refused to believe they were healthy, even when a blood test showed they were not infected.[19] Such was the onslaught of terrified heterosexuals in southern California that one of two Los Angeles test sites had to turn away people by the hundreds, and the other had an eight-week waiting list.[20] Other cities were reporting similar backlogs,[21] meaning that persons truly at risk for carrying the virus could not get tested. Said one doctor, "Our concern is that all of the people who are at low risk are taking up places for high-risk people . . . people who may be transmitting the virus."[22]

Some testing clinics did not complain about the added business but, in fact, drummed it up. One such center presented its advertisement as a mini-article, complete with footnotes. "Pace of Heterosexual Spread Surprises Scientists" was the title, which was pulled in turn from the title of a *Washington Post* article. The mini-article began:

A recent study of more than 4,000 people treated at a Baltimore sexually transmitted disease clinic found that one third of the men and nearly half of the women infected with the virus that causes AIDS, became infected through heterosexual contact. AIDS has infiltrated the heterosexual population, and a meteoric rise in reported cases of HIV infection is expected because of false assumptions that AIDS is a homosexual disease.[23]*

One issue of *Playboy* indicated that the beautiful "girl next door" was making no such "false assumptions." In the magazine's February 1989 special "Love" issue, six playmates were asked: "How well do you have to know a man before you're willing to get physical?" In their one-paragraph replies, five of the six referred to AIDS and said they would go as far as demanding a blood test.[24]

Horror Books

And then came the books. In the 1988–89 *Books in Print,* over 170 books were listed whose titles began with the word *AIDS.* Some were published by the giant houses like Simon & Schuster; some, by the smaller houses; some apparently self-published. The letters *A-I-D-S* in these titles were usually written much larger or in a different color so they could be read across the length of the store, but endnotes or bibliographies were in short supply. Also, the authors seemed to lack credentials. Often the writers were medical doctors; but since their expertise rarely had anything to do with epidemiology and etiology, they were not necessarily qualified to write about AIDS any more than a football player is to comment on hockey or handball. The doctors with expertise in AIDS were too busy fighting it to publish in popular journals, and left it to others to report their findings, fairly or otherwise.

At first, it could be assumed, many of these books made money. Some made lots and lots of money. But as time went on, the later titles, like the late joiners in a pyramid scam, found that they were lucky to break even.

Some of the books implied a conspiracy, as did *The AIDS Cover-up?* Some were touted as survival guides: *A Way to Survive the AIDS Epidemic, You Can Protect Yourself and Your Family from AIDS.* Many focused on personal relations: *When Someone You Know Has AIDS* and, by a different author, *When Someone You Love has AIDS.* Several grabbed readers with analogies to the plague: *Epitaphs for the Plague Dead, The Plague Years.* Some hinted at specialists looking to broaden their scope a bit: *AIDS and Other Sexually Transmitted Diseases and*

---

*The citation for this last sentence consisted not of a medical journal or journals but of two legal texts: *AIDS: A Legal Challenge of the Eighties* and *AIDS and the Law.* It was perhaps telling that a business that felt the need to cite authorities to convince readers would feel compelled to cite legal texts. Another curious aspect of the advertisement was that it ran in a Washington paper, not in Baltimore.

the Eye, AIDS: A Guide for Dental Practice, AIDS and the Dental Team. Many had safe sex as the theme and title: *Safe Sex in the Age of AIDS, Eroticizing Safer Sex.* Some gave instructions on nonstandard cures: *Healing AIDS Naturally, Psychoimmunity and the Healing Process* (published by Celestial Arts). Some spoke of AIDS in warlike terms: *An Emergency War Plan to Fight AIDS and Other Pandemics* (published by political extremist Lyndon LaRouche & Company), *The AIDS Fighters, Mobilizing Against AIDS.* Then there were the books that insisted that they were telling you the truth (and, by implication, that others were not): *The Truth About AIDS, AIDS: The Facts, The Essential AIDS Fact Book, The Real Truth About Women and AIDS.* The titles alone were enough to indicate that there must have been vast amounts of misinformation on the subject. When was the last time a book was entitled "The Truth about Raising Your Dachshund" or "Bird Watching: The Facts"?

Terror on Campus

Colleges began introducing AIDS into their orientations. "It's mandatory," said American University's president Richard Berendzen. "When you come in for orientation, you will learn where your classes are, you will be taken on tours of the campus, you will be taught where and how to set up a bank account . . . and one of the things is the AIDS orientation session. All go."[25] Other universities in the nation's capital also reacted to AIDS: Georgetown distributed copies of the U.S. surgeon general's report to incoming students, and George Washington University held AIDS workshops.

Many colleges, however, went beyond merely providing information. Dartmouth College began offering registering students "safer sex kits," containing condoms and latex pieces (approximately three square inches in size) called "rubber dams" to allow people to engage in oral-anal intercourse without making bodily contact.[26] According to a Dartmouth spokesman, Harvard, Brown, Cornell, Stanford, the University of California at Berkeley, Syracuse, and the University of Virginia had similar programs.[27] A Dartmouth group calling itself RAID, for "Responsible AIDS Information at Dartmouth," swamped the campus with AIDS reminders. Fluorescent orange posters inscribed "AIDS Kills— Use Condoms" were pinned on the walls of most campus buildings. Ads on WFRD, the campus radio station, parodied themes from "Star Trek" and "The Twilight Zone," warning students "to get safer sex or no sex at all." RAID members sponsored presentations, which included instruction on how to wear a condom and races in which audience members were timed to see how fast they could slip a condom onto the long end of a plunger held between their legs. All of which prompted the campus's celebrated conservative weekly, the *Dartmouth Review*, to blast RAID as "ridiculous, hyper-paranoid propaganda spouted by self-anointed busybodies." At the time, there was not a single reported AIDS case among Dartmouth students.[28]

Occasionally the purveyors of AIDS information became so zealous that a college administration felt compelled to act. At Pace University in New York, the school closed down the weekly *Pace Press* after it ran "Healthy Sex Guidelines" which included vulgar terms for oral-anal contact, oral-penile contact, and anal intercourse. Like the little boy who repeats for effect a swear word heard at school, the writer of the piece sought to surprise and shock his readers with his willingness to print obscenities. That was, of course, not the professed rationale, as the student wrote early in the article: "It is incumbent upon me to utilize the commonest mode of expression to facilitate making unmistakeably clear information of substantial import having the potential to mean the difference between life and death,"[29] thereby proving his vulgarity to be no match for his verbosity. (Indeed, many propagandists seemed to believe that using vulgarity somehow got the message across better. Booklets from Gay Men's Health Crisis in New York told readers that when applying a condom, "Keep the cock free of grease" and "place the condom against the erect cock"—as if they thought that if they used the word *penis* no one would have any idea what they were talking about.)

AIDS education also spread to public elementary and high schools. The New York Board of Regents narrowly voted to disapprove teaching condom usage to fourth-graders and went so far as to consider providing AIDS instruction to kindergarteners.[30] In Buffalo, ninth-graders were accidentally distributed material by and for adult homosexuals. The children found themselves being advised that urinating on one's partner's unbroken skin is "safe."[31]

Horror in the High Schools

The *Fairfax Journal* of Northern Virginia sent a reporter into local high schools to collect comments. Said Jennifer, age eighteen: "It's spreading to everybody now and it's just scary that anybody could get it." Rodrigo, age nineteen, "It's wiping out a whole lot of innocent people who don't know that the person they are sleeping with has the disease. They are just victims and it's a chain that keeps going on and on. Now anyone can get it." David, age eighteen: "Yes, I worry, especially when I get a cold and it lasts for more than two days. I think it'll never go away. I also think of all the people I've messed with two years ago when it wasn't such a big deal."[32]

The lead in the article was, "High school students in Northern Virginia know about AIDS and they are scared." The piece went on:

> Most of the students said they have heard AIDS discussed in class. Not only classes like the family life education [at one school], but government, history, English, biology, chemistry and physical education classes at the different schools and religion classes at [the] Catholic parochial school. None of the students questioned knew anyone who has contracted AIDS, but about half said they fear they might get the disease nonetheless. . . . None of the students labeled AIDS a disease limited to homosexuals.[33]

Safe Dating

The advertisement was smooth and blunt: "You can help prevent the spread of AIDS. Ask to see Care Card because you care about yourself. Show Care Card because you care about someone else."[34]

Around the United States, clubs and dating services sprang up to provide terrified singles with opportunities to date other singles certified as free of the AIDS-causative agent, the human immunodeficiency virus or HIV. Services—such as Care Card in Chicago, No AIDS in Cherry Hill, New Jersey, and the American AIDS-Free Association in Barrington, Illinois, and Peace of Mind in Bloomfield, Michigan—provided people who tested negative with cards to prove it. Others—such as the More-Health Institute in San Francisco, Safe Love International in Bethesda, Maryland, and Peace of Mind in Northern Virginia—actually acted as dating services for those certified as seronegative.

The problem with relying on such certification is threefold. First, there is a time lag between infection and when that infection shows up on the test, often six weeks or more. A person could become infected one week, join a club two weeks later, and be able to display a card saying he or she is negative. Second, as soon as one has intercourse after issuance of the card, that person would, strictly speaking, need to be recertified. Most clubs required retesting only every six months. Third, fake IDs are never hard to come by. Although insisting that one's sexual partner possess such a card reduces the chances of that person being infected, these people were not concerned with risk *reduction.* They wanted risk *elimination,* which the cards could not guarantee. But they could guarantee one thing: that the other persons in the club were looking for sex. Plus, it was a great way for the club operators to make a buck.

Regular dating services also claimed increased business from the heterosexual AIDS scare. One Washington, D.C., dating service attributed a 20-percent increase in business to an AIDS-generated increase in selectivity among single people looking for partners. "It's truly a sad reason for business to have taken such a good turn, but it's a fact," said the director of client services. "When people have money problems, they go to an accountant. Now, when they want to find safe dating partners, they go to a dating service."[35]

The Polls

A November 1985 Gallup Poll indicated that 27 percent of Americans thought it "very likely" that "AIDS will eventually become an epidemic for the public at large." By 1986, 36 percent thought it very likely, and 37 percent thought it "somewhat likely." Only 5 percent thought it "not at all likely."[36] A November 1987 Gallup Poll indicated that more than 40 percent of American adults were concerned they would contract AIDS. About 20 percent of American adults were "very concerned" that AIDS would strike them personally, and 22 percent were "a little concerned" that they would contract the disease. Sixty-eight percent said they believed AIDS to be the nation's most serious health problem, five times more than named cancer and ten times more than named heart disease, even though cancer that year killed over forty times (about 475,000 deaths) as many Americans as died of AIDS and heart disease killed seventy times (about 770,000 deaths) as many. Along with a significant percentage who said they were changing their sexual habits, 18 percent said they were avoiding public restrooms and 8 percent said they were no longer donating blood.[37] A 1987 poll by the *Atlanta Journal and Constitution* showed that AIDS was the number-3 concern in the nation, ahead of crime, taxes, education, the federal deficit—everything but drug abuse and drunken driving.[38] Polls also showed the public strongly favoring testing for drug users, homosexuals, and prostitutes (78 percent according to a mid-1988 poll); for couples applying for marriage licenses (78 percent); and for "critical" employees like health professionals, teachers, and food-service workers (75 percent).[39]

Panic in Great Britain

The fear was by no means limited to American shores. Indeed, panic was, if anything, greater overseas. Britain's advertisements were far more sensationalist than those in the United States. Included were such ads as a hideous-looking grim reaper knocking over terrified heterosexual men, women, and children with a bowling ball. On the other extreme, some of the British "adverts" were so sexually explicit as to be accused of being soft-core pornography. In one commercial, a sultry woman wearing black stockings and a low-cut blouse seductively asks her male dinner guest, "It is quite late—can you stay?"[40] A British print ad read: "IF YOU'RE PLANNING TO HAVE SEX IN THE NEXT 30 YEARS, SPEND 2 MINUTES READING THIS. Another warned: "It only takes one prick to give you AIDS." Although the accompanying photo shows a syringe about to be injected into an arm, the *double entendre* is obvious.

In 1987, the government sponsored AIDS Week, a massive publicity campaign that, according to an international survey by the *Financial Times,* put the United Kingdom in the forefront of the world's health-warning drive on AIDS.[41] Advertisements and billboards warned of AIDS; radio commercials implored listeners not to sleep around; one TV program after another discussed intimate sex; and government ministers spoke unabashedly about condoms.

All of this occurred at a time when but 686 cases of AIDS had been diagnosed in Britain, over 90 percent of them homosexuals and only 5 attributed to domestic heterosexual transmission.[42] All the more surprising in a country in which *No Sex, Please, We're British,* was going into its sixteenth year at the Duchess Theater. As one report put it, "the British government has swamped every home, every major newspaper, every TV station with words that would have been impossible a few years ago."[43] Every night during AIDS Week, on one channel or another, there was an AIDS program, the product of a joint effort by the British Broadcasting Corporation and the Independent Broadcasting Authority.

There were some complaints of overkill. A group of doctors testified before Parliament that the campaign was causing panic among heterosexuals, who could hinder medical efforts to fight the disease by swamping hospitals with unnecessary blood tests.

Solutions to the Problem—Or Problem Solutions?

In response to the AIDS terror, many people in the United States proposed solutions that were themselves terrifying. Mayor Ed Koch of New York proposed that foreign tourists be forced to undergo a blood test before entering the city (though he offered to grant an exemption to the Pope).[44] Others said everyone attempting to enter, or even to leave, the United States must be made to take the HIV blood test and declare "under forfeiture of property and liberty that they have not engaged in homosexual or IV drug abuse behavior since 1975."[45]

The chairman of a group called the Family Research Institute called for HIV-infected adults to be "semi-permanently tattooed on their right cheek," with no indication what "semi-permanently" might mean. "Hiding the mark would be a banishable offense"; and it was suggested that "Molokai, breeding ground of the hammerhead shark, might be suitable" as a location for banishment.[46]

AIDS Phobia: The "Worried Well"

If AIDS approached the level of a national obsession in several countries, it was clearly a full-fledged obsession with many individuals. For example, Brian (not his real name), a married man, began to suffer from irritation of the urethra in November 1982, a week after having sexual relations with a female co-worker. Despite administration of numerous drugs, his condition failed to improve, and he began to acquire other nonspecific illnesses. Robert, shortly after a sexual tryst with a bar pickup, began suffering from acute epididymitis (inflammation of the seminal tube). Ten days later he began to experience daily headaches, testicular pain, swollen glands, and splotches on his chest. Janet, a forty-one-year-old divorcée, began to suffer vaginal itching a week after a sexual encounter. Within months she became hoarse and chronically fatigued—symptoms that would not respond to treatment.[47]

All these persons had something in common. All were heterosexual, none was especially promiscuous—and all suffered from AIDS. But not the AIDS virus—the AIDS panic. "AfrAIDS." A combination of personal guilt and the public's mass hysteria caused each of these men and women to feel plagued with psychosomatic illnesses that did not even resemble the symptoms of AIDS.

A spokesman at the National Institute of Allergy and Infectious Diseases (NIAID) noted that many of the calls received there are "guilt-motivated—guys who saw a prostitute five years ago and are worried about giving it to their wives, really worried even though they have no symptoms at all."[48] Joyce Price began a *Washington Times* piece: "Doctors are seeing a growing number of patients with AIDS, but the numbers of patients with an unfounded terror of AIDS are growing much faster. They even have names for the debilitating fear: 'Pseudo-AIDS' or 'AIDSophobia.' The phobia leaves patients emotionally and physically disabled by a fear that is largely unfounded."[49]

Dr. Michael Jenike, writing in the November 1987 issue of *Medical Aspects of Human Sexuality,* said this "excessive fear of AIDS" occurs in both heterosexuals and homosexuals.[50] According to Dr. Peter Hawley, medical director of the Whitman-Walker Clinic in Washington, D.C., "There are some people who try to come back for testing almost every week." Even after testing negative for HIV several times and being counseled repeatedly that they are free of the virus, they refuse to accept the fact they are not infected. Dr. Hawley recalled one man so convinced he had AIDS that he spent at least two hours every day looking in the mirror for the telltale spots or lesions. "He became dysfunctional in his job with the federal government," Dr. Hawley said, "I wound up having to refer him to psychiatric treatment."[51]

Other symptoms commonly associated with the pseudo-AIDS, Dr. Jenike said, include depression, early morning waking, loss of sleep and appetite, loss of interest in work, malaise and isolation.[52]

Martha Gross, a Washington, D.C., psychologist who has counseled pseudo-AIDS patients, described them as the "worried well." Gross said these people are "emotionally riddled with anxiety and cannot rid themselves of fear" about getting AIDS. For many, the root of pseudo-AIDS may lie in feelings of guilt or vulnerability related to sexuality. Because of their concerns about sex, Gross said, they allow themselves to be overcome by fears about AIDS, which can be transmitted sexually. If they are convinced they are infected with AIDS, she said, they avoid sexual intimacy.[53]

Dr. Jenike said psychiatric symptoms resulting from fear of AIDS may mimic the early stages of AIDS itself and "lead to significant functional impairment"[54]—to say the least, to judge from some of the "worried well" dug up by television talkshows. One such person claimed to have been tested twenty times. "Why would anyone have themselves tested twenty times?" asked the host Geraldo Rivera. The man replied:

> When I was in college, which was just about three years ago—I was in my . . . freshman year, and as on most college campuses we were pretty wild. . . . [O]f course there's particular girls that got around, everybody knew

who they were. And we kind of—they made their numbers. And after a few years went by, friends of mine from college were coming down with strange things and a couple of the girls that we all knew and loved got very ill, and it seemed as though it was panic. There was this spreading all over the place throughout this college.[55]

Even after his test results came back negative, the man's worries continued. The worry led to diarrhea, which if chronic may be a symptom of AIDS. This begat more worry, which led to nightmares from which he would wake in a sweat. Night sweats are another AIDS symptom. A doctor had tried to convince him that if his sexual contacts were not homosexual he had little to fear, but to no avail. "I knew, you know, just convinced, you cannot tell me after what I've done in college you know—and I don't think I was too bad compared to most of my friends, but it's fairly normal, you know, you're at the age——"[56] The man's conclusion indicated that he felt cured, although his incoherent testimony may leave some doubt.

Next up on the Geraldo show was a woman who had stopped dating altogether but still moved out of New York City because "the [AIDS] statistics are incredible" there.[57]

A psychotherapist on the show, who started a "worried well" therapy program, confessed his mystification: "Why AIDS and not cancer? Why AIDS and not heart disease? AIDS is just another disease. We've got plenty of diseases."[58]

But the good doctor was wrong. AIDS is not just another disease. It is the most intensely reported-on, most metaphorical, most exploited disease in history. It is the ultimate triumph of politics over science. Indeed, it is the triumph of politics over reality, with what is "right" or "correct" determined not by what is scientifically right or correct, but by whatever happens to fit a specific agenda and whatever is socially acceptable. It shows the ability of the state, the media, and various special interests to shift an entire nation's perception—indeed, of several nations—of the spread of a disease. What was supposed to pose a greater threat than nuclear bombs has turned out to be more of a dud. The deaths of homosexuals and drug users were supposed to be a mere portent of things to come; instead, they would, for the most part, be all that was. Ultimately, the "epidemic of the millennium" would prove to be the hoax of the decade. Even as the actual epidemic was beginning to run down, the mythical epidemic was gearing up. Before it would run its course, this mythical epidemic would exact a severe price in wasted resources, squandered credibility, and sheer terror.

2

The Once and Future
Heterosexual Non-Epidemic

Nineteen eighty-seven was to have been the year of the heterosexual AIDS epidemic. Not heterosexuals infected through needle sharing, or blood transfusions, or clotting factor for hemophiliacs, or even through sex partners of any of the above. No, this was to have been a bona-fide epidemic, going from heterosexual to heterosexual, finding "fertile growth"—as *U.S. News* put it[1]—without need of the original connections to the risk groups. The debate on *whether* having ended, it was now all a matter of reaction, with *Time, The Atlantic,* and other magazines, newspapers, and television networks commissioning reports to write profound essays on how heterosexuals were coping with what they called "the new realities."

But a funny thing happened on the way to the apocalypse. By the end of the year, heterosexuals still were not dropping like flies, and it was looking more and more as if they were not about to start. Much of the media and the Public Health Service began to switch sides and state— cautiously, to be sure—that not only had there been no heterosexual explosion, but one was not imminent or even probable. In the course of that one short year, those who had created the fear—and to a great extent profited by it—were left standing on the dock, binoculars in hand, waiting for a ship that would not come in. Many of them would persist in their vigil, of course, screaming "It's here!" at the sight of any sail, or semblance of one, on the horizon. Yet time and again, they would be disappointed.

The "myth" of heterosexual AIDS consists of a series of myths, one of which *is not* that heterosexuals get AIDS. They certainly do get it, from shared needles, from transfusions, from clotting factor, which hemophiliacs use to control internal bleeding, from their mothers at or before birth, and sometimes through sexual intercourse with persons in these categories and with bisexuals. The primary myth, however, was that the disease was no longer anchored to these risk groups but was, in fact, going from heterosexual to heterosexual to heterosexual through intercourse, that it was epidemic among non-drug-abusing heterosexuals. As Dr. Robert Redfield, an infectious disease specialist at Walter Reed Army Hospital in Washington, D.C., articulated the myth (in which he believed) in 1985, "This is a general disease now. Get rid of the high risk groups, anyone can get it."[2]

Statistical Breakdown

Through August 1989, there were 106,000 AIDS cases reported to the federal Centers for Disease Control (CDC). Of these, 61 percent were homosexual or bisexual males presumed to be infected through sexual intercourse, 21 percent were intravenous drug abusers (IVDAs) presumed to have gotten infected through sharing needles with infected persons, 7 percent were both homosexual males and IVDAs, 1 percent were hemophiliacs, 2 percent had received blood transfusions infected with HIV, the cause of infection in 3 percent had yet to be determined, and 4.5 percent were listed as having probably been infected through heterosexual intercourse. Of this 4.5 percent, however, more than one third were "born in countries in which heterosexual transmission is believed to play a major role although precise means of transmission have not yet been fully identified"—a longhand way of saying "natives of Haiti and central and East Africa." (Patterns of transmission in those two areas will be discussed in a later chapter, as will the political considerations behind lumping these victims into the heterosexual transmission category.) Of native-born Americans, about 3,300 of the 106,000 AIDS victims, about 3 percent, were listed as victims of heterosexual transmission. The proportion had been just about 2.5 percent eighteen months earlier, but the new case definition of AIDS, which added such symptoms as wasting syndrome and dementia, caused a sudden jump in both heterosexually transmitted and IVDA cases.[3] About three fourths of these were men. Despite the media's and the various federal, state, and local public health services special targeting of the white middle class for "education," only 960 of those 3,300 were white. In fact, only about nine tenths of 1 percent of all AIDS victims are whites who are thought to have become infected through heterosexual intercourse, of which assuredly a much smaller percentage yet are members of the middle class. (Heterosexual transmission usually means the partner of an IVDA, and most infected IVDAs are lower-class.)[4] Thus, it is probably fair to say that this, the most heavily targeted of all groups, accounts for less than one half of 1 percent of all AIDS cases diagnosed in this country.

Further, there is evidence that even the 700 and 2,500 figures may include many persons who did not, in fact, become infected through heterosexual intercourse. In New York City, the heterosexual AIDS capital of the United States, out of 18,000 cases diagnosed by early 1989, only 7 males have been identified as having gotten AIDS from heterosexual intercourse.[5] Consider, on the other hand, that New York has slightly over one third of all female IVDA cases, and that male infections come almost exclusively from IVDAs. (After all, female bisexuals pose men no threat and female hemophiliacs are extremely rare.)* The explanation, it would seem, is that while some cities and states simply take a man at his word when he says he was infected by a woman, New York City thoroughly investigates each such claim, rejecting the vast majority as other risk factors come to light. Considering that New York City has about one third of all female IVDA AIDS cases, if other health departments interviewed patients as carefully as New York does, efficiently screening out those who don't admit to homosexual intercourse or shared needles but who have in fact done so, we would expect to find only about a score of such men in the entire country. As it was, in early 1989, 600 men were listed as infected through heterosexual intercourse throughout the nation.

The alarmists were highly distressed by the low number of men classified in New York as victims of heterosexual transmission. One of them, the author Chris Norwood, wrote that the figure

> was so incredible that the Commissioner of Health finally had to say he would appoint a special panel to review the city's casecounting methods. One reason the city "found" so few heterosexual men was, almost certainly, a refusal to look for them. When a man who said he was heterosexual didn't know for sure whether any woman he had slept with was at risk for AIDS, the Health Department made no attempt to test his present or past girlfriends for HIV infection. Instead, his case was simply assigned to the "no known risk" caseload.[7]

*As of January 1989, only 24 females were listed as having gotten AIDS in the United States through hemophilia clotting factor.[6]

Au contraire, according to Rand Stoneburner, director of AIDS research for the city, who told me the panel "found no bias involved that
would undercount significantly male heterosexual cases any more than
any other city in the country has. Ours was found as good or better than
any in the country."[8] In fact, speaking at a time when 8 men were in
the heterosexually transmitted category, according to the city's then-
chief interrogator, Anna Lekatsas, "I have doubts about seven of them,
but we couldn't prove anything."[9] Since she said that, one of the men
was found to have other risks and was dropped from the category.

Considering that the great majority of female heterosexual infections
come from IVDAs as well, and that New York City has about half of the
male IVDA cases in the nation (about 5,000 out of 12,000 at the end of
January 1989), yet less than one third of the female heterosexual transmission cases (about 500 out of 1,800 nationally), this also indicates that
female infections outside of New York City are being misclassified as
heterosexually transmitted. Thus, it is possible that even among that 3
percent, nearly one half of the cases had other risk factors they would
not admit to.

Nevertheless, let us assume for the sake of argument that all 3,300 of
those native-born cases were indeed heterosexually transmitted, as
were the 960 cases among whites. During the eight years those cases
were being racked up, about 380,000 Americans, the vast majority of
whom were white heterosexuals, were killed in automobile accidents.[10]
About 10,000,000 more suffered disabling injuries.[11] Almost half those
deaths and more than half of deaths and injuries combined could, according to the National Highway and Transit Authority, have been
prevented by the simple buckling of a safety belt, an act the victim
neglected because he or she did not think the risk was great enough.[12]
Indeed, a majority of Americans do not wear safety belts.[13] If we look
at AIDS in the short-term future, at the present rate of case reporting,
there will be somewhere in the range of 1,000 new native-born heterosexual cases reported to the Centers for Disease Control during 1989,
of which about 300 will be white and a significantly smaller portion of
these middle-class. During the same period, 475,000 Americans will die
of cancer and over 750,000 of heart disease.[14]

In fact, other than fairly spectacular rare occurrences, such as shark
attacks and maulings by wild animals, it is difficult to name any broad
category of death that will take fewer lives than heterosexually transmitted AIDS. In 1985, there were 19,628 murders,[15] 12,001 fatal falls,
5,316 drownings, 4,938 deaths related to fire, 4,091 accidental fatal
poisonings by solids or liquids,[16] 3,551 deaths by suffocation or ingested

objects, and 1,649 fatal firearms accidents.[17] Murder will claim perhaps twenty times as many heterosexual lives this year as AIDS; falls, eleven times; and so on. A middle-class non-IVDA heterosexual in the Chicago suburbs or Orange County, California—or, indeed, in almost any area of the country—has less of a chance of getting AIDS in the next year than of being struck by lightning or drowning in a bathtub (about 360 direct lightning strikes are recorded in the United States each year,[18] and about 350 Americans drown in a bathtub a year).[19] Most of us, while acknowledging the existence of these threats, be they murder or drowning, do not live in terror of them.

Indeed, if heterosexuals treated other risks as they have been told to treat the threat of AIDS, life as we know it would cease to exist. Heterosexuals have simply too many activities far riskier than sex that are nevertheless essential to conducting life or at least very important to a useful and enjoyable existence. Not so for homosexuals and IVDA. While I will discuss their individual risk factors later, suffice it for now to say that a homosexual having unprotected (without a condom) intercourse in most areas of the United States, or an IVDA sharing needles in an area where needle sharing is common, runs a risk of infection far, far greater than of dying in an automobile accident, much less of drowning or dying in a fire.

Asymptomatic Infections

One common objection to this line of reasoning is that one cannot look at present AIDS caseloads. After all, it often takes years before an infected person develops the full-blown disease. Thus, the sex therapists William Masters, Virginia Johnson, and Robert Kolodny declared in their controversial *Crisis: Heterosexual Behavior in the Age of AIDS* that there were probably 200,000 or more infected non-IVDA heterosexuals in the United States, and that the virus was therefore "running rampant in the heterosexual community."[20] The Hudson Institute fellows Kevin Hopkins and William Johnston, in their "preliminary report" *The Incidence of HIV Infection in the United States*, said there were anywhere from 200,000 to 500,000 such infections.[21] Unfortunately, none of these people bothered to show how they arrived at their figures.*

---

*The sex therapists conducted their own small study of volunteers but made no pretense that the study could be extrapolated in any specific way to the population as a whole.

The best answer to such fictitious estimates is to look at blood-testing figures, most of which to date are from military applicants and active duty personnel and from blood donors.

Military Testing

In October 1985, the Department of Defense began testing all applicants to the armed forces as well as active-duty servicemen. The first test results from the military were immediately interpreted as bad news, in great part because of the role of Redfield, the military's most outspoken AIDS doctor. The CDC announced in July 1986 that 15 out of every 10,000 applicants to the armed forces tested positive for HIV.[22] Much of the attention focused on New York City applicants, where the rate was 6 per 1,000. In Manhattan, it was 17 per 1,000, almost 1 in 50.[23]

It might have occurred to some reporters and doctors who were sounding the Klaxons that the fact that New York City has the largest number of IV drug users and homosexuals, and the highest level of HIV positivity in drug users, in the country was simply being reflected in the statistics. But no, declared the NBC science writer Robert Bazell in the *New Republic,* probably relying on Redfield (whom he quoted later in the article), "It appears that most of [the seropositive military applicants] are neither intravenous drug users nor homosexuals. They are just ghetto kids."[24]

Redfield's chief ally in the media, Ann Guidici Fettner, remarked, "Think about it: Six of every 1,000 young women from New York trying to enlist in military are carrying HIV," having just stated that "given the highly publicized policy of testing recruits for the HIV virus, it seems unlikely that swarms of 'at-risks' would be signing up."[25]

Some people were just a little less trusting of the Redfield interpretation than were Bazell and Fettner. In defense of a major article refuting the practicality of premarital testing (which Redfield continues to advocate), a group of Harvard Medical School researchers headed by Paul Cleary stated, "Army recruits are demographically different from the premarital population, and more likely to be sexually active homosexual men and drug abusers."[26]

But Redfield told his critics, "The Army population is the same as the population of the country."[27] In fact, he later told me that the army is almost certainly less likely to have members of risk groups than is the general population.[28] As an army veteran who left the service just three years before Redfield made that statement, I found it difficult to believe an Army officer could suffer such delusions. The two most obvious differences between the military and the civilian population are that applicants to the military are of the age category most at risk for AIDS and are several times more likely to be of races and ethnic groups (black and Hispanic) much more at risk for AIDS than are whites. Indeed, the rate among white applicants was only 1.0 per 1,000; while blacks were over four times more likely to be infected, at 3.9 infections per 1,000.[29]

In fact, it appeared that military applicants testing positive had the same old risk factors AIDS victims had. Writing in the *New England Journal of Medicine,* Stoneburner and others reported that 23, or about one fourth of the first set of rejected applicants to the military from New York City, had been located and interviewed. Of these, 10 turned out to be intravenous drug abusers, 7 were bisexuals, 1 was homosexual, and 1 woman knew that she had had contact with an infected man. Three of the infected men claimed no risk other than prostitute contact, a claim the report viewed with skepticism, especially because the only chance for interview was over the phone. The final infected person claimed no risk factors. Upon retest he was negative, which doesn't say much for military testing procedures.[30]

A presentation at the Fourth International AIDS Conference in Stockholm in June 1988 stated that while approximately 20 percent of active-duty male soldiers testing positive for HIV originally deny identifiable risk factors (intravenous drug use, homosexuality, and so on), an additional 60 percent of these are, upon further investigation, reclassified into traditional risk groups.[31]

Thus, researchers have estimated that the prevalence of HIV infection in military recruits not belonging to such high-risk groups is about 0.02 percent, or 2 in 10,000, or less.[32] Since then, the testing of recruits has not revealed increasing levels of infection, as Redfield and other alarmists declared they would; by the middle of 1988, infections were down significantly to 12 per 10,000.[33] The greatest percentage drop was among white males, who fell from 10 per 10,000 to only 5 per 10,000. This overall reduction in infections may simply represent a greater awareness on the part of applicants that they will be tested; hence, they are self-selecting out more efficiently than they formerly did. It may also mean that the level of infections in the general population is declining as persons with AIDS die off and are replaced by fewer newly infected people. Either way, it's certainly not bad news.

Blood Donations

Blood donations constitute the single largest blood-testing program in the nation. By the end of 1988, over 17,000,000 tests had been performed. In the first two years of such testing, 43 per 100,000 first-time donors proved to be infected.[34] In more recent testing, that figure has fallen to 40 per 100,000[35]—though, again, whether that represents better screening or a declining level of infection in the population is difficult to determine. Even though persons at high risk for HIV are meticulously screened through questionnaires, 80 percent to 90 percent of infected donors interviewed nonetheless turn out to be from high-risk groups. When members of high-risk groups are excluded, therefore, the level of infection falls to only 6 per 100,000.[36]

Thus, both the military and blood donor figures sound like wonderful news for sexually active heterosexuals. But not so said Hopkins and Johnston, whose report claimed that heterosexual infections were increasing dramatically. Responding to an article critical of that report (my own), which invoked the military recruit and blood donor figures, they stated "The Red Cross actively discourages donors with risk factors, and systematically excludes donors who have previously tested positive [and the] military does not test recruits until after they have already passed through a recruiting screen, including checks of school and police records . . . "[37] Likewise, Chris Norwood told her readers that, while "among more than 300,000 donors tested from late 1985 to late 1986, the Red Cross of Minnesota did not uncover one infected woman," this "encouraging fact loses significance when we remember that women who even suspect they may be at risk are no longer supposed to donate blood."[38] The point all three missed was that, while certainly IVDA women or men, and homosexual or bisexual men, might know to avoid blood testing, their unwitting heterosexual sex partners, whom Norwood and Hopkins wanted us to believe were being infected in massive numbers, would not. And they simply aren't showing up. If there were 200,000 to 500,000 non-IVDA-infected heterosexuals out there, as the Hudson Institute report claims, or 200,000-plus as Masters, Johnson and Kolodny claim, the majority of whom would be of eligible age to join the military, they would not know to self-select out and would undoubtedly start showing up in blood testing of either the military or the blood banks. They aren't showing up for the simple reason they don't exist.

A team of CDC scientists, writing in *Science* about these donor and military figures, has concluded, "These preliminary data suggest that the proportion of 'unexplained' heterosexual HIV transmission is not much higher than predicted from analysis of reported cases of AIDS."[39] In an editorial in the 7 October 1988 *Journal of the American Medical Association,* Dr. H. Hunter Handsfield, director of the Seattle-King County Department of Health, stated even more forcefully that, "even when the prolonged interval from HIV infection to overt AIDS is taken into account, it is likely that the classification of reported cases accurately reflects the actual patterns of transmission."[40]

More recently, CDC has begun numerous other testing programs, some of which are partially blind (no names are taken), fully blind (no names or even demographic information taken), and some of which allow identification of the individual. Where demographic information is kept, the results always reveal the same basic pattern: infection rates are much higher in inner cities and much higher among blacks and Hispanics than among whites.[41]

The largest of these studies (in terms of geographic area and size of potential pool) was a statewide survey in late 1988 in which for three whole months the blood was tested from all women giving birth in California. Of 135,762 tests, only 101 proved positive, for a rate of 7.4 per 10,000.[42] This is the land of east Los Angeles, Watts and Oakland— all high drug abuse areas—and these women are by definition heterosexual, sexually active, and of the ages during which IV drug use is most common. Yet purely random sampling found far fewer infections in heterosexual women than in the population of military recruits that many were saying was *underrepresentative* of the general population. Released in September 1989, it was wonderful news. Or should have been. The media greeted the release of the study with complete silence. More good news had come in May of 1989. A massive sampling of students on American college campuses revealed an infection rate in women of only 2 per 10,000. The media did make reference to this study, but failed to specify that even this low figure included needle-sharers and transfusion recipients as well as victims of heterosexual transmission. (This is discussed at greater length in chapter 19.)

The Future of Heterosexual Infections

As the heterosexual epidemic continued to fail to show up, either in actual cases or in infections, the alarmists took a series of fall-back positions. By early 1988, the alarmists had fallen back to Masters, Johnson, and Kolodny's, "The AIDS *virus* is now running rampant in the heterosexual community"[43] (emphasis added). By late 1988, the alarmists were couching their threats in the future, as with the Hudson Institute's concession that many middle-class heterosexuals were "at little immediate risk of catching HIV."[44] Thus, long after non-IVDA heterosexuals were supposed to be dying in droves, the warnings had gone from "they've got AIDS," to "they've got the virus," to "they're going to get the virus."

Somehow the alarmists failed to see (or at least claimed to fail to see) how the current low level of AIDS cases and infections in the heterosexual population was tied to a *continuing* low level. It was as if being spared the epidemic early on was simply a matter of luck, luck that could not hold out forever. No doubt this is how many people felt 150 years ago when they saw some cities devastated by the "Red Death" (cholera) while others were spared completely. Blind luck or the wrath of God or "miasma" (evil vapors) was blamed for epidemics back then, although we now know that the selectivity of cholera depended on the efficacy of a city's sewage system. Similarly, blind luck plays no part in accounting for the low levels of AIDS and AIDS virus infections in heterosexuals, especially white middle-class heterosexuals.

It can be said of the heterosexual AIDS alarmists that they have, with few if any exceptions, little idea of how epidemics work. This is no less true of the average person, the difference being that the average person does not broadcast his or her ignorance. The first point to recognize, in comprehending the heterosexual non-epidemic, is that *disease* and *epidemic* are not synonymous. In 1987, 14 cases of bubonic plague were reported in the United States,[45] yet no plague flags were flown, no red crosses painted upon the doors of quarantined households. For reasons that are unclear, there have been no plague epidemics since just after the turn of the century (the vaccine now used in some countries is a recent development); yet every year a few people will get plague, and a small percentage of those will die. Likewise, there is no reason simply to assume that because some heterosexuals are getting AIDS, there will be an epidemic of AIDS among heterosexuals.

In the hysteria surrounding the AIDS crisis, one of the tenets of epidemiology (the study of epidemics) which has been virtually ignored is that for an epidemic to spread, each case has to give rise to, on average, slightly more than 1 additional case. If, say, 100 cases give rise to 500 cases, the epidemic will spread quickly; if they give rise to 101, it will spread slowly, though inexorably. But if, say, 100 cases lead only to 100 more, the numbers will never increase; and if they lead to only 99, the incidence of disease will fall back upon itself or "implode" as some have put it. Of the aforementioned 14 plague cases, none spread to other human beings (they all originated with animals); hence, the disease quickly imploded. Nobody knows exactly how many cases 100 heterosexual AIDS cases will lead to; but for our purposes, all that must be figured is whether it is over 100 or under.

While extremely elaborate formulae can be concocted to try to give an exact answer to the $100 \geqq X$ problem, the basic formula depends on three factors: how long infected people remain infectious; how efficient is HIV transmission from men to women and women to men; and how often these men and women switch partners. There are no exact answers to these, but continuing research gives us figures that should suffice for our basic purpose.

Length of Infection

Although AIDS is no joke, there is good news and bad news about the length of HIV infectiousness. The bad news is that there's no reason to think that infectious persons will ever become uninfectious, short of death. As long as they are alive and well enough to have intercourse, they will be able to spread the AIDS-causing virus—human immunodeficiency virus, or HIV.

The "good news" here is actually terrible news for anyone infected. Originally, it was thought that only a small percentage of those infected with the virus would go on to develop the disease. While this was reassuring to infected persons, it made the long-term outlook for the spread of the disease look bad because it meant that large numbers of healthy persons would be spreading the virus to others indefinitely. But a consensus of opinion has now formed that the great majority, and perhaps almost all, of HIV-infected persons will develop debilitating symptoms or die.

For example, researchers at San Francisco General Hospital following a group of 288 HIV-infected homosexual men, who were originally recruited in the late 1970s to test their blood for hepatitis B (most of whom are believed to have been infected by HIV in 1981–82), have estimated that nine years from the date of infection, 50 percent of the group will have developed AIDS and an additional 25 percent will experience AIDS-related symptoms.[46] Interpreting the results, the lead researcher told reporters, "What we saw was that the number of those showing no effects from HIV infection is very small. This means that if you are infected with the AIDS virus, you will almost certainly go on to get AIDS."[47] Scientists at Frankfurt University in West Germany studied a group of 543 people and found that only 9.8 percent of the seropositives remained completely healthy after three years. A computer model found that 50 percent of the HIV carriers would develop AIDS within five years, and 75 percent within seven.[48] A study at the Walter Reed Army Medical Center in Washington, D.C., also found that about 80 percent to 90 percent of seropositives will experience some deterioration in their immune system over a few years—a finding that suggests that the vast majority of them, according to the National Institutes of Allergies and Infectious Diseases director Anthony Fauci, "will be adversely affected by the virus over time."[49] Still, it is possible that a small percentage of those infected with HIV will never develop full-blown AIDS or perhaps even develop symptoms.

While predicting average incubation time is still somewhat speculative, several studies based on the figures just presented can provide an idea. For example, one based on the San Francisco hepatitis-B cohort shows a median incubation time of almost eight years.[50]* In other words, eight years after infection one would expect half of the seropositives to have developed AIDS. Other studies have shown mean incubation times as high as 11 years.[52]

While it appears that HIV in homosexuals and hemophiliacs incubates at approximately the same rate, this may not be the case with transfusion recipients. Analysis of CDC AIDS surveillance data through July 1988, for persons presumed to have acquired HIV through blood transfusions, indicates a median incubation time of thirty-four months for children and thirty-six months for adults.[53] A Swedish study also showed accelerated incubation time for blood-transfusion recipients.[54] The most obvious possible explanation is the massive amount of HIV received during a transfusion, as opposed to a comparatively tiny amount during intercourse and through shared needles; but the accelerated incubation could reflect other factors, such as the generally older age of transfusion recipients.†

Thus, into the first part of the formula, length of infectiousness, one might plug a number of about nine years *except* that the development of symptoms indicating HIV infection tend to show up much sooner—in fact, on average about four and one-half years.[56] Thus, this will be a tipoff both to the HIV carrier and a potential sex partner that something

---

*Another analysis, using data on 114 men from a separate San Francisco group, indicated a median incubation time of 10.8 years. A third analysis of data from a German group of persons with hemophilia calculated a mean incubation time of nine years.[51]

†Children clearly progress much faster to full-blown disease than do adults: for example, a New York City study found that 42 percent of infected children developed symptoms in their first year of life; and of these, 73 percent developed full-blown AIDS.[55]

is wrong. The question, then, is how likely is one heterosexual to infect another before developing symptoms that will tend to negate the possibility of that transmission?

One way of measuring is to look at the possibility of infection on a per-contact basis, multiplying this by average number of sexual acts of a heterosexual couple in one year, about 100. The only such study to provide an accurate quantification of the per-contact risk was conducted by Dr. Nancy Padian, then at the Berkeley School of Public Health in California. She found that women in the study averaged about 1,000 sexual contacts with infected men before becoming infected.[57] Thus, according to this formula, a man would only have about a 50-percent chance of infecting a woman before becoming symptomatic.

But one problem with the Padian study, which she readily acknowledges, is that the risk may not be evenly distributed. It may be that some women will become infected easily, while others will become infected only after a period of many years or not at all. This, indeed, was the probable conclusion of a study by Dr. Thomas Peterman of CDC and Rand Stoneburner. In their study of transfusion victims and their female sexual partners, these researchers found a couple of women who became infected after only a few contacts each, and many women and men who remained uninfected after hundreds or even more than a thousand contacts.[58] This finding indicates that while as a crude measuring stick of a woman's risks it may be useful to use the 1-in-a-1,000 figure, to measure the spread of the epidemic it may be better to look at the overall chance an infected individual has of infecting a partner.

In the Peterman-Stoneburner study, about 20 percent of the men ended up infecting their partners, while 10 percent of the women did. These numbers seem to be about par for the course. Contrary to the assertion of *USA Today* in 1987 that "dozens of studies indicate that spouses spread the virus to each other more than half of the time by vaginal intercourse alone,"[59] a compilation of such studies from around the world in the 18 December 1987 CDC *Weekly Mortality and Morbidity Report* noted a total of only 22, of which only three showed partners seroconverting over half the time.[60] Another compilation of such studies—this one by the director of the CDC AIDS program, James Curran; the CDC chief AIDS epidemiologist, Dr. Harold Jaffe; and other doctors at CDC—in *Science* found that the great majority of AIDS carriers are unable to infect their steady partners heterosexually even over a period of years. Among female partners of bisexuals, about 25 percent become infected. Female partners of men who received HIV from transfusion have only about a 20-percent seroconversion rate.

Among partners of hemophiliacs, this rate falls to less than 9 percent. Only two categories show much higher seroconversion rates. One of these consists of both female and male partners of patients born in Haiti or Zaire, a subject to be discussed in a later chapter. The number of couples here, however, was so small (35, as opposed to 288 partners of hemophiliacs) as to make the results questionable. The other category comprised female partners of IV-drug abusers, of whom just fewer than 50 percent seroconvert; and male partners of female IV-drug abusers, among whom a full 50 percent seroconvert. Fewer than 15 percent of male partners of female transfusion recipients seroconvert by contrast (although both cohorts were small).[61]

This difference in transmission rates has puzzled some alarmists. Chris Norwood offers her bizarre explanation that "some unknown aspect of hemophilia may inhibit or retard replication of the virus, making sexual transmission less likely."[62] In fact, the hemophiliac-transmission figure is probably not so different from the blood-transfusion and bisexual categories as to require any explanation other than that they are all within the range of statistical error.[63] It's the extraordinarily *high* rate of IVDA transmission that needs explanation.

Higher rates of sexually transmitted diseases (STDs) among IVDAs and their partners may help account for this. But perhaps the best explanation is that it probably is not more efficient: that heterosexual partners of IVDAs are, in fact, also shooting drugs themselves and using their partners' needles. There is anecdotal evidence to this effect. In one reported case in New York, an AIDS victim kept denying risk factors other than heterosexual intercourse. But a wily investigator, excusing himself to go to the bathroom at the victim's house, found there syringes and needles.[64] This clearly has ramifications beyond establishing that partner studies overstate the risk of heterosexual transmission. Over three fourths of all heterosexually transmitted AIDS cases of native-born Americans occur in women, of whom over 80 percent are partners of IV-drug users.[65] If, as the partner studies would seem to indicate, a significant proportion of the women who claim to have gotten HIV sexually from their IV–drug-abusing male partners were, in fact, infected through needles, then that portion of AIDS cases attributed to heterosexual transmission among native-born Americans would be cut dramatically. This could well account for the disparity with New York City where, with over a third of the nation's IVDA AIDS cases, the city has less than one fourth of the national total of cases listed as being heterosexually transmitted—because of its excellent re-interviewing techniques.

Partner Switching

At a glance, then, from studies that show only 10 percent to 20 percent of heterosexuals infecting their steady partners over a period of years, one might assume that the "more than 100 cases for each original 100 cases" threshold could not be reached. Unfortunately, it's not quite that simple. Another factor that has to be figured in is nonsexual transmission: that is, to what extent is HIV entering relationships due to reasons other than sex? For middle-class heterosexuals, this is not a significant factor. As noted, intravenous drug abuse, especially with needle sharing, is largely confined to the lower economic class. Indeed, the needle-sharing aspect of it (and of course it's the sharing of needles, not the actual drug use itself, that spreads disease) tends to be much more of a black and Hispanic problem than a white one, as I will discuss in the chapter on minorities. The only other ways the virus is going to enter nonsexually into a relationship is through infection with hemophilia-clotting factor or blood transfusions. Yet only a small portion of the population has been infected this way (about 22,000, according to CDC estimates);[66] in addition, many, if not most, have been identified through testing and counseled to avoid infecting others. Finally, since testing of blood and heat treating of clotting factor were introduced in 1985, very few new infections have come about in these manners. Through attrition by death, the number of people infected through these methods continues to dwindle.

But this lack of outside infusion for white middle-class heterosexuals doesn't hold true for lower-class black and Hispanic ones living in America's inner cities. They have a constant infusion of new virus into their relationships because of the drug problem. This has also proved problematic in Africa, where tainted blood transfusions were and continue to be a much greater problem than in the United States and Europe, and where reuse of needles in hospitals has also contributed to, again, a constant infusion of virus into relationships. Even American homosexuals, at least those in the big cities, seem to have a much closer connection to the intravenous drug abuse culture than does the heterosexual middle class.

Another factor that has to be taken into account is anything that will increase the transmissibility of the virus. Specifically, some STDs have been linked to greatly increased transmissibility, as will be discussed in chapter 4. Once again this is not especially a problem for the white, heterosexual middle class, which has maintained low levels of these diseases for the past few decades. And once again, to look at black and Hispanic STD rates in the inner cities, this is very bad news.

The final important factor in gauging the possibility of spread is the degree of partner switching or promiscuity in a given group or "sub-population." If a man has sex only with his wife and his wife has sex only with him, the virus will never go more than that one step. But if a man has sex with three women, it is now theoretically possible for him to infect three women, although the chances of his infecting each woman is probably smaller than his chances of infecting a single monogamous partner.

The upshot is that the subpopulation that has more partner switching is going to spread the virus faster and farther than that which has less. Once again, this is a protective factor for the general middle-class population, which tends to have only a few partners a year. By contrast, prior to the appearance of AIDS, partner switching among homosexuals was practiced on a scale that would boggle the imagination of the most lusty heterosexual male. In their 1978 *Homosexualities,* the most thorough investigation of homosexual sex practices since the original Kinsey study, Alan Bell and Martin Weinberg found that—of homosexual men surveyed at just about the same time HIV was being introduced into the New York, San Francisco, and Los Angeles homosexual populations— 28 percent of white homosexual men claimed 1,000 or more partners, as did 19 percent of the black. Eighty-four percent of the whites and 77 percent of the blacks claimed 50 or more partners over the course of a lifetime.[67] A survey of the early homosexual AIDS victims found that they averaged almost 1100 lifetime partners each.[68]

Indeed, in one study, Dr. Warren Winkelstein and others reported on two randomly sampled groups of San Francisco men, one homosexual or bisexual and the other heterosexual. While Winkelstein found that by 1986 both groups had, apparently out of fear of AIDS, reduced their sexual contacts, the homosexuals *continued to have significantly more partners on average than the heterosexuals ever did.*[69] This is extremely important, considering that the dramatic decrease in new infections among homosexuals has been attributed in great part to this reduction in partners.

As to blacks and Hispanics in inner cities, the information is sketchier. Higher abortion rates, birth rates, and STD rates have all been cited to indicate that these groups tend to have more sexual partners; but the counter argument is that these things are only reported in higher numbers because inner-city minorities patronize public hospitals almost exclusively, and that's where the statistics are collected.

At this point, I have discussed the factors that go into determining whether 100 cases will equal more or less than 100, but have come to no solid conclusion other than of the absurdity of comparing the spread of the disease in the middle-class heterosexual population of the United States and Europe with the spread among homosexuals and Africans. In every way, the homosexuals and Africans had the odds stacked against them. If, for example, homosexuals had engaged in lots of partner switching but anal sex were a poor way of transmitting the virus, they would not have nearly the problem they do today. Likewise, even if anal sex were comparatively dangerous but homosexuals were essentially monogamous, they would not have had the same problem. But both of these factors were multiplied to create the homosexual epidemic. Similarly, in every way middle-class heterosexuals have the odds on their side.

While we just do not have enough data to make an exact statement of exactly what 100 cases do equal, as Dr. Alexander Langmuir, the founder of the modern epidemiology branch at CDC, has stated with all these facts in mind, "Everything I have seen says that outside of the high-risk groups, the spread is less than epidemic survival."[70] Indeed, the evidence for this goes right back to the case figures and blood-test figures given earlier. If there were heterosexual spread, after twelve years it would be showing up. It is not. As the New York City Department of Health paper presented at the Fourth International Conference in Stockholm stated in 1988, "In the city with the world's highest reported incidence of AIDS, these results suggest that HIV infection was primarily limited to known AIDS risk group members and their sexual partners."[71]

But again, what applies to white middle-class heterosexuals in the suburbs may not apply to their black and Hispanic brethren in the inner-city neighborhoods of New York, northern New Jersey, and perhaps southern Florida. As Stoneburner told me, "Between the IV-drug problem, the crack problem, and the high syphilis rates, there is a strong possibility of subpockets of epidemic in some areas such as the South Bronx. Over time, you could have serious problems."[72] Thus, it's important to be specific when referring to heterosexuals and their risks. Comparing the risks of a white person in the northern or western Chicago suburbs with that of a black or Hispanic person in the South Bronx is almost as inaccurate as comparing the risks of those suburbanites and homosexuals in San Francisco and New York.

It should be clear by now that there is no single "AIDS epidemic." There is an epidemic among homosexuals and bisexuals and their sex partners. There is an epidemic among intravenous drug abusers and their sex partners, which may widen slightly in some areas to include the partners of those partners. But among the great wide percentage of the nation the media calls "the general population," that section the media and the public health authorities has tried desperately to terrify, there is no epidemic. AIDS will pick off a person here and there in this group, but the original infected partner will be in one of the two groups in which the disease is epidemic. Most heterosexuals will continue to have more to fear from bathtub drowning than from AIDS.

Thus, the folly of slogans like "Everyone is at risk," or "AIDS doesn't discriminate," and of such broad-based educational approaches as sending a version of the Surgeon General's Report on AIDS to every household in the country. Such a mailing makes every bit as much sense as sending a booklet warning against the dangers of frostbite to every home in the nation, from Key West, Florida, to San Diego, California. But the slogans and the mailings did make sense in one very important way. They were essential to spreading the myth of heterosexual AIDS.

3

A Primer on a Pestilence

AIDS is a disease* brought about by a deficiency in the body's immune system, which fights infections in the body caused by foreign organisms, including viruses, bacteria, and fungi.

As to the cause of AIDS, the consensus in the medical community is that AIDS is caused by HIV, short for human immunodeficiency virus.† HIV was originally called HTLV-III in the United States and LAV overseas; then later HTLV-III/LAV. They all mean the same thing, however, and will be referred to in this book as HIV or, simply, the AIDS virus. Recently, a second distinct strain of HIV has been discovered, and it is called HIV-II. When HIV-II is referred to, the first-discovered strain will be called HIV-I. Both strains of HIV are re-troviruses, a type of virus only recently discovered in humans.‡

---

*The debate continues over whether to call AIDS a disease. The purists say that it is not a disease in and of itself, but rather a condition that allows disease to flourish. But it has now been found that the AIDS virus itself may have direct effects on the brain and thus may qualify as a disease in its own right. Purists may consider my usage of *disease* a form of shorthand.

†The consensus is just that. A handful of holdouts, most notably Dr. Peter Duesberg, continue to insist that HIV is not the causative agent;[1] and the journalist Katie Leishman has also popularized the view that HIV is not the causative factor.[2]

‡A primer on retroviruses: A virus (from Latin *virus*, "poison") cannot reproduce outside living cells; it enters into another organism's "host" cell and uses that cell's biochemical machinery to replicate itself. These replicant virus particles then infect other cells; this process is repeated until the infection is either brought under control by the host's immune system, or the infection overwhelms and kills or debilitates the host, making it susceptible to other infections (as does HIV). Alternatively, virus and host may reach a state of equilibrium in which both coexist for years. The virus's initial entry into the host cell may cause symptoms of viral infection. Certain viruses can remain inactive, or latent, inside the host cell for long periods without causing problems. They can remain integrated with the cell's DNA (genetic material) until triggered to replicate (typically when the organism is compromised by old age, immunosuppressive drug therapy, or infection by another virus or by bacteria). At this point, the DNA is transcribed to RNA, which in turn becomes protein.

A retrovirus replicates "backward," transferring genetic information from viral RNA

HIV is normally detected in the blood through use of tests for anti-bodies to the virus. People whose blood tests positive are called "HIV-positive," "seropositive," or, often in medical literature, "antibody posi-tive."

HIV's ability to "hide out" in the body for years before striking is characteristic of its being a slow virus—the literal meaning of *lentivirus*. Part of the awe that has come to be associated with HIV is that it is the only lentivirus yet found among humans, although sheep, goats, and horses all suffer from lentiviruses. There is also *kuru*, a slow-acting transmissible agent that is fatal and incurable in humans; but kuru is transmissible only by eating human brains and only affects a single tribe in New Guinea.[4] Diseases that cause AIDS-like conditions are also known in the animal world. Feline leukemia virus, one of the prime killers of house cats, can cause immune deficiency similar to AIDS, as does a virus in monkeys which is known as SAIDS ("simian AIDS").

The Humble Origins of AIDS

The history of AIDS and HIV prior to its development into epidemic is of more than academic interest to this book. Many readers are famil-iar with the assertion, based on Randy Shilts's book *And the Band Played On,*[5] that a Canadian airline steward, Gaetan Dugas, was, to use the *New York Post*'s banner headline, "THE MAN WHO GAVE US AIDS."[6] In fact, while Shilts did portray Dugas as a modern Typhoid Mary and a highly efficient spreader of the virus, he made no assertion as to him being the source of the American epidemic, either in his book or elsewhere.[7] Dr. Harold Jaffe, chief of AIDS epidemiology at CDC, thinks the very labeling of Dugas as "Patient Zero" (the label was CDC's but was made public in the Shilts book) was foolish in that it allowed such an implication.[8] In part because of the misinterpretation

---

into DNA, the opposite of previously known viral actions. The retrovirus carries RNA (instead of DNA) as its genetic material along with a unique enzyme, reverse transcriptase (whence the name *retro*). This uses the RNA as a template to generate (transcribe) a DNA copy. This viral DNA inserts itself among the cell's own chromosomes. Positioned thus to function as a "new gene" for the infected host, it can immediately start producing viral RNAs (new viruses) or remain latent until activated. In the case of HIV, the latency period can be as short as a few weeks or as long as fifteen years or more. Activation is followed by a sudden explosion of replication activity that may directly kill or otherwise immobil-ize the host's cell—depletion of T-lymphocyte, a white blood cell that regulates the body's immune response. The rapid depletion or immobilization of T4-cells, characteristic of AIDS, leaves the human host vulnerable to many infections that a normal immune system would repel. The HTLV isolated by Robert Gallo in 1980 was the first identified retrovirus associated with human disease.[3]

of Shilts's writings, it is commonly believed that AIDS first became epidemic in Africa, later struck homosexuals in America and became epidemic among them, then only much later began infecting American heterosexuals. This belief, propagated by the media and the heterosexual AIDS alarmists, was a linchpin of the myth of the heterosexual AIDS epidemic. Books like James I. Slaff and John K. Brubaker's *The AIDS Epidemic,* among the most quoted of the earlier alarmist texts, stated, "It is believed that the first Americans infected were tourists vacationing in the Caribbean. The virus came to the Caribbean from Africa in the middle 1970s."[9] With such a time line established, it was easy for *Newsweek* to proclaim: "AIDS in Africa: The Future is Now";[10] or for the Associated Press to headline a piece "Spread in Africa Provides Glimpse into Future."[11] Similarly, throughout the epidemic, we would hear that AIDS just happened to hit the homosexual population first but that it was only a matter of time before heterosexuals bore the full brunt of the epidemic. Yet the Africa-to-American-homosexual-to-American-heterosexual time line is quite simply wrong.

The first medical report of what was soon to be named AIDS appeared in the Public Health Service (PHS) Centers for Disease Control (CDC) publication *Morbidity and Mortality Weekly Report (MMWR)* in June 1981. Entitled simply, "Pneumocystis Pneumonia—Los Angeles," it told of five young men, all active homosexuals, all previously healthy, who were struck by a disease that previously had been almost exclusively limited to patients receiving immunosuppression therapy in order to prevent rejection of donor organs and the like.[12] A few months later, the phenomenon made it into the medical journals as *"Pneumocystis Carinii* Pneumonia and Mucosal Candidiasis in Previously Healthy Homosexual Men."[13] Meanwhile, in 1981 doctors in Kinshasa, the capital of Zaire, began to document dozens of cases of unexplained immune dysfunctions. The dysfunctions were accompanied by infections and the appearance of a new, more aggressive form of Kaposi's sarcoma, a skin tumor that had been fairly common in Africa before but was rarely fatal until then.[14] It was the appearance of this new type of sarcoma, along with the underlying immune deficiency, that led a physician working in Zaire to consider that the African and American diseases might be related.[15] African patients suffering the same baffling symptoms also began turning up in Europe at about that time.[16]

By 1982, CDC was reporting these afflictions in American heterosexual intravenous drug abusers (IVDA),[17] in Haitians residing in the United States,[18] in persons with severe hemophilia,[19] in persons without the preceding risk factors who had received blood transfusions,[20] and in newborn babies.[21] The mothers who were available for interview admitted to being IVDA, or were Haitian.[22]

During the first week of 1983, CDC reported that two women had been afflicted with what was now being called AIDS. Neither of the women admitted to being in any of the preceding groups. But one had had a long-term sexual relationship with an IVDA; the other had had one with a bisexual; and both of their sexual partners had previously contracted AIDS, one of whom had already died.[23] This was the first publicity given to heterosexual transmission, although the media and the U.S. surgeon general, C. Everett Koop, would persist in announcing it as though it were something new through as late as 1987 (as discussed at length in chapter 19).

In fact, infection of heterosexuals in the United States goes back much further than 1983. Researchers for the New York City Department of Health have found records of children who appear to have been infected at birth as early as 1977, and thus concluded that "the presence of AIDS in the children studied provides evidence of the existence of HIV infection as early as 1977 in heterosexually active women using intravenous drugs in New York City."[24] Other doctors in analyzing this data set the date of introduction into the drug-using community at "around 1975 or 1976, or perhaps even earlier."[25] In fact, when investigators began combing through medical histories of past patients, they found a small number of probable cases on three continents going back nearly thirty years. Working back in time, they found AIDS-like symptoms in patients as early as 1959:

- 1977: a twenty-seven-year-old Rwandan mother developed the novel immunodeficiency symptoms.
- 1977: a thirty-four-year-old Zairian woman sought treatment in Belgium: she died in Kinshasa, Zaire, in 1978.
- 1977: a forty-seven-year-old Danish surgeon, who had worked in rural Zaire, died in Denmark. (Shilts tells her story in his book.)[26]
- 1976: a thirty-year-old Norwegian, his thirty-three-year-old wife, and their nine-year-old daughter all died after their health had deteriorated for seven to ten years.
- 1975: a previously healthy seven-month-old black infant developed *pneumocystis carinii* pneumonia (the prime killer of AIDS victims) in New York City.
- 1969: a fifteen- or sixteen-year-old black male in St. Louis, Missouri, died of a condition brought on by severe immune deficiency. Autopsy revealed Kaposi's sarcoma.

- 1959: a British sailor with Kaposi's sarcoma (the second leading killer of AIDS victims) died in Manchester, England.
- 1959: a forty-five-year-old U.S. man born in Haiti died.[27]

As the search continues, even earlier cases may be found. Notes the Harvard medical historian Dr. Allan Brandt, "We could have had a historical epidemic of disease caused by HIV but we wouldn't have recognized it like we do today." He points out that in the late nineteenth century, due to improvements in medical science, many symptoms formerly attributed to other causes were recognized as symptoms of secondary and tertiary syphilis. This news touched off tremendous public reaction which would last until the discovery of penicillin, even though actual levels of syphilis were probably no higher than they had been for centuries.[28] With AIDS there is a similar problem because even with today's diagnostic procedures, it can be difficult to look at symptoms and make a positive AIDS diagnosis with no other information, such as a test for HIV. Cases now attributed to AIDS would have been in the past (indeed, were) attributed to pneumonia, cancer, fungal infections, and other diseases today recognized as being part of the HIV syndrome. If, in fact, AIDS killed Egyptians during the time of Cheops or Romans during the reign of Claudius I, we would probably never know. The age of the virus is still a matter of extreme controversy, with estimates ranging from millions of years to thirty, and many points in between.[29]

Something New Out of Africa?

Besides the older cases I have just discussed, detected primarily by analysis of symptoms, frozen blood samples allow HIV to be traced back all the way to 1959. A sample collected that year in Kinshasa has proven HIV positive by various tests.[30] In the 1 March 1985 *Science,* an international team of scientists reported on frozen blood samples taken from 42,000 Ugandans between August 1972 and July 1973. The report created quite a sensation. Of seventy-five blood specimens sampled randomly, it was found that an amazingly high number showed HIV infection, with about 65 percent of the children and 48 percent of the adults carrying antibodies to the virus.[31] The fact that there was no outbreak of anything like AIDS reported at the time led the scientists to conclude that the virus must have mutated to a more malignant form sometime in the middle to late 1970s, roughly when it began to show up in Africa as AIDS.[32]

When the early cases I have discussed came to light, this hypothesis appeared to crumble. Further, the extraordinarily high infection rate— especially in children—was completely at odds with the results of tests being done fourteen years later on fresh samples. When Dr. J. W. Carswell and others tested healthy adults in Kampala, Uganda, in 1986, they found seropositivity rates of only (as compared with the earlier figure) 15.4 percent. These would appear to have been fairly recent infections, because Carswell's testing of older (mostly seventy years and over) people in Kampala revealed no seropositives in the ninety-six samples tested. Of those living in the West Nile district where the early 1970s blood was taken, there was only 1.4 percent seropositivity among healthy adults in 1986.[33] So what happened to all those early seropositives? It turned out they were false positives, triggered by something other than HIV antibodies such as antibodies to the malaria causing agent.[34] Thus, the international Panos Institute could assert in its 1988 book *AIDS and the Third World*:

> A series of serological studies, using sensitive and specific blood tests, subject to experienced interpretation, has failed to find high prevalences of the AIDS virus in Africa before the mid-1970s [excluding the 1959 sample], exactly the same situation as in the United States and Europe.[35]

Meanwhile, in 1978, the San Francisco Health Department began a study to monitor hepatitis-B infections in homosexual men (henceforth to be called the San Francisco hepatitis-B cohort). When stored samples were later tested for HIV, it was found that of 283 men tested, only 0.3 percent were infected as of 1978.[36] This finding indicates that there were probably very few homosexual seropositives in the country before 1978.

Unfortunately, the news that the early African testing was faulty seems to be practically a state secret. It continues to be the common wisdom that high levels of both AIDS and HIV existed in Africa for a considerable time before they were present in the United States.

Nonsexual HIV Transmission

There are many ways by which infectious agents are transmitted. Some are transmitted by insect vectors, like bubonic plague (rat fleas) and malaria (mosquitoes); some are airborne, carried in droplets of sputum expelled during coughing, talking, or sneezing, like cold viruses, measles, smallpox, influenza, and pneumonic plague; some are transmitted by physical contact, like the sexually transmitted diseases (STDs), warts, and impetigo; some, only in bodily fluids like blood and semen, including hepatitis B. Some contagions are extremely easy to contract (colds); some extremely difficult such as leprosy, which usually requires contact and to which most persons have built-in immunity.[37]

There is absolutely no relationship between symptoms and transmission. Smallpox and cold viruses are transmitted in the same way, yet their symptoms are entirely different. Further, one is often fatal in a previously healthy person; the other, virtually never fatal. This all seems elementary enough; but unfortunately when the topic of AIDS comes up, these basic principles have often been forgotten. Thus, some people have assumed that because AIDS has symptoms similar to that of a sheep virus that is airborne, AIDS may be transmitted by coughing.[38] Others think that because mosquitoes can carry diseases in blood, they can transmit HIV.[39] One alarmist stated, "The original doubts about heterosexual transmission become only more astounding with the knowledge that syphilis, the classic venereal infection, also needs to reach the bloodstream to cause disease and is often transported there by the same T-4 lymphocytes that transport the AIDS-causing virus."[40] What is truly astounding is that one could infer from the fact that because two types of contagion both need to reach the bloodstream to cause disease, their transmission efficiency is similar.

In fact, HIV is what is called a blood-borne virus: that is, it can be transmitted through blood-to-blood contact or through contact of some other bodily fluids containing HIV with the blood of a recipient. In the *scientific* community, there is no serious debate about this. Several studies have been conducted of the family members of both children and adults with HIV infection. Despite extensive and prolonged household contact with an infected person, none of over four hundred family members has ever been infected with HIV except sex partners, children born to infected mothers, or persons with independent risk factors (that is, factors outside the home).[41]

While HIV can survive for several hours to days in insects fed blood with high concentrations of HIV or injected with HIV-contaminated blood, no evidence of HIV replication in insects or insect cells in laboratories has been reported, and epidemiological studies show no patterns of HIV infection by insects.[42]

Nor is HIV about to mutate into a more easily transmissible form as some observers, including the editorial staff of the *Wall Street Journal,* have suggested it might.[43] One sometimes hears this possibility bandied around, often prefaced with a remark that since it happened with

bubonic plague, it can happen with HIV. At a conference sponsored for
Congress by Representative Dan Burton (Republican of Indiana), a
woman claiming as her credentials a B.S. in microbiology testified:

> Mutation could possibly change the mode of transmission [of HIV] as hap-
> pened during the bubonic plague. In the first one-third to one-half time
> period, the plague was transmitted by the rat flea through the blood but
> converted its mode of transmission in the middle of the plague to be transmit-
> ted by a cough. Thus, the new nomenclature pneumonic plague.[44]

For one thing, plague is a bacillus—it's hardly fair to compare viral
mutation to bacterial mutation. At any rate, bubonic plague did not
mutate. The Black Death appears to have been a complex combination
of bacterial strains, sometimes taking only the bubonic form; while, at
other times, the bubonic, pneumonic, and even a third form, septica-
emic, appeared simultaneously.[45] Sometimes a person with bubonic
plague would become infected in the lungs and spread the bacillus by
coughing, thus leading to contagious pneumonic plague. But this is no
more a form of mutation than the flu mutating into pneumonia, simply
because pneumonia sometimes strikes flu patients.

Bacilli aside, no virus known has ever mutated so much as to change
its mode of transmission. I asked Dr. Harvey Fineberg, dean of the
Harvard School of Public Health, about the possibility of such an evolution with HIV. He replied that his researchers had considered the
question carefully but concluded it was "as likely as a pig growing
wings." In fact, if anything the virus will probably tend to mutate in the
direction of benignancy since viruses that kill their hosts also kill themselves; therefore, they are less likely to spread than viruses that live
longer.* (Such a benign mutation was the final outcome of Michael
Crichton's deadly but fictional "Andromeda strain," to which HIV has
sometimes been compared.)[47]

In sum, HIV is transmitted only by *direct* contact with bodily fluids.
Breathing in coughed droplets or being bitten by a mosquito are not
enough. The questions, then, are: *Which* bodily fluids transmit HIV?
How do those fluids enter the body? And how much of those fluids are
necessary to infect?

To some extent, the response to the last question answers the first,
since it raises the matter of the efficiency of HIV transmission. Despite
assertions that all that is needed for HIV infection is one virion (one

---

*Such a mutation to virtual benignancy has occurred with another virus, the Myxoma,
introduced into the Australian rabbit population.[46]

particle of virus), researchers have learned that, in relation to other viruses that plague mankind, a comparatively large dose of HIV is needed to infect a person. One study in the *New England Journal of Medicine* found:

> The risk of HIV transmission from a single needle-stick accident [which occurs when someone is giving an injection or drawing blood from a patient, and inadvertently jabs himself or herself with a contaminated needle] appears to be approximately 0.35 percent [about 1 in 300] on the basis of a composite analysis of eight seroprevalence studies of parenterally exposed [that is, having received injections below the skin] health care workers.[48]

By contrast, hepatitis B infects about 12 to 17 percent of those accidentally stuck with needles containing that virus:[49] that's 1 in 6 for hepatitis B versus 1 in 300 for HIV. The Hepatitis Branch of the CDC has estimated that 200 to 300 health-care workers die each year from the direct or indirect consequences of occupationally acquired hepatitis B; as many as 12,000 become infected with the virus.[50] As of March of 1989, only 18 Americans are thought to have contracted HIV by this method (25 persons world-wide).[51] One study of almost 800 homosexuals found that hepatitis B is probably transmitted ten times more efficiently sexually than is HIV.[52]

Dr. Albert Sabin, developer of the oral polio vaccine and more recently a consultant to the National Institutes of Health (NIH), put it this way: "It's not a question of one particle. It's not just that the virus is present, virus is absent. That's not good enough. From everything we know about infectious diseases, it's not just the presence, it's the quantity, and what happens when it multiplies." He added, "Surely a trace of the virus somewhere, in tears, saliva, the vaginal mucosa, doesn't mean the disease is transmitted that way."[53]

The Fear of Tearing and the Kiss of Death

Reports that even such fluids as tears could transmit HIV caused alarm in the offices of ophthalmologists everywhere; but, in fact, it is unusual for virus to be found in tears of a seropositive person, and there is no evidence of transmission of HIV to health-care workers or other persons by ophthalmological procedures or contact lens fitting.[54] Likewise, saliva has never been shown to contain enough virus to cause infection. In one study, for example, virus was isolated from the saliva of only one of 83 infected patients, compared with isolation from the blood of 28 of 50 infected patients.[55]* Nor has HIV-infected saliva been implicated in bite wounds. In one West German case a bite was suggested as the route of HIV transmission between two young brothers, but the bite did not even break the skin.[57] Other studies have shown no transmissions through biting, including a CDC one in which 48 health-care workers were bitten through the skin or into a mucous membrane surface by a seropositive individual, yet none became infected.[58]

Recently it was reported that saliva can actually inhibit infection with HIV. A study published in 1988, in the *Journal of the American Dental Association,* reported that "the ability of HIV to infect human peripheral blood lymphocytes (white blood cells, the usual abode of HIV) can be completely inhibited by incubation of the virus in unstimulated whole saliva" in the test tube at body temperature for one hour.[59] This is good news not only for those who like their kisses wet, but also for those on the "giving" side of oral sex.

Needle Sharing

Needle sharing has accounted for the second largest category of AIDS cases. After purchase, drugs in powdered form are commonly placed in a "cooker" consisting of a bottle cap. The powder is then diluted in tap water, heated to go into solution, and withdrawn into needle and syringe. A vein is identified and punctured, blood is withdrawn into the needle and syringe, and the solution is injected. Often small quantities of drug are injected repeatedly, with intervening blood withdrawals. It is common in the IVDA subculture, especially in the East Coast, for needles, syringes, and "cookers" all to be shared. The place where IVDAs gather to share these needles is called a "shooting gallery." After use, the contaminated "works" (to use the vernacular for the assorted equipment) are loaned or rented to another user. The needle and syringe may be reused repeatedly until they are no longer serviceable. Thus, sequential anonymous sharing of blood-contaminated needles and syringes occurs among large numbers of persons. It would be hard to design a system more efficient in transmitting a blood-borne virus.[60]

*One report did suggest infection from kissing. The case of an impotent man who apparently transmitted the virus to his wife sent tremors through the heterosexual world. It was gleefully seized upon by persons seeking to establish that the government had conspired to understate the AIDS threat. But while the woman was initially reported to be seronegative (no HIV antibodies) yet positive for the virus itself, subsequent tests have shown her to be both antibody negative and negative for the virus.[56]

(*Blood-borne* means the virus can be transmitted only in body fluids, including blood, semen, and sometimes secretions from cervix or vagina.) Indeed, surveys in some parts of the country, such as New Jersey and Puerto Rico, have found seropositivity levels among IVDAs as high as 59 percent, although areas where needle sharing is unusual will report rates in the single digits or indeed no IVDA infections at all.[61]

Blood and Blood Products

Although any AIDS case is a tragedy, acquisition of HIV through blood products seems all the more horrible since that which was intended to save lives ultimately destroys them. Prior to 1985 there was no test for screening blood to detect the presence of antibodies to HIV. As a result, an estimated 12,000 persons received HIV-tainted transfusions,[62] although many of them died from complications of the medical emergencies that made them require transfusions in the first place. Because hemophiliacs use clotting factor, which is made up of the blood product of many donors mixed together, there are extremely high rates of infection among hemophiliacs, depending on the type and severity of the hemophilia. HIV prevalence ranges from 15 percent to over 90 percent, with the highest being for persons with severe hemophilia A and the lowest for those with hemophilia B and mild or moderate hemophilia A.[63]

Both infected transfusion recipients and hemophiliacs, being representative of the population as a whole, are predominantly heterosexual and hence may be a source of contagion for other heterosexuals, although a large percentage of both groups have been notified of their seropositivity and thus can be presumed to be less likely to pass the infection on. Transfusion recipients also tend to be elderly, and thus less likely to spread the virus through sexual intercourse.

In this chapter I have intentionally skirted the most usual method of AIDS transmission—sexual intercourse. To it I now turn.

4

The Risks of
Heterosexual Intercourse

Although there is much to be learned from the AIDS epidemic and our reaction to it, for many of us the interest in AIDS comes down to one question: What are *my* risks? Robert Redfield answers the question simply by saying that anyone is at risk who has sexual intercourse with anyone else who has the virus.[1] Such a statement essentially keeps a person from figuring out any way to reduce risks other than abstaining from all sex—as it is intended to do. The answer is, in fact, both more complicated and more simple.

Like all sexually transmitted diseases (STDs), HIV is more difficult to spread than, say, the common cold or the flu, both of which are carried by airborne droplets. All STDs are comparatively inefficient: that's why they need close bodily contact. But even by STD standards, HIV is extremely inefficient in traveling from host to host. Mere juxtaposition of genitalia is enough to transmit syphilis, gonorrhea, herpes simplex II, and chlamydia, all of which require only direct contact with the mucous membrane.* (Gonorrhea, and herpes are not even restricted to genitalia, but sometimes infect the mouth or throat.)

Some doctors and texts have claimed matter-of-factly that HIV also penetrates through an intact mucosal membrane: for example, Dr. Margaret Fischl of the University of Miami School of Medicine has declared "that this virus [HIV], when it comes into contact with any mucous membrane, is going to be transmitted."[2] Redfield backs up this theory

---

*Mucosal membranes are, in simple terms, very thin skin areas on various parts of the body, including rectum, vagina, penis, areola around the nipples, and lining of the mouth.

by pointing out that chimpanzees have been inoculated with swabs in their vaginas.

In fact, things are not nearly so clear on this as they would have us think. Different STDs penetrate the body in different ways. Like hepatitis-B virus, however, HIV is bloodborne—the most inefficient type of transmission an STD can have. As Dr. Katherine M. Stone of the STD section of the Centers for Disease Control explained it to me, "Hepatitis B and AIDS don't bore through intact skin. It's not really clear what's going on, but it probably takes a small abrasion from trauma."[3] Mucous membranes, in consisting of very thin layers of skin, require far less trauma for penetration than other areas on the body. A sore, even an undetectably small one such as often accompanies herpes, would also offer a passageway for these viruses.

But in addition to its apparent need for an opening, HIV's relative inefficiency in heterosexual transmission is a result of the need for a heavy dose, as attested by the differences in infection rates between HIV and hepatitis B. This probably explains Redfield's chimp vagina. What he doesn't point out when he uses this example is that no one inoculates an animal using blood or semen; rather, the virus that is swabbed into the vagina has gone through a centrifuge that multiplies the virus concentration by 50,000 times. If one takes a virus that is difficult to transmit because it needs high concentrations, and then concentrates that virus by 50,000 times, it shouldn't be surprising that modes of transmission that were extremely inefficient before centrifuging suddenly become efficient.

That HIV is a bloodborne virus needing extremely efficient means of transmission explains the high incidence of AIDS among hemophiliacs and intravenous (IV) drug users who share needles, since putting HIV-infected blood, or blood extracts such as hemophilia clotting factor, directly into the bloodstream is an extremely efficient way to transmit the infection. Less obviously, the bloodborne nature of HIV also explains its prevalence among homosexuals. The overwhelming risk factor associated with sexually transmitted AIDS is anal sex—especially for the passive or recipient partner.

Receptive Anal Intercourse

The reason for the danger of anal sex in the era of AIDS is in part the difference between the tissue construction of the male urethra and rectum and the female vagina. While the vagina is constructed of tough platelike cells that resist rupture and infectious agents, and are designed to withstand the motions of intercourse and childbirth, the urethra and rectum are constructed primarily of columnar cells which tear or rupture easily. This allows semen to enter the more readily accessible blood vessels of the rectum or, conversely, allows blood from a ruptured rectum to seep into the urethra of the insertive partner in anal intercourse.[4] One major study found that "men who reported rectal or penile bleeding on five or more occasions during or immediately following sexual exposures were considerably more likely to [have become infected] than men who had not noticed any bleeding at all."[5]

There are other factors in the AIDS–anal sex connection. The vagina provides natural lubrication, whereas there is little in the anus. Anal douching, a practice many homosexuals engage in prior to anal intercourse, can remove what lubrication the anus has, and has been shown to increase the risk of transmission.[6] Nonlubrication not only increases the chance of ruptures but at the same time reduces the efficiency of the condom, which many have touted as the way to turn unsafe homosexual sex into safe sex. The condom has a considerably higher breakage rate during anal sex, as will be discussed in chapter 12.

Finally, since HIV has been found in the epithelial cells lining the bowel, it appears that while a tear in the anal wall would facilitate HIV transmission, HIV can directly penetrate blood vessels below the surface of the anus even without such trauma.[7]

In study after study, receptive anal intercourse has consistently been reported as the sexual behavior most strongly associated with HIV infection.[8] According to the late Dr. B. Frank Polk, director of the Johns Hopkins University component of the Multicenter AIDS Cohort Study, "In gay men, 95 percent or more of the infections occur from receptive anal intercourse."[9] A study published in the April 1987 *American Journal of Public Health (AJPH)* found that, of 240 men in the test group who became infected over the course of the study, all but 4 had engaged in receptive anal sex.[10]* In fact, some studies have found anal intercourse, along with associated rectal trauma (as evidenced by bleeding), to be the *only* important risk factor (and one found that even the number of partners was not a significant risk factor).[13]

---

*Another study that year found that unprotected receptive anal intercourse could account for nearly all of the 95 new infections detected among 2,507 initially seronegative men after six months of followup. The degree of risk accelerated in proportion to the number of receptive anal partners, from about threefold for one partner, to eighteenfold for those with 5 or more partners in the six-month period.[11] In a more recent study, of 85 seropositives all but 2 reported engaging in receptive anal intercourse.[12]

(It is important to remember that, while the comparative efficiency of HIV transmission through anal intercourse as opposed to vaginal is very significant—compared with transmissibility of other STDs such as syphilis, gonorrhea, or herpes—even with *anal* sex, HIV is difficult to transmit. HIV may be a "super virus" in the sense that it virtually always kills once it infects; but compared with most germs, either bacterial or viral, HIV outside of the body is a real wimp. This explains why the figures bandied around a few years ago by such sources as Slaff and Brubaker's *The AIDS Epidemic* and *U.S. News & World Report* that said 70 percent to 90 percent of all homosexuals in San Francisco and New York were infected have turned out to be greatly exaggerated.[14] If this *were* the case, then AIDS might well have developed into a very serious problem for heterosexuals as well.)

The best evidence that receptive anal intercourse is more dangerous than vaginal intercourse, however, comes from a growing number of studies showing that anal intercourse significantly increases a woman's chance of becoming infected if she has an HIV-infected partner. The Padian study, for example, found that women who engaged in anal sex had 2.3 times greater chance of infection than women who did not.[15] (This should not be misconstrued as indicating that anal sex is only 2.3 times more efficient than vaginal sex, however, since the women who engaged in anal sex in the study did so together with vaginal intercourse.) A Brazilian study presented at the Fourth International Conference on AIDS in Stockholm found that, of female partners of bisexual men, only 19 percent of 42 women engaging in strictly vaginal intercourse seroconverted; while out of 33 women engaging in both vaginal and anal intercourse, almost three times that percentage, or 54 percent, become positive for HIV. The doctors concluded that anal intercourse was significantly more risky than vaginal intercourse.[16] Finally, a New York heterosexual partner study presented at the same conference found that "the number of episodes of anal intercourse was the only significant independent predictor of HIV seropositivity."[17]

Heterosexual Transmission

The best method for measuring HIV transmissibility is, unfortunately, for couples to engage in unprotected (no condoms or infrequent condom use) intercourse with a person known to be seropositive. Efforts to analyze this situation are called partner studies. Why someone would want to have unprotected intercourse with someone known to be infected, despite repeated warnings from those who conduct the partner studies, is an interesting question (many, in fact, are enrolled after both parties have become infected); but the data provided is invaluable.

In 1987 Dr. Padian and her fellow researchers at Berkeley released the results of a partner study in which, aside from showing the increased risk of anal sex as noted earlier, Padian was able to calculate the risk of HIV infection as less than 1 in 1,000 to one going from men to women. (These figures are not just for vaginal intercourse: the study included women who also engaged in anal intercourse. Therefore, excluding anal sex would drop the odds ever further.)[18]

Of the 97 women in the Padian study who had had intercourse with a total of 93 infected male partners (some of the men had sex with more than 1 woman), 22 of them, or 23 percent, became infected themselves. The study found that rates of infection for partners of bisexuals, hemophiliacs, and blood-transfusion victims were statistically identical (22 percent, 21 percent, and 25 percent, respectively); but that partners of men who were intravenous drug abusers were infected at a much higher rate, 42 percent. The study found a clear correlation between increased contacts with an infected man and increased risk of HIV infection. Infected women were 4.6 times more likely than uninfected ones to have had more than 100 sexual contacts with an infected man. Nonetheless, of 25 women with 600 or more contacts each with infected men, 14 remained uninfected.

Dr. Redfield, amazingly, has declared male-to-female vaginal HIV transmission to be 50 percent *per contact,* in an interview with Ann Guidici Fettner.[19] He referred to a letter published in *Lancet* in which it was reported that, of 8 Australian women inseminated artificially with sperm, 4 seroconverted.[20] Redfield asserted: "The bottom line for women is that half of them get infected in spouse studies [and] very few viruses are effectively transmitted even 50 percent of the time. It's a very efficient virus."[21]

The explanation for the high seroconversion rate associated with the artificial insemination study lies, aside from the tiny sample size, in the mechanics of artificial insemination, of which both Redfield and the reporter, Fettner, appeared ignorant. During normal vaginal intercourse, the male ejaculates into the vagina, whence the sperm swim through the woman's cervical fluid into the blood-lined wall of the cervix. Cells found in the lining of the cervix (the narrow lower end of the uterus) may be highly susceptible to HIV in semen.[22] HIV is contained in the semen, which normally does not make contact with the cervix—*except* during the most common technique of artificial insemination. It was later verified that, indeed, in the Australian inseminations the semen was placed directly into the cervical os (opening).[23] A five-minute phone call to any of several public interest groups or medical facilities dealing with artificial insemination would have revealed this distinction, but apparently neither Redfield nor Fettner bothered to make that call. When I asked Redfield some time later if he knew the mechanics of artificial insemination, it turned out that, indeed, he did but that he didn't think the difference between laying semen on the cervical wall and on the vaginal wall "was necessarily that important."[24] Which it isn't if one assumes, as he does, that HIV even in low concentrations penetrates right through intact vaginal mucosa.

The notion that HIV is transmitted just as efficiently vaginally as anally is one the alarmists hold dear. In a 1986 letter to Representative Dan Burton, A. D. J. Robertson, later to become an advisor to Gary Bauer, director of policy development in the White House, declared that "it is important to remember that it is only recently that it has become clear that the risk of heterosexual transmission is roughly equal to the risk of homosexual transmission."[25]*

While anal sex appears to put a woman at much greater risk of HIV infection than vaginal sex, it is highly improbable that most non-IVDA women infected heterosexually are infected via the rectum, as many heterosexuals seem to want to believe. It is certainly correct to state that many seropositive or AIDS-diagnosed women who deny anal sex are lying, for the same reason men lie about their homosexuality or drug abuse. However, it would be very difficult to explain why studies such as Padian's[28] would show a positive correlation between women admitting to anal sex and HIV infection if, in fact, *all* the HIV-infected women had participated in anal sex. This would make the act of *admitting* to anal sex a risk factor. (Perhaps it could be argued that women who admit to anal sex engage in it more frequently, but this is tenuous.)

While the vaginal wall is far more rugged than the anus, the science

---

*Some homosexuals also did not want to believe that the rectum could be more vulnerable. Indeed, the special vulnerability of the rectum has, strangely enough, turned this orifice into an ideological battleground. Militant homosexuals have bristled at the suggestion that the anus could somehow be inferior to the vagina as a receptical for the male sex organ. "Is the Rectum a Grave?" asked the title of one provocative essay.[26] Their concern was understandable. Homosexuals generally don't say that they know that homosexuality is unnatural, but they wish to practice it nonetheless. The general line is that it is as natural as heterosexuality, only different. This being the case, pointing out that at least with respect to AIDS the anus is clearly a more dangerous place for a sexual rendezvous is seen as an indictment of the naturalness of homosexuality in general. Indeed, writers like Patrick J. Buchanan and Norman Podhoretz have argued exactly that.[27] But this is a battle for another day.

writer John Langone notes that the former is far from impervious to the sort of damage that might allow transmission of HIV:

> Trauma during sex—say, a bruise of the vaginal wall—may . . . play a role in transmission, along with any of a number of other diseases and conditions. . . . the probability of infection can also be increased by any condition accompanied by vaginal bleeding, related or unrelated to menstruation—vaginitis, pelvic inflammatory disease, fibroid tumors, herpes, serious yeast infections, and even the stress associated with diabetes and ulcers—as well as by the use of IUDs and birth control pills. Some post menopausal women bleed during vaginal intercourse unless they use a lubricant; and . . . the wall of the vagina becomes more fragile as a woman ages.[29]

In short, vaginal transmission is, while possible, far less likely than anal transmission. This difference significantly contributes to the greater likelihood of HIV spread among homosexuals than among heterosexuals. It explains why the odds are so much against transmission of HIV from an infected man to an uninfected woman in a single act of even unprotected intercourse.

Female-to-Male Transmission

But if the odds against HIV going from men to women are high, how about women to men? Dr. Redfield has stated, "This infection goes as easily from a man to a woman as from woman to man and from man to man."[30] Dr. Margaret Fischl of the University of Miami School of Medicine has also maintained that men and women are equally vulnerable,[31] and A. D. J. Robertson advised members of Congress that just as the risk of heterosexual transmission was virtually identical to that of homosexual intercourse, the risks of female-to-male transmission were equivalent to those of male-to-female.[32] Said Redfield:

> The argument of the purists that all sexually transmitted diseases are more efficient from man to woman is valid. But to me, that's not significant. What the purists are talking about is the difference between 30 percent and 40 percent, and that's giving people the wrong message, and it's not enough to make any difference in your risk.[33]

In fact, there is every reason to believe that transmission from women to men is significantly less efficient than the opposite way.

If we first look at the numbers of men and women listed by the CDC as infected through heterosexual intercourse, we find that the ratio of female to male cases (among native-born Americans) is about 3 to 1.[34]

At a glance, this might seem to provide strong evidence for increased male-to-female efficiency. But this is not necessarily the case, because it also happens that there are far more potential sources of infection for female heterosexuals than there are for men. The great majority of female heterosexual transmission cases come from sex with male IVDAs, and there are about four times as many male IVDAs as there are female ones.

Further, women can also get infected by bisexual males. Since HIV is not spread among lesbians, without other risk factors bisexual women pose little risk to a man. Still, if one looks at New York City, where the heterosexual figures are far more accurate than federal figures for reasons noted earlier, one sees that while the ratio of male-to-female IVDA cases is again about 4 to 1, the ratio of female to male heterosexual partners of IVDAs who have AIDS is over 50 to 1.[35] Even factoring out cases in which a bisexual was the transmitter, there is an overwhelming disparity. Thus, the New York figures do seem to indicate that a man is far safer having sex with an infected woman than vice versa.

Strong evidence for the relatively low risk to men of vaginal intercourse comes from some of the aforementioned homosexual studies, which indicated that while receptive anal intercourse was by far the most hazardous act, penetrative anal intercourse seemed to carry little or no independent risk.[36] Some studies, however have found there could be some risk for the penetrating partner. For example, in the *American Journal of Public Health* study I have described, three of the four seropositives who denied engaging in receptive anal intercourse engaged in penetrative anal sex.[37] The two seropositives in the *American Journal of Epidemiology* study had likewise engaged in penetrative anal intercourse. Further, since many of the men in the study engaged in both insertive and receptive anal intercourse, it is possible that some of the men classified as anal-receptive seropositives actually were infected through an insertive act. Yet, if we compare men who engaged *only* in receptive intercourse or in both activities versus those who engaged *only* in insertive intercourse, we find significant differences. Thus, in the *AJPH* study, while only 22 percent of those engaging in strictly insertive intercourse became infected,[38] 66 percent of those who did both became seropositive.[39]

In light of the comparatively small risk to homosexuals who are the penetrating partner in anal sex, it stands to reason that the risk to a man from vaginal penetration would be smaller than that of a woman vaginally penetrated. In fact, it is probably much smaller, because one factor in seroconversions of insertive homosexual men is that penile bleeding may result from the lack of natural lubrication and the tightness of the anus in comparison with the vagina.[40]

More evidence of low risk for the penetrating partner comes from partner studies. For the last few years, Padian has been following 20 men who have had either regular or intermittent intercourse with seropositive women. None of these men have become seropositive,[41] although she cautions about reading too much into the results from such a small sample. The results of other partners studies also show women less likely to infect men than vice versa.[42] For example, the Peterman/Stoneburner study found 18 percent of wives becoming infected but only 8 percent of husbands.

Dr. H. Hunter Handsfield, however, says that the difference might be greater than it appears, and thus indirectly challenges Redfield's assertion about other STDs. Handsfield has noted that while one study suggests a 50-percent risk of transmission of gonorrhea from men to women following a single sexual exposure,[43] other studies have estimated the risk at 80 percent or even higher.[44] By contrast, the risk of female-to-male transmission of gonorrhea is reasonably well documented to be 20 percent to 25 percent. The prevalence of gonorrhea nonetheless appears to level off at 80 percent to 90 percent in men (and probably in women), regardless of exposure.[45] Uncontrolled but extensive experience in STD clinics tends to confirm this pattern for gonorrhea and also for chlamydial infection, as in figure 4.1. If HIV transmission is similar, says Handsfield, the prevalence of infection in the regular sexual partners of infected persons may give an inflated estimate of female-to-male transmission efficiency.

The mechanics of decreased risk for female-to-male transmission are fairly easily explained. "Think of viral load," said Dr. George Galasso, a member of the NIH task force on AIDS:

> Even during normal [vaginal] sex, the male is putting lots of cells into the female, so the possibility of infecting in that direction is greater. You can't exclude the other way, of course, because if the virus is in the female, abrasions on the penis make it possible. But the odds are that it's going to go male to female rather than the other way.[46]

HIV, unlike some viruses such as hepatitis B and herpes simplex II, is only infrequently found outside of cells. For example, in studies conducted by Dr. Jay Levy at the Cancer Research Institute Department of Medicine in San Francisco, only 20 percent to 30 percent of semen specimens had detectable virus that was not in cells; and to the extent

FIGURE 4.1

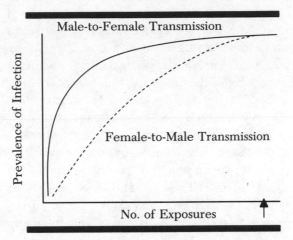

NOTE: Hypothetical transmission patterns for sexually transmitted diseases dependent on exposure to semen or cervical secretions. Similar prevalences of infection in men and women beyond number of exposures denoted by arrow do not necessarily imply equal efficiency of transmission in both directions. Thus, while eventually the infection rates for men and women may equal out, it may take much longer for those men to become infected, indicating greater facility of transmission from men to women.

SOURCE: H. Hunter Handsfield, "Heterosexual Transmission of the Human Immunodeficiency Virus," *JAMA* 260 (13 [7 October 1988]): 1944.

that the virus was present, it was in extremely low levels.[47] In one study of cell-free cervical secretions, a similarly low level of virus was found in about half the specimens examined,[48] and in yet another study, of vaginal/cervical fluid from 18 seropositive women, no virus could be found.[49] In the absence of venereal infection, vaginal/cervical fluids usually carry few cells and are therefore capable of carrying little virus. According to Levy, levels of hepatitis-B virus in such fluids will be 100 to 1,000 times greater concentration than HIV.[50] Semen, however, normally contains an average of 3,000,000 white blood cells per milliliter. Thus, while a seropositive woman is usually shooting blanks, the average seropositive man is firing a loaded submachine gun.

Relative Transmission

When they weren't telling untruths by saying that there is no difference in transmissibility between homosexuals and heterosexuals, the alarmists simply avoided the issue altogether. Instead, they would often choose simply to state over and over that HIV is indeed transmissible heterosexually, portraying it as an "either-or dilemma." When pressed, they would simply say, "It is transmissible from man to woman and

woman to man as well as man to man."* It is as if two arms salesmen
are plying their wares to a third party, and the one trying to sell ninety-
year-old British Lee-Enfields keeps insisting, "A bolt-action rifle can kill
a man and an automatic rifle can kill a man." Yes, yes, yes. Nobody
doubts that both rifles can kill; the potential buyer wants to know which
rifle can kill more efficiently. Similarly, persons interested in the spread
of AIDS, whether for personal reasons or for sake of the nation or the
world, already knew full well *how* it *could* be transmitted; they needed
to know the likelihood or comparative efficiency of the various means
of possible transmission. Was it safer to have sex with a woman than a
man, all other things being equal? Was oral sex safer than vaginal sex,
vaginal sex safer than anal? This is what they wanted to discuss, and this
is what the alarmists kept trying to avoid with their tireless invocations
of "It goes from a man to a woman and a woman to a man."

The Role of Sexually Transmitted Diseases

Studies in both Africa[53] and the United States[54] have found that
certain STDs can dramatically increase the probability of transmission
of HIV. This increased probability appears whether the STD is in the
HIV carrier or in his or her sexual partner. In respect to carriers, an STD
raises the level of white blood cells in genital secretions, whether semen
or cervical-vaginal fluid.[55] In the HIV negative partner with an STD, on
the other hand, the body sends white blood cells to the infected area
to fight off the STD, which allows HIV a much better chance of taking
root in the blood system. But probably more important is that many
STDS cause genital ulcerations. For a micro-organism that bores
through the skin, the presence or absence of such ulcerations is probably of little consequence. But for one like HIV that appears unable to
penetrate intact skin, a genital ulceration is the equivalent of throwing
open the castle gates for the invading hordes.

The increased efficiency of HIV transmission in the presence of other
STDS seems to occur regardless of the sex of a partner.[56] For homosexual men, the risk appears to be increased if they engage in unprotected
anal intercourse (without a condom). In Africa, research suggests that
STDs play a role in the transmission of HIV independent of how many
different partners one has.[57]

The importance of this last factor, the irrelevance of the number of

*Those who have used virtually these exact words include Dr. Jonathan Mann of the
World Health Organization,[51] and Kevin Hopkins and William Johnston.[52]

partners, is that one could argue that the STD-HIV connection is *casual* and not *causal*. Casual means that they have HIV because they're more promiscuous and thus they also have STDs. Causal means the STD contributed to the contraction of HIV. The previously cited studies indicate that while we might expect some casual relationship, STDs do appear to *lead to* HIV infection rather than just come along with it.

Women infected with genital ulcer disease or other STDs, which damage the genital mucous membranes, appear much more likely to contract HIV during sexual intercourse with an infected partner than women without such ulcers, according to a study carried out in Nairobi. Chlamydia infection also was associated with some increased risk.[58] In one group of women in Zaire, the risk of becoming infected with HIV tripled for those with a history of genital ulcer disease.[59] Another study found that a woman with genital ulcers was four times as likely to contract the AIDS virus from an HIV-infected partner as a woman without ulcers.[60] According to one of these researchers, "genital ulcer disease not only makes a woman more susceptible to acquiring the AIDS virus, it also probably makes her more infectious for her sexual partner."[61] Another pointed out, however, that "in patients who already have the AIDS virus, immune deficiency can predispose them to picking up infections which cause genital ulcers."[62]

Oral Intercourse

Oral sex, by contrast, appears to carry with it comparatively little risk of infection. Again, this finding is explainable by looking at the orifice involved. The anus is not made to take anything in, while the vagina is made to occasionally receive the male organ. But mouths are built to take in regularly all manner of things, hot and cold, hard and soft, animate, formerly animate, and never previously animate. Nevertheless, bleeding gums are not uncommon during brushing of teeth or eating[63] and may be present at other times. Further, the inside of the mouth can, as a mucosal membrane, be comparatively easily torn. Thus, in theory infection via oral sex would appear to be comparatively safe but not risk-free.

One indicator of whether receptive oral sex may transmit HIV is whether children have been infected through breast feeding, since the breast milk of infected women may contain HIV. The problem here is that 25 percent to 50 percent of seropositive mothers will give birth to a seropositive child;[64] and so it is difficult to tell whether the child was infected before birth or after. Still, to the extent it has been possible to make a determination, breast feeding seems to have been a likely mode of transmission in only a few cases, if at all.[65]

Penile-Oral Intercourse

As of this writing, there are no confirmed cases of AIDS caused by insertive penile intercourse with the mouth, and the practice is almost certainly less hazardous than other sexual activities.[66] For example, one study of seroconversion among homosexual men not practicing receptive anal intercourse found seroconversion among men practicing both insertive anal intercourse and oral intercourse but not among men practicing only oral intercourse.[67]

The problem with such studies is what could be called a masking effect: that is, more hazardous activities will mask those that are less hazardous. For example, if activity A results in infection 10 percent of the time and activity B results in infection 1 percent of the time, those engaging in both activities might actually have fewer infections than those engaging in just A (to the extent that engaging in activity B displaces some occasions of engaging in activity A), yet it is wrong to conclude that B is necessarily completely safe. Thus, the only way of measuring how risky, if at all, a less risky activity is would be to look at those who engage only in such activities. Among homosexuals, engaging in oral sex alone is infrequent. In an *American Journal of Public Health* study, only 18 out of 359 men in the study did not engage in receptive anal intercourse; and of those, an unspecified smaller number engaged only in oral intercourse.[68] Thus, positively identifying oral intercourse as the culprit is difficult, while trying to come up with an exact risk ratio on the order of the Padian figure is downright impossible. It is because of this masking effect that Masters, Johnson, and Kolodny, and Kevin Hopkins and William Johnston of the Hudson Institute, were wrong when they cited a study by Margaret Fischl as indicating possible infection through oral intercourse.[69] All the Fischl study showed was that those women practicing both oral and vaginal sex had higher rates of infection than those who practiced only vaginal intercourse.[70] To interpret this finding as meaning anything about the hazards of oral transmission would be to say that oral sex must be *more efficient* than vaginal intercourse in transmitting HIV; otherwise, it would be masked and so would not show up in the overall rates. No one, including these people, have ever claimed that oral sex is more infective than vaginal. Unfortunately Fischl, who is not an epidemiologist, contributed to this confusion by also misinterpreting her own data, stating that the higher level of seropositivity among women engaging in oral sex suggests "that this may be a potential mode of heterosexual transmission."[71]

One study has been published in which the authors purported to show direct evidence of HIV transmission through fellatio. The authors claimed to have identified five seropositive men, four of whom supposedly had ceased participating in anal intercourse for at least three months before they seroconverted, and one of whom claimed never to have engaged in anal sex.[72] This study must, however, be qualified in several ways. First, it was presented only as a letter, which means it bypassed the peer review medical journal articles must go through. Second, it was conducted in France, which makes outside investigation difficult. Third, the authors didn't bother to state the size of their entire cohort. When groups of hundreds of men show no fellatio-related seroconversions, it might be interesting to know how many were in this French group. A small number would be very suspicious. Yet the study is extremely suspicious already, insofar as two of the seropositive men claimed to have engaged in only *insertive* oral sex. Between the utter lack of documented salivary HIV transmission through kissing, and the evidence showing that cervical fluid, with its higher concentration of HIV than salivary fluid, seems to be a very inefficient transmitter of HIV through the penis, the possibility of being infected during insertive oral intercourse would seem staggeringly low. Insertive oral intercourse, according to numerous studies of both homosexuals and heterosexuals, appears to carry no risk.[73] For two men in one study to claim this as their only possible mode of infection clearly stretches the bounds of credulity.

Indeed, several physicians strongly protested the conclusion of the French doctors, pointing out that merely abstaining from anal sex for three months before seroconversion does not mean the subjects had not been infected earlier, since it is not uncommon for seroconversion to take more than three months.[74] But probably a better explanation lies in human nature. Men who have been severely warned against participation in anal sex, as had all of these, will have a tendency to deny that activity. The problem of a patient lying about his risk factors is one of the most pervasive in understanding the spread of AIDS, and I shall deal with it at length in chapter 7.

A final piece of evidence relevant to the transmission efficiency of HIV through penile-oral sex is that while hepatitis B is a far more infectious virus than HIV, there are no confirmed cases of hepatitis B ever being transmitted in this manner, according to Dr. Niu Manette of the hepatitis-B section of the CDC. "They've tried inoculating chimpanzees with hepatitis B through the mouth," she says, "but it just didn't work."[75]

Vaginal-Oral Intercourse

Despite the presence of dental dams in "safe sex kits" to keep a man's (or a lesbian's) tongue and mouth from direct contact with a woman's vagina and vaginal fluids, the risk of infection this way is virtually or entirely nonexistent. There was a flap in early 1989 over a letter to the *New England Journal of Medicine* in which two doctors reported the case of a man suffering from HIV-related dementia and fatigue who claimed to have been impotent for the previous several years due to an underlying diabetic condition. The man denied drug use and homosexual contact, but did claim to have had a two-year relationship consisting entirely of oral-vaginal sex with a prostitute whom he claimed had injected drugs on at least one occasion.[76] The seemingly obvious conclusion, and the one the doctors came to, was that the man had been infected through the mouth by vaginal fluid. Certainly this is the way the media portrayed it.

The strength of the assertion, however, begins to break down when one learns that the great majority of men who originally claim prostitute contact as their only risk for HIV infection admit later to either homosexuality or IV drug abuse. What makes this case all the more suspicious is that, even though the man claimed to have had sex with the same prostitute over a two-year period and obviously knew where she could be located, the doctors mentioned no efforts to test her. If she tested positive, it would not necessarily verify the man's story, but a negative test would disprove it. In addition, since the man was suffering dementia, his ability to relate information was reduced—thus further weakening this as a bona-fide case of vaginal-oral transmission.

There have also been two cases of lesbian-to-lesbian transmission, but neither has been considered a likely candidate for demonstrating oral-vaginal transmission. For example, in the one on which good information is available (the other was reported from the Philippines[77]), the early conclusion drawn by the researchers was that the second woman contracted HIV from the first through sexual contact that included oral sex during the first woman's menstruation, oral-anal contact, and vaginal sex that produced bleeding in both women. It then developed that the second woman had had sex with four other partners in the seven years before being diagnosed as antibody positive in 1984—including intercourse with a bisexual man (although she claimed they used condoms). She also had sexual contacts with two other men, one of whom proved seronegative while the other refused testing.

One possible way of determining whether this may be a possible means of transmission is to ask again whether it is a means of transmission for hepatitis-B virus (HBV). "We've never had clear evidence that hepatitis B is transmitted that way," Dr. Mark Kane, a medical epidemiologist at the CDC hepatitis branch, told me. "The oral route is not an efficient mode of getting HBV."[78] Dr. Robert Rolfs, an STD specialist at the CDC, added, "I think whether or not transmission occurred in that one instance [the man and the prostitute] is probably not that relevant. HIV is transmitted by a number of routes. I think if that was an important route it would have showed up in other instances."[79]

Relative Efficiency

The point Rolfs made is important when discussing *all* modes of HIV transmission. The public and the media, led by the alarmists, were virtually obsessed with the question of whether HIV *can* be transmitted in this manner or that manner, when the question should have been *how efficiently* or, to put it another way, how much do we have to worry about this? As Kane put it to me, "When you have millions of people doing millions of things, anything that can happen will."[80] Numerous other epidemiologists, including Dr. Jaffe,[81] have made similar statements.

Yet there was an additional impetus for the alarmists' lack of desire to discuss transmission efficiency. The Harvard microbiologist Myron Essex, when asked the probability of AIDS being transmitted during a "one-night affair," replied:

> That is simply a statistical probability. I would say that no one can give you an exact figure; it is dependent on the degree of exposure. It is dependent on which partner was infected and the type of sex that went on and whether there were other enhancing factors, such as other venereal disease. All of these things have to be factored in. The bottom line is that it is absolutely certain that a one-night stand is enough to allow transmission.[82]

Assuming one already knew there was *some* chance of transmission in one sex act, does Essex say a single thing of any utility to any reader? The alarmists as a general rule were not in the business of providing useful information for risk taking. But it either did not occur to the alarmists, or did not matter to them, that some people are going to venture out in deep water, muddy or not; and that by refusing to provide information about what persons and activities were especially risky, the alarmists could be robbing the risk takers of life-saving information—even as the alarmists bandied about slogans to the effect that education is the best defense against AIDS.

With the caveats that no immoral act is made moral by its comparative safety in preventing viral transmission, and that there are no guarantees in life, I have sought in this chapter and elsewhere to unmuddy the waters that others have dirtied.

5

The "Perils" of Promiscuity

A man espied a particularly lovely young lady in a singles bar. He bought her a drink, one thing led to another, and the woman spent the night in the man's apartment. When the man awoke that morning, the woman was gone. But as he lathered up his face and looked in the mirror, he beheld a terrifying message. Written in lipstick was "Welcome to the wonderful world of AIDS."

I first heard this tale from a friend in Illinois who said it happened in the Chicago area. Two days later, I heard it from a woman in Washington, D.C., who said it happened around there, and that the woman involved was a prostitute. In her story the man had actually developed AIDS. Like the story of the ghostly hitchhiker or the white alligators in the sewers of New York City, the urban legend of the man welcomed to the "wonderful world of AIDS" has been told and retold, the facts changing slightly each time. Each time it is told in deadly earnest by someone who claims to be no more than two or three persons removed from the hapless young man, as in "a friend's cousin," "a cousin's friend," or "the friend of a cousin's friend." As far as some moralists were concerned, if it wasn't true perhaps it should have been. Even the evangelist Billy Graham told the story: in his rendition, the man was a married Hollywood actor.[1]

Just as it was a given that AIDS had become epidemic in the general heterosexual population, so, too, was it that promiscuity was behind AIDS, and that the legendary "one-night stand" was tantamount to rolling dice with the grim reaper. Promiscuity has been called "the major transmission factor."[2] It has also been treated as a form of transmission in and of itself.

• HIV is transmitted through "shared use of needles by drug abusers, and promiscuous sex of any kind," one book states.[3]

• "If you have multiple sex contacts, you're going to be at greater risk," Dr. Robert Redfield states flatly.[4]

• Declares "The Surgeon General's Report on Acquired Immune Deficiency Syndrome," considered by many to be the most trustworthy publication on avoiding AIDS, under the heading "Multiple Partners": "The risk of infection increases according to the number of sexual partners one has, *male or female.* The more partners you have, the greater the risk of becoming infected with the AIDS virus" (original emphasis).[5] Masters, Johnson, and Kolodny proceeded to make this statement of the surgeon general's a linchpin of their report.[6]

• "Risky behavior" consists of "sex . . . with someone you know [who] has several partners"; thus, even if your *partner* has had multiple partners, you are at increased risk, according to the version of this report that was to have been mailed out to every household in the nation.[7]

There was also little dissent about denominating "casual sex" as the demon of heterosexual transmission.

• A zealous editor at the *Washington Times* slapped the headline "AIDS Risk for Women Rises with 'Casual' Sex" over an article that barely touched on the subject and said no such thing.[8]

• "Casual sex and one-night stands are now for daredevils," announced Geraldo Rivera.[9]

• "If you're a single woman, remember no casual sex ever again," wrote the sex therapist Dr. Helen Singer Kaplan.[10]

• "For the sake of health, casual sex and multiple partners must be abandoned,"[11] declared Theresa Crenshaw, then president of the American Association of Sex Educators, Counselors, and Therapists and future member of the President's AIDS commission.

The surgeon general also laid the heterosexual transmission problem right at the door of casual sex. Addressing the presidential AIDS commission, Koop began the segment on heterosexual transmission: "People engage in casual sex."[12]

If nothing else, the admonition against multiple partners always had a definitional problem. To wit: How many partners is multiple? More than one in a lifetime? A year? A month? A week? *U.S. News & World Report,* in a question-and-answer sidebar, urged readers to be tested for HIV if they "have had more than three or four sexual partners in any of the last five years."[13] According to that formula, someone with four partners in one of the past five years but no partners in any of the others is at risk, but someone with three partners a year for five straight years is not.

It was as if something magical occurred between that first and second partner. One partner, good; two to two thousand, bad. Thus, *USA Today* advised its readers that persons at risk are those women whose sexual partners are bisexual or homosexual men, who use intravenous drugs, or "who have more than one male sex partner."[14] Again, no time frame was given, such as more than one partner per year or even more than one partner since 1978.

The first indicator that something is amiss with the multiple partners rule can be seen in the extreme example of comparing a person who has 1,000 seronegative partners with another person who has 1 seropositive partner. Who is at greater risk?

In fact, the importance of reducing partners either to monogamy or at least to a lesser number depends on two variables: infectivity or transmissibility; prevalence of HIV in the population of potential mates. With most STDs, which is to say most of the ones we all know about—syphilis, gonorrhea, herpes simplex II, chlamydia—infectivity is high, so high that the cumulative probability makes it more likely than not that the partner is infected after the first few contacts. Conversely, for a germ like HIV, the cumulative probability of becoming infected does not approach equilibrium until the number of contacts is in the hundreds—over five hundred according to the Padian study. Put another way, having sex one hundred different times (the number of times most young couples have sex in a year[15]) with one person who is already infected carries nearly the same risk of HIV infection as having sex one time each with one hundred different partners, each of whom is infected.

To the extent that limiting one's partners reduces the total number of acts of intercourse, limiting partners would be beneficial in reducing risk, but it does not necessarily follow that a person having sex with more people is necessarily having more sex. Whatever one thinks of the morality of one-night stands, from the standpoint of avoiding AIDS they do have one advantage: by definition, they consist of only one to two sexual contacts (that night and the next morning). Unlike one night in a bathhouse, where it's possible for homosexuals to have ten or more contacts, that one-night connection for heterosexuals entails a certain amount of time and effort which tends to limit severely the number of such stands. In fact, the heterosexuals Masters and Johnson chose for their AIDS study as being the most promiscuous of the promiscuous still averaged only about 11 partners a year.[16]

Consider, then, the case of the "loose woman" on campus. According to the media, campuses are a fertile breeding ground for AIDS because college is considered to be a period of great sexual experimentation.[17]

As noted in chapter 2, sampling of blood on select college campuses revealed that about 2 female students per 10,000 tested were positive. While female heterosexuals are far more likely to be infected than male ones, let's assume that on one hypothetical campus, 1 in 1,000 infections is among heterosexual men. Our loose woman has a one-night stand with a man each month of the school year and one during orientation, meaning she has had 10 sexual partners that year. Clearly by the standards of most of us, this woman is promiscuous, even highly promiscuous. Yet her statistical chance of having had coitus with that 1 seropositive heterosexual man per 1,000 is only about 1 in 100. Assuming her chance of infection to be 1 per 1,000 (the Padian figure), she has just

TABLE 5.1

Cumulative Probability of HIV Infection from 1,000 Sexual Exposures Assuming 1 Infection per 1,000 Contacts with an Infected Individual

Prevalence of HIV Among Potential Partners	Frequency of Condom Use		
	Never	Half-time	Always
One partner			
0.001	0.0001	0.0001	0.00006
0.01	0.001	0.001	0.0006
0.05	0.005	0.005	0.003
0.25	0.025	0.025	0.016
0.50	0.050	0.050	0.032
Five partners			
0.001	0.0004	0.0003	0.00009
0.01	0.004	0.003	0.0009
0.05	0.020	0.016	0.004
0.25	0.070	0.060	0.021
0.50	0.094	0.087	0.038
Ten partners			
0.001	0.0006	0.0004	0.0001
0.01	0.006	0.004	0.001
0.05	0.028	0.019	0.005
0.25	0.082	0.067	0.021
0.50	0.098	0.091	0.039
Fifty partners			
0.001	0.0009	0.0005	0.0001
0.01	0.009	0.005	0.001
0.05	0.037	0.023	0.005
0.25	0.090	0.073	0.022
0.50	0.099	0.093	0.039

SOURCE: Adapted from Harvey V. Fineberg, "Education to Prevent AIDS: Prospects and Obstacles," *Science* 239 (4840 [5 February 1988]): 593.

over 1 chance in 100,000 of contracting HIV with unprotected intercourse, just over 6 in 1,000,000 if she always uses a condom (see table
5.1). But if she chooses just 1 of those men as a steady partner and has
100 acts of intercourse with him during the upcoming year, her chances
of infection are almost ten times as great, about 1 in 10,000 with unprotected intercourse, or 6 in 100,000 if she always uses a condom.
Already promiscuous by anyone's standard, this woman could increase
her one-night stands to 50 a year, almost 1 per week, and still have a
far smaller chance of infection (9 chances out of 100,000 with unprotected intercourse) than if she chooses one of those men as a steady
partner and forsakes polygamy.

Thus, the media portrayal of the singles bar as the heterosexual version of a bathhouse was grossly exaggerated. "I think people believe
that a straight man going to a singles bar for purposes of having sex is
like a gay man going to a bathhouse," says Harold Jaffe. "That simply
isn't true."[18] Several epidemiologists told me categorically, "AIDS is not
being transmitted in the singles bars."

Of course, the message to heterosexuals was not always to avoid
multiple partners. The less alarmist often simply admonished heterosexuals to *reduce* their numbers of partners. It was a recognition that
there was no magical difference between one partner and more than
one, and also that risk reduction can make a good compromise between
risk elimination that consists of sacrifices some people won't agree to,
on the one hand, and conducting business as usual, on the other. The
message to "limit your partners" was intentionally kept ambiguous, in
recognition of the fact that heterosexuals have different numbers of
partners to begin with, and that heterosexuals have different numbers
of partners than homosexuals. But was heterosexual-partner reduction
a valid risk reducer? Was it comparable to homosexual risk reduction?
The answer to both is, perhaps surprisingly, no.

Consider again the promiscuous woman on campus with her 10 one-
time contacts per year, giving her 6 chances in 100,000 of infection per
year. (Keep in mind that figure is for unprotected intercourse; if she
were fairly careful—but not absolutely fastidious—about using condoms, she could cut her risk to 1 in 1,000,000.) Let's say this woman
begins to worry about AIDS and cuts her number of partners in half the
next year. Now she has only 4 chances in 100,000 of being infected
without using condoms, and 9 chances in 10,000,000 of being infected
if she uses condoms.

At a glance, this might appear to be an important risk reduction.
Two notes, however. First, even before she cut her odds by a third—

compared with her chances of being raped (about 1 in 1,500 a year in a metropolitan area),[19] murdered (about 1 in 11,000),[20] or killed in an automobile accident (about 1 in 4,500),[21]—her odds of getting AIDS are slim.

Second, while she has cut her odds on paper, in real life there is no measurable difference. Let's say there was a warehouse of golf balls in which 99,999 were normal and one was irregular. The Society for the Discovery of Unusual Golf Balls has offered you a reward for finding the irregular one, the catch being that you are only allowed to examine five balls a year and upon examining them you must return them to the pile so that the total number of balls always remains at 100,000. But then the Society decides to make it easier for you. In the future, it will now allow you to look at 10 balls a year. Are you jumping for joy? Are you already fantasizing about how you're going to spend the reward money? Of course not. If you had the least amount of sense you declined the first offer and stated, "You *are* crazy" after hearing the second. Put another way, this woman could have sex with 10 men a year for 50,000 years before the odds would start to turn against her. If she cut the number of her partners in half, she could have sex with 5 men a year for 75,000 years before the odds would turn against her. Despite slashing her number of partners in half, this woman has not appreciably reduced her risk, since—tart though she may be in the eyes of some— she is not at high risk for AIDS.

Is the same true of homosexual promiscuity? No. The importance of multiple partners directly relates to two factors: the efficiency of transmission and the probability of contact with an infected person. The higher the efficiency of transmission and the higher the percentage of seropositivity in the potential partner pool, the more important is the role of partner reduction in significantly reducing risk. Consider the case of the homosexual male who, like an average member of the first cohort of homosexual men with AIDS to be studied, had 70 partners a year. Let's say he made all of these contacts at a bathhouse and that the seropositivity level of this bathhouse was 20 percent—a figure probably not too high for bathhouses in major cities around 1981 as indicated by San Francisco Cohort Studies.[22] Based on studies showing that receptive anal intercourse results in infection on average 1 time in 100 contacts with a carrier, this man has 14 chances in 100 of being infected in one year. After just four and one-half years of sexual activity at the same level, the odds will be against him. If, however, *he* cuts his number of partners in half, he will have over nine years before the odds are even that he will be infected—a real difference.

Cutting that number in half again will give him about fourteen years before the odds become even.

In short, the best risk-reduction advice for heterosexuals is not that they should limit the number of their partners but rather that, to the extent they have a continuing sexual relationship with one partner, they should carefully evaluate the risk that that partner might be infected.

This has been shown in a study conducted by researchers at the University of California at San Francisco (UCSF). The study sample consisted of over 500 sexually active heterosexual women over the age of eighteen, of whom 100 were prostitutes. The study found that the number of partners was irrelevant to the risk of infection; rather, it was the "character" of those partners that determined a woman's risk. A UCSF researcher, Judith Cohen, told *Science News* that personal intravenous drug use raised a woman's risk. So did having sex with IVDA men, as did having sex with men identified as seropositive. Nevertheless, having multiple sex partners from no known risk group—whether 5 or more than 50 over a three-year period—does not make a woman more likely to become infected than a woman who is not "sexually adventurous."[23]

This was the thesis of an article that appeared in the *Journal of the American Medical Association* in 1988 with the subtitle "Are We Giving Our Patients the Best Advice?" The article was a landmark one in that it represented the best effort to date to answer the universal question: What are *my* risks? The article revolved around the following chart (see table 5.2) set up by the authors, Drs. Norman Hearst and Stephen Hulley, to determine the risk of penile-vaginal intercourse with ejaculation. In order to do this, they looked at three variables: infectivity (with and without condoms), likelihood of the type of sexual partner being infected, and number of sexual encounters with that type of partner.[24] For the first variable, the authors used a constant figure of 1 infection on average for 500 acts of intercourse, whether male-to-female or female-to-male.[25] Considering the Padian partner study figures indicating 1 infection per 1,000 contacts male-to-female and apparently significantly less female-to-male, this figure is probably extremely conservative. But since other factors may increase infectivity, such as STDs, it might be a good ballpark figure even though it probably overstates the risk for the white suburban heterosexual and understates it for the inner-city minority heterosexual. For the second variable, prevalence, these researchers relied on blood testing from blood donations, military applicants, and other studies.[26] The doctors

TABLE 5.2
HIV Infection: What Are the Risks?
Chances of HIV Infection from Heterosexual Intercourse

	Estimated Risk of Infection[a]	
	One Sexual Encounter	500 Sexual Encounters
Partner never tested for infection		
Not in high-risk group*		
Using condoms	1 in 50,000,000	1 in 110,000
Not using condoms	1 in 5,000,000	1 in 16,000
High-risk groups		
Using condoms	1 in 100,000 to 1 in 10,000	1 in 210 to 1 in 21
Not using condoms	1 in 10,000 to 1 in 1,000	1 in 32 to 1 in 3
Partner tested negative for infection		
No history of high-risk behavior†		
Using condoms	1 in 5,000,000,000	1 in 11,000,000
Not using condoms	1 in 500,000,000	1 in 1,600,000
Continuing high-risk behavior		
Using condoms	1 in 500,000	1 in 1,100
Not using condoms	1 in 50,000	1 in 160
Partner tested positive for infection		
Using condoms	1 in 5,000	1 in 11
Not using condoms	1 in 500	2 in 3

[a]Assuming 1 chance of infection per 500 contacts with infected individual.
*High-risk groups include homosexual or bisexual men, intravenous drug users, hemophiliacs, female prostitutes, heterosexuals from countries where heterosexual spread of HIV is common and patients who received multiple blood transfusions between 1983 and 1985 in areas with high prevalence of HIV infection.
†High-risk behavior is sexual intercourse or needle-sharing with a member of one of these groups.
SOURCE: Susan Okie, "Heterosexuals Told to Avoid Risky Partners," *Washington Post,* 22 April 1988, adapted from table in Norman Hurst and Stephen B. Hulley, "Preventing the Heterosexual Spread of AIDS," *JAMA* 259 (16 [22–29 April 1988]): 2429.

also used an arbitrary figure for condom efficacy of 90 percent, relying on the commonly used 10-percent failure rate.[27]

As the authors noted, the most striking feature of the table is the tremendous variation in the risk of HIV infection under different circumstances, anywhere from 1 in 5,000,000,000 to 2 in 3. Certainly, it didn't do much for such sweeping statements as "we're all at risk." By far the most important cause of this variation was the risk status of the sexual partner. Choosing a partner who is not in any high-risk group provides almost four orders of magnitude (5,000-fold) of protection compared with choosing a partner in the highest-risk category (a male homosexual or IVDA from the areas of the country with the highest HIV prevalences). By contrast, condoms are estimated to provide only one order of magnitude of protection. Even a negative HIV blood test provides only about two orders of magnitude of protection (because of the possibility of false negatives).

The authors singled out specific pieces of advice given by the Public Health Service and other agencies, such as the admonition to wear condoms. In many cases they said this may be good advice, but in many others it may not. If one is regularly having intercourse with a known seropositive person, even use of condoms can allow a risk of infection that many of us would consider intolerable. Conversely, if one is having sex with someone in no risk group, the risk of infection per act is only about 1 in 5,000,000. While condom usage can reduce that to 1 in 5,000,000,000, for those who object to condom usage, this hardly seems worthwhile. Thus another epidemiologist, Dr. King K. Holmes, has declared, "It would be crazy to tell *all* sexually active Americans to start using condoms."[28] Although taking note of that segment of the alarmists who declare that any chance of death is too high, the authors pointed out that such a standard is unworkable in the real world, and that the 1-in-5,000,000 chance of being infected in a single encounter "is about the same as the risk of being killed in a traffic accident while driving ten miles on the way to that encounter."[29]

The authors also criticized the notion that partner reduction for heterosexuals somehow equates automatically with risk reduction, and used arguments similar to those outlined above.

As to what *is* good advice, obviously it is to choose one's partners carefully. As the authors noted, "Many victims of heterosexually acquired AIDS knew all along that their partners were drug users or bisexuals; what they may not have known was how dangerous this was for them personally."[30] Of course the risk factors of a partner are not always known, and there is no foolproof way of determining what they are. But as the chart makes clear, the risks for most heterosexuals are quite low at any rate. Reducing those risks even further may involve giving advice different from that which would be given to someone who starts out at very high risk. As the authors noted, "Giving people advice they decide not to follow (e.g., to use condoms) may make them disregard other advice that is more important and could be more acceptable."[31] The less drastic the action required by a doctor's advice, the more likely the patient is to take it. The best advice in the world is, if untaken, worthless. This is something that many of the alarmists, endeavoring to reduce risks to zero, could not comprehend.

Thus, the answer to the question of the article's subtitle is that *no*, the Public Health Service and the powers-that-be are not giving the best advice. Whoever followed Redfield's advice to "abandon the risk groups" was in fact abandoning the single best method they had of protecting themselves. Further, telling heterosexuals to "limit partners," or "avoid multiple partners" or "no casual sex ever again" as a shorthand way of saying "avoid high-risk sex," is the equivalent of shortening "Don't drink and drive" to "Don't drive."

Not only was the advice to heterosexuals to limit partners of no value; indeed, to the extent it was accepted it may have proven harmful. The problem with the misemphasis on multiple partners is the same as with any misemphasis: it detracts attention from where the real problem lies.

When you drill "promiscuity, multiple partners, promiscuity, multiple partners" into heterosexuals' heads, they naturally think that if they are monogamous they are safe. But it has proven to be the case empirically as well as mathematically that, as Dr. Stoneburner told me, "Where you look at a steady relationship, that's where your risk is the highest."[32] In fact, the epidemiologists, from Stoneburner to Jaffe[33] to Padian,[34]* told any reporter who was willing to listen that it is the steady relationships one has really to worry about. One of the most tragic and ironic casualties of the heterosexual AIDS myth was the number of poor women trotted out by the media or government who swore up and down that they had been monogamous yet had still gotten AIDS. Telma Luft, a woman suffering from HIV illness, displayed (for lack of a better term) at a Health and Human Services media briefing, emphasized to reporters that she was not an IVDA and not sexually promiscuous.[36] This woman was also displayed in various women's magazines,[37] and other such magazines also featured women victims (usually unnamed) who continually denied promiscuity.[38]

In the ultimate irony, the reason these women were trotted out was to show how great the threat to heterosexuals truly was. The idea was that if even monogamous heterosexuals could get AIDS, what possible chance could a promiscuous heterosexual have? To some extent, the propaganda no doubt worked. Some promiscuous non-IVDA heterosexuals probably became somewhat less promiscuous. Some probably became temporarily celibate.

But what of the other side of the equation? Because of the false message, for example, IVDA have reported more changes in sexual behavior with casual sexual contacts (for example, use of condoms) than with partners with whom they have a long-term relationship.[39]

---

*In Padian's own partner study, infected women actually had significantly fewer partners on average than those uninfected.[35]

How many monogamous women—black, Hispanic, and some white—were falsely reassured by the intense campaign against multiple partners? How many rolled over in bed, looked at their IVDA boyfriends or husbands, and said how glad they were that they had been faithful these past five years? There is no way to know how many have died and will die. The monogamous AIDS victims so grandly displayed were not so much evidence of general heterosexual mortality; instead, they were the poster children of the victims of government and media ignorance and disinformation, sacrificed on the altar of sloganeering and democratization.

6

"Russian Roulette," and Other Fearsome Fallacies

Several epidemiological fallacies arose with AIDS. Some, recalling President Franklin D. Roosevelt's admonition that it matters not so much for whom you vote but *that* you vote, were pseudo profundities that had a pleasant ring to the ear but fell apart under any degree of scrutiny. Others, such as laying heterosexual AIDS transmission at the feet of bisexuals, played with man's (or, more aptly, woman's) fear of the unknown. Another one, tertiary transmission, involved the single greatest fallacy of the heterosexual AIDS scare. Like all of the heterosexual AIDS fallacies, it was blindly accepted, blindly relayed, and blindly reaccepted. Still, others, like the idea of an "explosion," made such beautiful metaphors that they quickly seized the imagination of the press and the public. Let us look at a few of the fallacies that spread the epidemic of heterosexual fear.

Heterosexuals and the Explosion that Wasn't

Surgeon General C. Everett Koop said in April 1987, "If the heterosexual explosion follows the homosexual explosion, then we are in for unbelievable trouble."[1] From that moment on until the end of the year, Koop was identified with the words *heterosexual AIDS explosion.* "Heterosexual AIDS May Surge, Koop Says," ran one headline.[2] "Koop Warns of an 'Explosion' of AIDS Among Teen-Agers," blared another.[3] Thanks in part to Koop's use of the term, *explosion* became something of a sine qua non of any discussion of heterosexual AIDS.

The explosion allegory is very much the sort of thing Susan Sontag criticized when she declared in *Illness as Metaphor,* "My point is that illness is *not* a metaphor, and that the most truthful way of regarding illness . . . is one most purified of, most resistant to, metaphoric thinking."[4]

The basis for the explosion theory was the delayed incubation time of the virus, which meant that an infection might not be diagnosed as full-blown disease for many years. The explosion metaphor was a way of turning apparent good news (few cases of heterosexual transmission) into bad news. It evoked the idea that the low number of cases so far was actually a sign that pressure was building. After all, volcanoes apparently explode only after years of building pressure. We say people "explode" because they fail to let off steam. So the explosion theory could be used to invoke imagery of a pressure buildup. In a similar fashion, heretofore-hidden HIV infections contracted in 1980 might suddenly show up in 1987 or even later. As Redfield put it, "If we simply look at AIDS cases, we are ten years behind."[5] He claimed, "Today's AIDS cases represent an historical account of the magnitude of this epidemic in the late 1970s, . . . four or five years before we had even recognized AIDS. This tells us nothing about heterosexual transmission today."[6]

It was a wonderful argument for the alarmists. First, it could be used to counter the assertion (even while granting the main point) that the number of AIDS cases among heterosexuals was still extremely small.[7] Second, it was a way of saying, "We really have no idea what is going on." If the alarmists couldn't convince you that things were going terribly, they at least wanted to convince you that nobody knew how things were going. That way they could then say, as many did, "since we don't know what's going on we have to err on the side of caution and presume the worst."[8]

Redfield and the explosion proponents made their theory sound plausible by confusing incubation time with *average* incubation time and with *maximum* incubation time. Likewise, the alarmists could leave you with the impression that every incubation time was equal to the maximum incubation time—that, for example, all individuals infected in 1982 might suddenly show up as AIDS cases in 1992. In fact, as noted earlier, average incubation time for HIV-I is thought to be about eight years, while incubation time itself can range anywhere from two months[9] to at least eleven years and probably much longer. According to Nancy Hessol, supervisor of the ongoing San Francisco hepatitis-B cohort study, some positive members of the cohort have yet to develop AIDS after eleven years.[10] (One of the characteristics of HIV-II is that

its incubation time may be longer; at this writing, no one yet knows.[11])
While few infections develop into full-blown AIDS in the first two years,
after that more and more will develop each year. The case load will
increase gradually. Some 1982 cases will show up in 1984, with more
and more showing up each year thereafter. That the *average* case is not
diagnosed for eight years, and that it may take *as long as* eleven years
or more for a case to show up, by no means leaves us with an eight-to-
ten year blind spot. There was no possibility of seeing a very low level
in 1986 and suddenly a very high level in 1987.

Eventually even Koop saw the lack of writing on the wall. The explosion had not materialized; and toward the end of 1987, he was admitting as much.[12] One year later, he told a magazine flatly, "From the
very beginning, I've said there does not appear to be any chance that
there will be an explosion in the heterosexual [community]."[13] Unfortunately, the mischief he did lived after him, and alarmists can still be
heard proclaiming that a heterosexual explosion is imminent.[14]

Bisexual Boogeymen

"Is There a Man in Your Man's Life?," asked the article in *Mademoiselle* magazine.[15] In the era of AIDS, this was every sexually active
white suburban woman's worst nightmare. Her man is dead, and now
she lies dying, due to a past that he kept from her either over fear of
losing her or because he didn't feel it to be of any importance.

The media, especially Hollywood and the women's magazines, were
utterly fascinated with male bisexuals. One television show, "Midnight
Caller," had an extremely handsome, masculine-acting bisexual flitting
from singles bar to singles bar, infecting women everywhere he went.
Such portrayals prompted one homosexual writer to exclaim bitterly
that "the bisexual is characterized as demonically *active*, the carrier,
the source of spread, the sexually insatiable."[16]

In light of all the attention given to bisexuals, one might never
know that only a small portion of female heterosexual transmission
victims were infected by such men. By early 1989, of 2,130 woman
listed in the CDC's heterosexual transmission category, only 244 or
about 11.5 percent received the virus from bisexual men.[17] The majority of female heterosexual transmissions come from IVDAs, about
60 percent of the 1989 figure.[18]* In all, of adult women diagnosed

---

*Of the 2,130 women, in addition to partners of bisexuals and IVDA, 313 were Hai-
tians or central Africans, 29 were sex partners of hemophiliacs, 21 were sex partners of
natives of Haiti or Africa, 37 were sex partners of men who had received HIV through

with AIDS, only about 3.5 percent have been infected through sexual contact with bisexuals.[19]

Further, as one article in the *British Medical Journal* reported:

> [Even in] San Francisco, where the epidemic among male homosexuals dwarfs the epidemic among intravenous drug users [97 percent of San Francisco AIDS cases are in the homosexual/bisexual category], three cases have been attributed to heterosexual transmission from intravenous drug users and three to bisexuality. Thus, the rapid spread of HIV in drug users appears to be the main source for any future heterosexual epidemic.[20]

Indeed, the national figure of 11 percent of women infected by bisexuals is down from 16 percent two years earlier[21] and can be expected to drop even farther as the percentage of cases attributable to homosexuals and bisexuals continues to decline.

The overemphasis on bisexuals went right along with the media's efforts to portray AIDS not only as a tremendous heterosexual problem but as a *middle-class* heterosexual problem. Intravenous drug abusers are both much more easily identified than bisexuals and much more likely to belong to the lower classes. Thus, the average middle-class white woman—that is, those who buy the women's magazines and are most likely to be watching "Midnight Caller"—could identify more with dating a bisexual than with dating an IVDA.

But bisexuals were useful to sell more than just individual shows and periodicals. The selling of the entire concept of a heterosexual AIDS epidemic hinged to a great extent on convincing the middle-class white woman. It was clear from the statistics that women were and are at considerably higher risk for heterosexually transmitted AIDS than men. Authors from Dr. Helen Singer Kaplan to Chris Norwood aimed entire books at women. But one could not hope to bring these women under the fear umbrella by emphasizing the IVDA man.

Thus, Norwood tormented her readers by telling them, "Plenty of men in the 'homosexual and bisexual' category [in the CDC's AIDS statistical breakdown], for example, had only a few homosexual experiences, usually when they were teenagers. They may have acquired AIDS then, but they could hardly be described as homosexual or bisexual." The "current AIDS education in the United States will do little to alert them—or the women they love—to the danger."[22] What Norwood ignored was that the fewer homosexual acts they engaged in, the lower

---

blood transfusions, 183 were sex partners of men with unknown risks, and the risks of 14 risk women were still under investigation.

their risk. It may be easier to get infected with a "few" homosexual acts than with a few heterosexual ones, but it's still extremely difficult. Obviously there would be exceptions, but dwelling on the exceptions was more an appeal to fear of the mysterious than a practical way of warning women of their risks.

Yet dwelling on the exceptions was the stock of the women's-magazine heterosexual-AIDS fear trade. They loved to terrify their readers with stories of white, middle-class women whose husbands or boyfriend got AIDS, often passing it on to the woman. Generally the names and locations were changed, and the stories all went pretty much the same way. Woman meets wonderful man, knowing little or not caring about his past. Man gets sick. Woman takes loving care of him, notwithstanding surprise revelation he formerly had sex with men or shot drugs. Sometimes woman gets sick; sometimes not.

But one story really stood out. It was tagged on the cover of the magazine *Ladies' Home Journal* as "AIDS & Marriage: What Every Wife Must Know," sharing space with Vanna White's face and figure. Inside we read the story of Tommy, a faithful husband who suddenly sickened and was diagnosed with AIDS. Three things made the story unusual even for the typical women's magazine piece: it featured female-to-male transmission; transmission from a nonmember of a high-risk group—Tommy allegedly got the virus from a woman who got it from her bisexual husband; and the transmission was from a single act of intercourse. The writer was explicit on this point, having the wife recall the night before they got married when she and Tommy had argued and Tommy had stormed out. "When Kathy saw him the next day, she knew he had been with another woman."[23] From an alarmist's viewpoint, the story was just too good to be true.

It was. The article had listed Tommy and Kathy's location, and I called the Houston Department of Health to see if I could get the facts on Tommy. But even though the department is required to document all area AIDS cases, it had no report of such a man. In fact, only two males were listed under the heterosexual contacts category. One of them was Haitian. The other matched the victim in the story in every way except that the relationship with the HIV carrier was "ongoing." The single incident so carefully described in the story was fictitious. I also asked about the woman's risk factors. Did she get it from her bisexual husband? "That's the story," I was told, by a skeptical-sounding health official. And was this ongoing relationship really premarital? He began to speak but then caught himself, saying that was private.

"What every wife must know," the article implied, was that, since most husbands these days enter marriage as nonvirgins, your husband could be a time bomb just ticking away. This is the case even if he doesn't do drugs, have sex with men, or cheat on you and even if he had sex with only one other woman one time before he married you. The real lesson is that every reader should know that a magazine with a hot heterosexual AIDS story isn't going to take particular care to get its facts straight if that means watering down the story, even to a point of simply making the characters appear less sympathetic.

Monogamous Sex as "Group Sex"

While he was the nation's top health official, Health and Human Services secretary Dr. Otis R. Bowen, stated, "when a person has sex, they're [*sic*] not just having it with that partner, they're having it with everybody that partner had it with for the past 10 years."[24] Surgeon General Koop made similar pronouncements;[25] while Redfield has said that having sex with a prostitute who has had sex with 5,000 men is "as if you've had 5,001 partners."[26] The sex therapist Dr. Theresa Crenshaw simplified it by saying that when two people sleep together, "it's group sex."[27] The group-sex shibboleth appeared over and over, with few people bothering to question its validity.

As Allan Brandt has pointed out, this is a metaphor with a range of meanings:

> At a moment when the dangers of promiscuous sex are being emphasized, it suggests every *single* sexual encounter is a promiscuous encounter. . . . As anonymous sex is being questioned, this metaphor suggests that no matter how well known a partner may be, the relationship is *anonymous.* Finally, the metaphor implies to heterosexuals that if they are having sex with their partner's (heterosexual) partners, they are in fact engaging in homosexual acts. In this view, every sexual act becomes a homosexual encounter.[28]

The absurdity of the group-sex fallacy is brought out in the warning that "L.A. Law" 's socially conscious producers had the show's resident playboy deliver to an office mate upon revelation that his fellow attorney has been having unsafe sex:

> She's, what, 30, 35. That's 15 years of sexual activity, average a dozen guys each year, each with a dance card of his own. Twelve times fifteen is one hundred and eighty. One hundred and eighty to what, the 20th power. Face it, any time you hit the sheets with someone new, you link yourself up virally to about half the world population.[29]

Why, then, don't we get half the world's germs every time we have sex with someone? Because transmission is far less than 100 percent. Using Padian's 1-infection-per-1,000-contacts figure and assuming (for this purpose only) that this figure is equal female-to-male and male-to-female, having sex once with an HIV carrier gives a person 1 chance in 1,000 of infection. But a person who then has intercourse once with that second person has only 1 chance in 1,000,000. That's quite a difference in odds. It also helps illustrate why having one-night stands with other heterosexuals whose only risk is a one-night stand puts one at so little risk of HIV infection. And it certainly dissolves the group-sex fallacy.

The sensible thing to do, then, is not to worry about your partners' partners' partners' partners, but to worry about your own immediate partner and what you do with him or her. If one's immediate partner has not had a long-term relationship with a member of a high-risk group, the chance of becoming infected from that person is virtually nil.

Tertiary Transmission

One key indicator of whether AIDS was becoming epidemic among heterosexuals would have been the amount of tertiary transmission. Yet, at the height of the media heterosexual AIDS flap, the concept of tertiary transmission was ignored by both the media and public health authorities. Primary transmission is to a member of a high-risk group—homosexual, bisexual, IV-drug user, hemophiliac, recipient of a blood transfusion. Secondary is when the primary virus recipient passes the virus heterosexually to a non-high-risk member. Most secondaries are steady female partners of IV-drug abusers. Tertiary transmission occurs when the secondary recipient passes the infection on. The media simply assumed the existence of such transmission.

One of the more prominent of the AIDS videos had a lecturer who summed up the media belief nicely:

> Let's say that a gay man has intercourse with a bisexual man. Now, that gay man is infected, and he infects that bisexual man who, over a period of time, has intercourse with a completely heterosexual young woman. And she becomes infected, and that young woman has intercourse with a young man. And that young man becomes infected. And you go down the list, one, two, three, four, five, six, seven, eight, nine, ten, and you say to yourself, how did this nice, young Catholic girl get AIDS?[30]

When I set out to document tertiary transmission or lack thereof in 1987, I found that the CDC kept no figures on it. So I contacted the health officials of the four cities with the highest numbers of AIDS cases. The concept was so unheard of at that time that at least one of the public affairs officials had at first no idea of what I was talking about. As was the case with most of the media, it did not occur to him to distinguish between secondary and tertiary transmission. Three public health departments kept no such records on this, but their numbers of heterosexually transmitted cases were so small—18 in San Francisco of 3,661 cases, 30 in Los Angeles of 3,459 cases, and 12 in Houston of 1,344 cases—as to leave little room for tertiary transmissions. New York has by far the largest number of heterosexual AIDS cases of any American city. The New York epidemic is also thought to be slightly more mature than that in San Francisco or Los Angeles. At that time at least, New York's tracking and identification of cases was probably also the best in the world, as evidenced by its "no identified risk" category of less than 1 percent. New York reported that of 11,217 AIDS victims, "zero" had been definitely traced to tertiary transmission. After seven years of epidemic, zero cases? "None," the spokesman reiterated.[31]

Naturally, there is no physical law saying tertiary transmission *cannot* happen. Rather, it is extremely rare—so much so that when it does happen the media is likely to make the very most of it. Such was the case with the famous Swedish sailor, Lars. He was a big hit with the media, becoming the showpiece of front-page newspaper articles with such titles as "Data Shows AIDS Risk Widening."[32] This was because Lars represented what they claimed HIV was regularly doing—going from heterosexual to heterosexual to heterosexual with no drug users or homosexuals in sight. According to Swedish researchers, Lars picked up the virus from a Haitian prostitute. Subsequently he infected three of his six female partners. Of these three, one infected her husband while another infected her child perinatally.[33]

Possible explanations for Lars include his passing on an extremely efficient strain of HIV, his proclivity for sex in a manner unusually conducive to HIV transmission, or the explanation alarmists wanted us to believe: Lars wasn't really unusual. While answers one and two may have some merit, the best explanation is "none of the above": Lars simply represented a lesson in the laws of probability.

For example, 977 of 1,000,000 persons tossing a coin ten times will flip ten heads in a row. If we looked only at those 977, we might be tempted to conclude that coin tosses aren't nearly as fair as they have traditionally been held to be. But our puzzlement comes to an end when we find out that 977 persons also flipped ten tails in a row. Now we understand it was simply an effect of the laws of probability. So, too, with Lars. In a large enough group of anything, there will occur events that seem at first too strong to be coincidence unless one looks at the entire group as a whole.

Indeed, nothing was more obvious from the hysterical reactions of the AIDS alarmists—including their willingness to compare odds of perhaps 1 in several million or more with Russian roulette's odds of 1 in 6—than that we as a people are grossly unfamiliar with the concept of relative risk. Dr. Gary Noble, AIDS coordinator for the Public Health Service, tells us, "Having unprotected sex with a man you don't know well is like playing Russian roulette";[34] but Dr. Bruce Voeller, one of the nation's leading experts on STDs, says, "The safe-sex message just isn't true. You're still playing a kind of Russian roulette."[35]

The concept of relative risk is grounded in a basic and obvious point, which doomsayers nevertheless fail to grasp: *everything* in life carries a risk. Driving to the drug store to get a candy bar entails a risk. We all have known people who have died in car accidents, and at some level appreciate that there is some danger in being in an automobile. Yet we take that risk daily because we consider it small enough to be justified by the likelihood of even such trivial gains as being able to enjoy some chocolate.

Inherent in our everyday judgments about risk taking is the concept that the risk is not considered alone; rather, it is weighed against the potential reward. How many risks would you refuse to take if someone offered you a dollar, but would readily accept if someone offered you a million dollars? Note that when a state's lottery jackpot increases dramatically, the number of persons buying lottery tickets also shoots up, even though their chance of winning drops accordingly. Similarly, a low risk can make a low reward tolerable. Driving to the store to pick up a candy bar doesn't sound like much of a reward if there is a risk of death by automobile accident, but the probability of risk is so low that it's tolerable.

The willingness to take a risk varies not only with the size of the reward but also with the values and temperament of the person contemplating it. What is too high a risk for some people even to consider taking is low enough for others to take. A rich man would probably never consider playing a round of Russian roulette for $10,000, but a poor man whose wife will die without a $10,000 operation might consider the opportunity a gift from heaven.

When the president of Americans for a Sound AIDS Policy (ASAP), Shepherd Smith, referred to sex as "a few moments of pleasure" (see page 84), he was telegraphing exactly his group's perspective.[36] People who enjoy sex and value it for reasons above procreation would never think of referring to it in those disparaging terms, any more than would a gourmet refer to caviar as "fish eggs" or a rock music aficionado to the sounds of a rock band as "noise." It's easy to see how a person who calls sex "a few moments of pleasure" might declare that even a 1-in-10,000,000 risk of death for those "few moments" was still too high.

There have always been risks associated with sex. Pregnancy, contracting a sexually transmitted disease (including back when syphilis was untreatable and often fatal), being caught by one's spouse or one's neighbors, dying of a coronary, punishment in the afterlife: all of these are risks associated with illicit and sometimes even licit sex. But some people have always taken them and always will, and the same is sometimes true of those who run a high risk of catching AIDS. Hard though it may be for most of us to believe, there are those who engage in unprotected anal intercourse with a partner whom they know is infected with HIV. Conversely, there are those who, knowing exactly what their odds are, feel that even vaginal intercourse with a person who has recently tested HIV-negative remains too risky even if a condom is used. Both of these situations involve people who know their risks and have made their decisions based on their individual evaluation of them.

What the AIDS alarmists wanted us to think was that a risk's inexorably fatal outcome somehow negated the whole nature of risk taking. When the World Health Organization's director, Jonathan Mann, was asked to put an exact figure to the risk of heterosexually acquired AIDS, he conceded that it was low in numerical terms but said that this was beside the point: "If the risk were one in 10,000 of acquiring not gonorrhea, which can be treated with an injection, but a fatal, life-long infection . . . how many people would take that risk?"[37] The answer is: fewer. But we take risks involving death all the time; we simply demand that when death is at stake either the reward be higher or the probability lower. For most heterosexuals, which is to say those heterosexuals targeted by the media and the government's national advertising campaigns, the probability of death from AIDS was and is extremely low.

Said one female doctor who studies HIV-infected prostitutes, "It's true that in the dating situations I find myself in, the chance [of HIV infection] is slim. But it's 100 percent if you're the one who gets it."[38]

Temple University mathematics professor John Allen Paulos cites a virtually identical statement as an example of what he calls "innumeracy" in his best-selling book of the same name. (Innumeracy is the inability to understand mathematics and probability.) The speaker, writes Paulos, will "then nod knowingly, as if they've demolished your argument with their penetrating insight."[39] Indeed, the statement sounds profound, until one realizes that this is true of any risk taking. How about: "It's true that the chance of being mauled to death by a tiger in Manhattan is slim. But it's 100 percent if you're the one mauled."

One problem with risk taking is that to do it rationally, proper information is necessary. Neither the media nor the alarmists seemed to have the desire or the ability to convey that information about AIDS. When they weren't giving information that was false, they were giving information that was useless. For example, the media's favorite technique of conveying AIDS information appeared to be through anecdote as in the following quotes that began an article in the *Washington Post:*

> *The last guy I slept with gave me an infection. Nothing serious, fortunately. But . . . I haven't slept with anyone for almost a year. Maybe I'm overreacting.*—A 33-year-old attorney.

> *I've done a lot of fooling around—slept with dozens of women—and for me, this is a real change. I'm more cautious now and ask plenty of questions before I make my move.*—A 30-year-old advertising executive.

> *Much as I don't like doing it, I put every man I meet [and am interested in] through the third degree. I still like sex and want to find a husband—without dying in the process.*—A 29-year-old merchandise manager.

Restating what from the quotes appears to be the obvious, the reporter then begins, "People have worried about sex since man first crawled out of the primordial swamp, but the specter of AIDS has given the subject a deadly urgency."[40] While the quotes—assuming they weren't made up—tell us people are scared of AIDS, they tell us nothing about whether they *should be.*

Let's say that every day you walk across a fairly busy street to get your morning newspaper at the local Quickstop. But then one day you read that the number of pedestrians killed crossing the street has suddenly doubled and is expected to double again shortly. You begin reading this everywhere. The statistics are false, but you don't know it. Then you begin reading stories of people who used to cross the street every day but are now terrified to do so. "Sally S. says she used to cross the street once or twice a day, but she's sworn off it now. 'I'd rather just stay home and knit,' says Sally. 'In a way, I like it more this way, anyway, and what with all those pedestrian deaths I've been hearing about . . .' Mark, however, is quoted as saying, 'Hey, when your time comes, it comes. Until then, I'm going to cross streets and have fun!' " You shake your head as you read this. Boy, that Mark has it coming. You still haven't seen for yourself any evidence of this increase in pedestrian deaths, but you read about it in the newspaper's headlines. You don't know it, but in fact *every* pedestrian death is now a big story. You're considering giving up your walks across the street. How important is that paper to me anyway? you think. But then you hear some reassuring statistics on how low your chances are of getting hit while crossing the street. You feel better about your walks now. But then you hear the rebuttal to this reassuring news. "I don't care if your odds are one in ten million!" booms the voice. "Is that little newspaper really worth your life?" You look at the newspaper in your hand. Worth my *life?* you think. Of course not. And so you give up crossing the street.

The Risk-Free Society

Clearly, one of the most influential factors in the heterosexual AIDS hysteria was the quest for what has been called the "risk-free society"— an obsession with protecting life and limb over everything else. This obsession is of only recent development. One writer in the *New Republic* contrasted the nation's reaction to the deaths of three astronauts in the first *Apollo* spacecraft with the deaths of seven astronauts in the *Challenger* space shuttle nineteen years later. In the first instance there was a congressional hearing and some delay, but "the Apollo program went smartly ahead, with the full understanding and support of the nation, and within 18 months Apollo 11 landed on the moon, ahead of the deadline set by John Kennedy." After *Challenger*, "the prevailing mood in America so panicked NASA that it took almost three years to send up another shuttle." Commented the writer, "In the 19 years between those tragedies, the idea that our individual lives and the nation's life can and should be risk-free has grown to be an obsession, driven far and deep into American attitudes."[41]

Another AIDS-era example of such obsession was the Great Sun Tan Scare of '88. It began when the popular news commentator Ted Koppel checked into a hospital for treatment of a cancerous condition that had probably resulted from a severe burn decades before. Suddenly the papers were filled with stories about the evils of the sun *tan*. Doctors were quoted asking how having darker skin could possibly be worth the chance of death. Fashion designers were quoted as saying the tan was "out" and pale, white skin was "in." One would never have guessed from all this that people have been getting tans since the beginning of time, that sunscreens are better than ever, that skin cancer survival is better than ever (Ted Koppel is alive and well), and that in that very year there was made widely available a new ointment, Retin-A, that was shown not only to reduce the possibility of developing skin cancer but cosmetically to improve overexposed skin as well.[42]

"Erring on the Side of Caution"

As the horrific projections of the alarmists were first called into question, then discredited, the alarmists invariably responded that even if we couldn't accept their arguments on the basis of their evidence, we should still act as if their conclusions were true so as to "err on the side of caution."

• Gary Bauer, the White House chief of policy development: "We ought to err on the side of caution, until we know for sure whether heterosexual transmission is a big risk or not."[43]

• Mathilde Krim, Co-chairperson of the American Foundation for AIDS Research: "Given that we're dealing with a deadly disease that could cause enormous disruption in society it is justifiable to assume that the worst scenario is the right one. If we're mistaken, we'll have a few hospital beds too many and we can congratulate ourselves."[44]

• Dr. Robert Redfield: "The worst that could happen was that we would have had to admit we were wrong."[45]

• W. Shepherd Smith, Jr.: "If we are wrong . . . then we will have cautioned people in a way which may have limited their opportunities for a few moments of pleasure. However, if we are right, then many people will be at risk of contracting the virus and ultimately dying."[46]

If they could get you to buy into it, "erring on the side of caution" was an irrefutable argument. First, there was a strong element of circularity. By the time Bauer made his statement in early September 1988, for example, there probably wasn't a single public health official in the nation who would go along with the heterosexual-breakout position that his office and the Department of Education were continuing to push. Shepherd Smith made his statement half a year later in a confused and bitter denunciation of public officials who had once spoken in terms of a heterosexual explosion but had now switched sides—against him. All Bauer and Smith were saying was, "As long as there is dissent on this issue, we should do things my way, and I'm dissenting"; or, to put it another way, "If I win the argument, we do things my way; if I tie in the argument, we do things my way; if I so much as *say* there's a tie in the argument, we do things my way."

The alarmists wanted us to think that "erring on the side of caution" would at worst be inconsequential. But all actions have consequences. Implementing an AIDS policy is a major action and will have major consequences, one way or another. Melvin Grayson and Thomas Shepard, in their 1973 book *The Disaster Lobby,* recount how time and again in the 1960s and 1970s alarms were raised over the ecology, from mercury in fish to DDT.[47] Each time an alarm was raised, drastic action was taken, even though it was later discovered that the alarm was in great part, if not completely, false. We erred on the side of caution, and the result was severe hardship for fishermen and inconvenience to consumers who wouldn't eat swordfish for years, even though it was discovered in a matter of months that the levels of mercury in swordfish and other fish were no higher than they had ever been.[48] In some areas, erring on the side of caution was utterly disastrous. Sri Lanka stopped spraying its mosquitoes with the insecticide as a result of warnings in Rachel Carson's landmark 1962 book *Silent Spring.*[49] Consequently, the incidence of malaria jumped from nearly zero to 2,500,000 cases and 10,000 deaths before the country began spraying again.[50]

Another difficulty with issuing too many warnings is that eventually they lose their impact, particularly among people who need them most. We have been so beset by studies purporting to show that this or that can cause cancer that a few years back the American Cancer Society had to run commercials mocking the notion that, as an actor on the commercial put it, *"Everything* causes cancer." So many people have made their reputations by crying "Wolf!" in the area of food or drug or environmental causes of disease that many of us have become convinced there are no wolves. *But there are.* Cigarettes are a perfect example. One can't help but wonder how many cigarette smokers comfort themselves by thinking, "Well, they say *everything* causes cancer." When one is addicted to nicotine, such feeble excuses are more than enough.

When the AIDS alarmists told us "everyone is at risk" and ignored relative degrees, the threat was beneficial for fund raising and destigmatization, but disastrous as a source of information. Persons at low or zero risk were told that they should spend time and energy reacting to a nonthreat. Worse, each person who was truly at high risk was reassured that he or she was simply one among many. Sure, homosexuals with multiple partners are at risk, but so are heterosexuals with multiple partners. Never mind that the first might be having high-risk sex with a hundred such partners a year, thirty of whom are seropositive, while the second might be having lower-risk sex with two partners a year whose chance of being infected is virtually nil. Sure black women dating IVDA men in Brooklyn are at risk, but so, we're told, is the white female yuppie who has an occasional one-night stand with a white male yuppie who never had anything injected into his veins that wasn't a vaccination.

It is one of the greatest ironies of the AIDS alarmists that in their obsession with reducing the risks of contracting HIV to zero, they were oblivious to the risks of overreacting. Somewhere out there, in the white upper-middle-class areas of New York City or New Jersey or Los Angeles, there may be a man or a woman who, but for the cries of the AIDS alarmists, would be infected with the AIDS virus. But how many in the black and Hispanic ghettos of those same cities, and how many homosexuals in areas outside of high-information places like New York and San Francisco, *became* infected because they absorbed the same message? Everything causes cancer, everything that you eat is bad for you, and everybody is at risk for AIDS. The alarmists call it "erring on the side of caution." They should have shortened it to just "erring."

7

To Tell the Truth

While epidemiology is probably a more exact science than some of the alarmists would wish us to think, it clearly has weak points. One of these is that often it must rely upon disease sufferers to find out the source of their infection. If public health authorities interview victims of an outbreak of salmonella, for example, it's important for the accuracy of the epidemiology analysis that victims carefully recall everything they've recently eaten.

Whatever problems lapses of memory may bring, disease victims rarely have cause to deceive their interviewers. One historical exception to this, however, has been sexually transmitted diseases. As one health care provider at the turn of the century recalled:

> I may be told by some that men may contract syphilis by sitting in a public privy; to this I can only answer that I have never witnessed a single instance; nor did the late Mr. Obre, who had been for many years extensively engaged in treating venereal disease; for on asking him if he believed that the disease was propagated in this manner, he shrewdly answered, that it sometimes was the manner in which married men contracted it, but unmarried men never caught it in this manner.[1]

Denial may even become an institutional phenomenon. During the First World War, the navy removed doorknobs from its ships and installed swinging doors instead, on the assumption that many of its sailors were getting infected with syphilis by touching doorknobs with their hands instead of others' sex organs with their own.[2]

One seldom cares to admit to strangers that one engages in illicit activity. One sees little to be gained by it, since it won't speed recovery, and much to lose, since it could cost them reputation, family, or job. A victim may comprehend that an honest answer will help protect others, but when sick one tends to think of oneself.

When investigating transmission of a disease that carries with it the stigma of illicit activity, the epidemiologist must, therefore, be careful not to be led down the alley of virtue and accident. Syphilis can infect anyone engaging in intercourse with anyone; and while one may be understandably reluctant to identify all the sex partners who could have given one syphilis, its stigma can hardly compare to that of the much more socially deviant activities of homosexual intercourse or injecting illegal drugs. Thus, as much incentive as there is to deny activities leading to syphilis, the incentive is far greater with AIDS.

When interviewed about the source of their infection, AIDS patients will often try to lie. If they feel they can get away with blaming a doorknob or toilet seat, they will do so. But if they feel they have no choice but to blame a somewhat stigmatic activity (going to a prostitute) or a highly stigmatic activity (having sex with other men), they will choose the lesser stigma over the greater. Degrees of resistance to admitting AIDS risk factors vary. For an openly homosexual man, there are probably none. For a completely closeted bisexual husband and father, the stigma is so great it may prove impossible for him to admit having sex with other men. Often, however, the chances of getting an honest answer will depend on the skill of the interviewer. One who asks an AIDS victim, "So tell me, are you queer? Have you been letting some other man put his penis where it doesn't belong?" is less likely to get an honest answer than one who says, "I know you're not feeling well, but what you tell me here is very important if we are to keep others from getting sick, too. Please tell me if ever, on any occasion, you have shared a needle with someone else or ever had a single, perhaps quick act of sex with another man?" John Tierney, writing in *Rolling Stone* magazine, told of an investigator for the AIDS Surveillance Unit of the New York City Department of Health named Anastasia Lekatsas and the case that he says "set her on the way to becoming America's most dogged snooping street detective of AIDS."[3] The patient was a middle-aged Hispanic maintenance worker, a widower with children. The year was 1984, and researchers were anxiously looking for the first signs of the Heterosexual Breakout, realizing that if it occurred anywhere, it would do so first in New York City. The Hispanic man was classified as "no identified risk" (NIR) because he had denied homosexual acts, intravenous drug abuse, hemophilia, having had a blood transfusion, or having a sex partner of someone in a risk group.

Lekatsas went to the man's hospital room and shut the door behind her. She recalled the following conversation:

"I have this terrible problem," she began.
"What's your problem?" he said.
"I've come here to make you feel bad."
"What do you mean?"
"You told your doctor that you got infected by having sex with female prostitutes, and I don't believe you."
"Why not?"
"I don't believe you can get it that way."
Silence from the man.
"Do you think," Lekatsas asked, "that one of those prostitutes might have been a man?"
"No."
"It's really important that you share the truth with me."
"Why?"
"Does the nurse's aide bring your food to your bed?"
"Yes."
"Does your doctor come to see you?"
"Yes."
"The reason these people aren't afraid to come near you is that we think we understand the way this is transmitted. That's why my research is important. Now, do you think one of those prostitutes could have been a man?"
"I don't think so."
"Look, I'm not going to share this information with your doctor. It's just a number at the health department. Do you think one of those prostitutes could have been a man?"
"I don't remember."
"Why don't you close your eyes—you don't have to look at me. I'm not here to make a judgment. And I'm not going to think you're a homosexual if you've had sex with a man one time. Do you think one of those prostitutes could have been a man?"[4]

The man closed his eyes, replied yes, and started to cry. For the next two hours, he told Lekatsas how a woman had taken advantage of him after his wife's death and how in bitterness he started snorting cocaine at a social club and ended up having sex with men. Lekatsas started crying as well. But the NIR case was solved.[5]

I discovered a couple of crucial things that afternoon about getting people to admit they're lying [Lekatsas told Tierney]. One is that you have to give them a reason to tell you the truth. The other is that you have to free up the person. You have to give them a chance to say that it happened once, or that it might have been a man in drag. I don't believe anyone who ever confessed to me that he had a one-time [act of oral sex] really did have only that one.

... But you can't say to him, "Come on now, you were anal receptive, weren't you?" You can't take away all his cards.[6]

While as the epidemic progressed some researchers got more savvy, many still relied on standard questionnaires which were of little value. "They use the questionnaires because it's easier," Lekatsas says.

> You can go down the list and not really confront the person with these painful issues—you can withdraw into the questionnaire. But it's not the way to get the truth. In my experience, only once did someone really get something from a questionnaire. There was a young guy from the Navy, and his doctor reported that he was a heterosexual. So we sent a worker over, and the guy said no to the questions about homosexuality or bisexuality, and the worker kept going through the forms. There was a question, "What percentage of the time during sex did you or your partner insert a fist in the rectum?" He answered, "Fifty percent." I think he didn't realize that heterosexuals don't do that. So we kept investigating, and eventually we found out that he was homosexual.[7]

Sometimes people will carry their secrets to their death. Rand Stoneburner told me of one man who had been interviewed and reinterviewed and continually denied sex with men or IV drug abuse. After his death, however, when his home was cleared out, a videotape was found that "made it apparent he had been with other men and that that was his sexual preference."[8]

The lying factor goes a long way toward explaining the belief that prostitutes are spreading the disease. While chapter 8 is devoted to this subject, suffice it for now to point out that since it is popularly believed that prostitutes spread the disease, and because many of them are in fact seropositive, they serve as a handy excuse for men who are infected and don't wish to admit to homosexuality or drug abuse. In many states, men who claim prostitute contact are taken at their word and classified under the "heterosexual transmission category," and this figure is then relayed as such to the Centers for Disease Control. But New York City officials are not so trusting. Thus, according to Stoneburner, as of January 1989, "Of 63 men with AIDS who reported prostitute contact but denied other exposure, 42 were later found to have a history of contact with homosexual men or had engaged in intravenous drug abuse."[9]

Dr. Joyce Wallace, president of the Foundation for Research on Sexually Transmitted Disease in New York, in a study of clients of prostitutes (discussed later), once had to interview a seropositive man four times before he finally admitted to engaging in receptive anal intercourse. Another admitted to homosexual coitus, but said it was only "once, in an orgy setting." Says Wallace, "In my experience, many men will say they've had sex with a dog before they'll admit to sex with another man."[10]

One case of lying created considerable alarm. A retired Methodist bishop, who ministered to Houston AIDS patients, himself died of the disease, leaving behind a wife and son. His son told reporters, "There has been no homosexual or extramarital sexual contact," adding also that his father had not been a drug user and had received no blood transfusions. "He helped to plan and conduct funerals, provide transportation to the hospital and clean the apartments of AIDS victims," said the son, and expressed his belief that family members may never determine how he contracted the virus. The Houston Health Department assigned the case to the "undetermined" category.[11] Between the clergyman's continual close contact with AIDS patients, the fact that he had married and raised a family (working against suspicion of homosexuality), and his family's strong denial of his having had risk factors, the obvious conclusion was that this was a bona-fide case of casual transmission. Fortunately, within days reporters had discovered that the bishop's connections to homosexuals had been closer than had been let on. In fact, the bishop had been a frequent patron of local gay bars and, by all accounts, also appeared to be extremely promiscuous.[12] The case was closed.

Risk Factors Are in the Eye of the Beholder

Two investigators can look at the same group of individuals and classify them entirely differently. An investigator who assumes a high likelihood of heterosexual transmission will readily believe a man who blames prostitutes for his infections. A more skeptical investigator, like Stoneburner or Wallace, will interview and reinterview, with the result that most men originally denying homosexual or intravenous-drug-use risk factors will eventually concede them. Stoneburner also explains that part of the problem is "the old clinician's perspective: 'that my patients wouldn't dare to lie to me.' I used to be shocked when my patients told me they weren't drinking and it turned out they were alcoholics. I was very hurt. Doctors aren't in the business of determining if patients are lying or not."[13]

Stoneburner learned his lesson the hard way; others did not. Robert Redfield, who would become the single greatest advocate of a heterosexual breakout, started down this path in October 1985 when he announced in the *Journal of the American Medical Association* that 8 soldiers with AIDS under his care at Walter Reed Army hospital had been infected through prostitutes, and 1 through sheer heterosexual promiscuity.[14] Other doctors, including those with the New York City Department of Health, were far less trusting than Redfield, noting, among other things, that in West Germany (where 6 of the men claimed they had been infected), none of the AIDS cases reported indicated female-to-male transmission.[15] If German men weren't getting infected by women, it was unlikely that so many GIs stationed there were.

Two years later, another skeptical team of researchers hypothesized that since drug use and homosexuality are both dischargeable offenses in the military, these men might have been hiding their risk behavior from Redfield. The El Paso County, Colorado, Health Department interviewed 20 seropositive servicemen, of whom 15 originally claimed no high-risk activity. After reinterrogation, all but three admitted either to homosexual acts or IV drug abuse.[16] Redfield, however, continues to insist that at most 2 of the 9 men in his cohort had risk factors other than promiscuity or prostitute contact.[17]

One of the most interesting aspects of the lying factor is that it allows an alarmist to make his or her own prophecy self-fulfilling. A researcher who believes that heterosexual transmission is widespread will readily believe the patient who claims to have gotten it from sheer promiscuity or prostitutes.

Dr. Thomas Quinn, another AIDS alarmist, tested blood samples at a Baltimore STD clinic and came up with a tremendously high proportion of infected heterosexuals. This study was the one which the for-profit HIV testing clinic discussed in chapter 1 used to terrify heterosexuals into shelling out their money for useless tests. Indeed, many trying to play up the spread of heterosexual AIDS relied upon it. The Baltimore study showed that "as many as 40 percent of seropositive men and 62 percent of seropositive women may have acquired HIV through heterosexual activities."[18] But not only was the allegedly heterosexually transmitted percentage in Baltimore far higher than in any other study in any other city, it was also anomalous in one other important respect: there were no interviews of tested individuals, nor reinterviews of seropositives. The study relied entirely on anonymous self-administered questionnaires.[19]

But would these Baltimore seropositives lie even when guaranteed anonymity? Certainly. Shortly after the Baltimore study was completed, federal officials announced that plans to do survey testing around the country had bogged down because up to one third of those contacted refused to participate despite the government's guarantee of anonymity.[20] Further evidence of the fallaciousness of the Baltimore study lay in Baltimore's AIDS statistics. A look at the 331 total Baltimore cases as of 30 November 1987, a few months after the Quinn study closed, revealed that only 11 (3.3 percent) could be attributed to heterosexual activity. Even though there is a lag between seroconversion and development of AIDS, it is ludicrous to think that, in a city where only 3 percent of the AIDS cases are heterosexually transmitted, 50 percent of all HIV carriers got the virus through heterosexual activity.

Further, in an ongoing study in the Jamaica section of New York City, the latest figures at the time of the Baltimore study had only 5 of 440 seropositive men (slightly over 1 percent) claiming no risk factors other than sexual contact with an IVDA. (Two others also claimed no risk factors at all, but one was suspected of having homosexual relations and the other of abusing drugs.)[21] Why would the city with the highest number of IVDAs in the country, and consequently the highest number of heterosexually transmitted AIDS cases, have so much lower heterosexually transmitted seropositivity than Baltimore?

Why, indeed, was Baltimore's seropositivity so much higher than in any other study in the nation? Because Thomas Quinn didn't bother to set up a procedure for reinterviewing seropositives. To be fair, he did note, in the second-to-last paragraph in the article, that the "acknowledgment of high-risk behavior may have been different if the patients had been intensively interviewed by an experienced professional. In a recent study of blood donors in Los Angeles, Baltimore, and Atlanta, 87 percent of 152 seropositive subjects acknowledged high-risk behavior in person-to-person reinterviews, even though they had initially denied such behavior before serologic testing."[22] That's one hell of an exception. Yet the media and everyone who cited the Quinn study ignored it, including Quinn himself when I debated him and Dr. Helen Singer Kaplan on television.[23]

The only STD study which showed results anywhere close to that of Quinn's study did so because it was conducted—or misconducted—the same way. Those tested were screened only by a self-administered questionnaire, and there was no reinterviewing. Sure enough, a high rate of seropositivity, 3.4 percent, was found among non-IVDA heterosexual men.[24] Unlike Quinn, however, the author, Charles Rabkin, made no attempt to exploit the study as a basis for a claimed heterosexual explosion. Dr. Stoneburner told me that before reinterview the Jamaica study had similar results to the Rabkin study, and that it was only after reinterviewing and weeding out reluctant homosexuals and IVDAs that the much lower Jamaica figures were arrived at.[25]

In the alarming seropositivity study to end all alarming seropositivity
studies—that conducted by Masters, Johnson, and Kolodny—there was
also no follow-up interviewing of those testing positive. So sloppy was
the sex researchers' presentation of their results, however, that the only
way the reader could discern the lack of follow-up was from the authors'
profession of surprise that so few of the study subjects bothered to even
find out their serostatus.[26] In this study, out of 400 ostensibly non-IVDA
heterosexuals recruited who claimed at least 6 different partners a year
for the last five years, 7 percent of the women and 5 percent of the men
were found to be seropositive.[27] On the basis of this finding, Masters,
Johnson, and Kolodny declared, "The AIDS virus is now running rampant in the heterosexual community."[28]

But what would have happened if the trio had bothered to reinterview? One gets a good idea from Joyce Wallace's aforementioned study.
Wallace and other doctors recruited New York men who claimed to
have had sex with prostitutes in the last decade. As with the Masters,
Johnson, and Kolodny study, it was made clear that those who had used
intravenous drugs or had homosexual sex with men need not apply. The
size of the cohort was even similar to that of Masters, Johnson, and
Kolodny—in this case, 340 men. Of these 340, 6 tested positive. But
upon reinterview, half of the 6 men admitted to homosexual acts or
intravenous drug use.[29] So the answer to what would have happened
if Masters and Johnson had bothered to reinterview is simple: No book.
And no royalties, no *Newsweek* cover, no sudden resurgence of fame.

Truthfulness is also a factor in the partner studies that are important
in determining modes of and efficiency in transmissibility. All we know
for sure in partner studies is who is infected. Sometimes we know for
sure which partner was infected first, but often partners are enrolled
in a study after both are already seropositive so that not even that is
certain. Beyond that, in assessing specific risks, the researcher is at the
mercy of whatever the partners agree to say. I have already noted the
tremendous disparity between the IVDA-partner infection rates and
the low partner infection rates in studies in which the index case was
either a hemophiliac or a transfusion victim. I have discussed the real
possibility that much of the higher infection rate in the former studies
is due to clandestine needle sharing. Again, it is only reasonable to
assume that victims will prevaricate in the direction of less stigma. A
woman who is infected through needle sharing may deny it, instead
saying intercourse was her only risk factor. Furthermore, as Dr. Robert
Gould pointed out in his controversial *Cosmopolitan* piece,[30] anal sex

is often perceived as stigmatic, and no doubt some women who claim vaginal intercourse as their only risk are too embarrassed to admit to being sodomized. Redfield's partner study showed 5 out of 7 partners infected, or a rate of 71 percent.[31] One simple explanation for this percentage being so much higher than all 22 of the partner studies presented in a special CDC report in December 1987[32] is that it's such a small group, which allows the figures to be more easily skewed in either direction. Another possible explanation is that all of the index partners had full-blown AIDS, and there is some evidence that such persons are more infectious.[33] But as to the role of surreptitious needle sharing, we really don't know, because while Redfield lists 2 index partners who infected their spouses as IVDAs, the other 3 are listed either as simply "heterosexual promiscuity" or "none identified."[34] Those are terms other partner studies just do not use. Instead, they make certain they can classify that index partner as an IVDA, bisexual, hemophiliac, or transfusion victim. Redfield, however, was so ready and willing to believe these men had simply been infected through sheer promiscuity that he eschewed the kind of tough questioning that an unbiased epidemiologist would have pursued.

It is difficult to overstate the importance to the cause of the alarmists of the faulty methodology of these researchers. Without the studies of Redfield, Quinn, Margaret A. Fischl of the University of Miami, and Masters, Johnson, and Kolodny, the alarmists, already long on rhetoric and short on empirical evidence, would have had little basis for their arguments. By the end of 1987, 18 STD clinic studies had been conducted in 7 different U.S. cities or states, some of which showed zero non-IVDA heterosexual infections.[35] But the alarmists would step past every one of these and go straight to Quinn's Baltimore study, sometimes throwing in Rabkin's study as well. For example, Kevin Hopkins and William Johnston of the Hudson Institute ignored all of the STD clinic studies save Quinn's.[36] Kirk Kidwell in his defense of the Masters, Johnson, and Kolodny study, in the *New American,* cited only Quinn's study and the Rabkin study.[37] If you wanted (ersatz) evidence of oral sex transmitting HIV, Fischl was your lady.[38] If you wanted to show widespread heterosexual tertiary transmission,[39] if you needed a heterosexual partner study showing an extremely high rate of transmission,[40] or if you wanted to show that prostitutes were becoming infected for reasons other than using intravenous drugs or being infected by steady, nonpaying partners,[41] you turned to Fischl's isolated studies as well.

To be sure, even the most reassuring of statistics could be twisted by the alarmists to their own use, as I will later document. But these are the doctors who provided the "empirical evidence" vital to a group otherwise bankrupt of such material. They were doctors who didn't ask too many questions, who didn't bother to think things through, with a loyal band of followers who shared these same traits.

8

Prostitutes:
The "AIDS Assassins"

"We call them the AIDS assassins," says Geraldo Rivera. "Having the virus and passing it on to an unknowing partner is about as callous and reckless and immoral an act as we can imagine, yet [they] do this repeatedly."[1]* To drive home the point, he conducted a dialogue with a seropositive prostitute:

> GERALDO: How many do you go with every day when you're out there on average? Any idea?
> PROSTITUTE: About 10.
> GERALDO: But what if they're married, what if they bring it home to their wives or something?
> PROSTITUTE: It's not my problem.[3]

Often revered in ancient times, prostitutes have continually been the objects of both attraction and derision from generation to generation. Many men profess to loathe them, yet that so many also seem to require them is as apparent as the numbers of women in short skirts lining strips in virtually every major city in the world. It may be that those who date them and those who desire them are fairly exclusive, yet one suspects that just as the ranks of those demanding temperance have more than their share of alcoholics, many of those who are the harshest on purveyors of sex for money are probably among their best customers. The TV

---

*Rivera also pushed the prostitution spread line on other, considerably later, occasions. In response to the assertion that HIV rarely goes from women to men, he said, "That's why people are so worried about female prostitutes and their high HIV-positive rate in this country, because they're giving it to the johns who take it home to suburbia."[2]

evangelist Jimmy Swaggart's fixation with prostitutes included railing against them on TV and patronizing them personally. Branding him— or anyone obsessed with outlawing something they themselves practice—a blatant hypocrite may be unfair. A desire to control the vices of others may be considered simply a reaction to inability to control oneself. Whatever the case, the hostility expressed toward this group of generally downtrodden women has often seemed to transcend their actual culpability.

As with many aspects of AIDS, the proposition that prostitutes (*prostitute* in this chapter referring only to females*) are the Typhoid Marys of AIDS, as Rivera put it, was simply accepted by the media and then the public at large. And why not? If casual sex and the one-night stand were the prime risk factors for heterosexual AIDS, then prostitutes, who make their living by these practices and have more casual sex and one-night stands than most heterosexuals can even fantasize about, were clearly at the greatest risk for both contracting and spreading the dread virus.

Thus Judy Mann of the *Washington Post* wrote matter-of-factly, "Prostitutes are spreading it to their customers, who then spread it to their spouses or girlfriends."[4] This while *U.S. News* was declaring, "Many [AIDS victims] will be men infected by prostitutes."[5] The ABC news correspondent George Strait told "Nightline" viewers: "Who gets infected? Everyone is at risk. Heterosexual cases of AIDS in the United States doubled last year. Prostitutes are the major route for heterosexual transmission here."[6] (Actually, *all* cases of AIDS doubled that year.)

"Prostitution Isn't Victimless with AIDS Here," declared an opinion piece in the *Wall Street Journal*.[7] Some writers even declared that prostitutes had been added to the "high risk" or "at-risk" statistical groupings[8]—something the Public Health Service never did. Hollywood also joined the crusade. Home Box Office aired, during National AIDS Awareness Month (October 1987), a British film about an Englishman who contracts AIDS from an American prostitute.[9]

With prostitutes branded as AIDS carriers, action was taken to pre-

*Of course, many prostitutes are males, most of whom solicit other males for sex but some of whom, *à la American Gigolo* or *Midnight Cowboy*, service women. As a rule, however, these are not what people think of when they hear "prostitute" or what the media refers to, unless specifically stated. Gigolos are too uncommon to be a major factor in the spread of HIV. Males who service men may be a different matter. It is reputed that many of the customers of these prostitutes are married, or, at any rate, bisexual. Thus, not only does their behavior put them in the same category as any male having sex with males, but they will be more unlikely to admit it. It is probably reasonable to assume that a certain percentage of men claiming female prostitute contact as their only risk are at least telling a half-truth.

vent their ability to spread the disease. Both prostitutes and their clients were put on the list of those barred from donating blood for transfusions.[10] The city council of Newark, New Jersey, unanimously passed an ordinance requiring AIDS tests for convicted prostitutes, their pimps and customers—the first city in the nation to do so. Customers of prostitutes, if convicted, would be required to pay for both their own test and that of the prostitute.[11] Since the ordinance did not specify any steps to be taken if someone tested positive, it wasn't clear what the purpose of the test was, except a simple additional disincentive to engage in prostitution. A wide variety of measures to control this alleged spreading of AIDS from prostitutes to customers were implemented or proposed, from testing convicted prostitutes,[12]* to testing any woman ever even arrested for prostitution,[13]† to legalization and regulation (to allow customers to know which were uninfected, as is done in Germany and the Netherlands),[14] to police crackdowns.[15]

The Statistical Game

Some commentators tried to put exact numbers on prostitute transmission. Said Rivera, "The government estimates that in this year alone, 500 to 5,000 heterosexual men, many of them married, will get AIDS from hookers."[16] In the preceding *Wall Street Journal* opinion piece, the writer stated that "between 1,000 and 10,000 American men will become infected with the AIDS virus this year by having sex with female prostitutes." He also threw in tertiary transmission saying, "They will continue to have other sexual relations, putting their partners (and their partners' partners and children) at risk."[17] Another writer made national news with his model indicating that in five years a single prostitute could be expected to infect about 20 men.[18]

Actually, the government never made any estimate on how many infections prostitutes would produce. When I asked Dr. William Darrow at the Centers for Disease Control about the Rivera figure, he said, "I don't know of any basis for a statement of that kind." Darrow, who is chief of social and behavioral studies at the CDC's epidemiological branch, added, "Certainly we have not done [such a study] in the AIDS program . . . and we're the ones doing research in that area."[19] A call to the office of the surgeon general revealed that they had never heard of any such study either.[20] Whatever the CDC's shortcomings in deal-

*At least thirteen states had enacted such laws by September 1988.
†Colorado has enacted such legislation.

ing with heterosexual AIDS, pinning blame on prostitutes has not been among them.

As to the 1,000 to 10,000 figure in the *Wall Street Journal,* a conversation with the writer revealed they were based strictly on a mathematical formulation which, like all mathematical formulae, was no better than the estimates that went into it. Obviously at least one of the estimates was far off, since the total number of men in the CDC's "undetermined" category, at the time the opinion piece appeared (June 1987), was only about 800 cases.

Similarly, the model showing 20 infections for each infected prostitute was absolutely divorced from reality. By early 1989, the New York City Department of Health reported only 21 New Yorkers who *claimed* to have gotten AIDS through prostitute contact and were not later found to have other risks. Thus, the 1-for-20 figure would indicate that a few years earlier there was only 1 infected prostitute in the city. Not likely.

Were Prostitutes Spreading AIDS?

But were prostitutes spreading AIDS? Strictly speaking, yes. Since there are estimated to be more than 200,000 professional prostitutes in the country, performing 300 million sexual acts annually,[21] it would be amazing if no one ever got AIDS from a prostitute. The better question is to what extent are they spreading the virus, and do they deserve the attention and reputation they have gotten? In short, do they really fit the "Typhoid Mary" image that has been created for them?

Even aside from traditional animosity toward sex for pay, it's easy to see how the image came about. Prostitutes in some areas of the country had extremely high HIV-infection rates; they have traditionally been treated as a threat during VD epidemics; and many men who contracted AIDS claimed no other risk factors than sex with prostitutes. This was regarded as not only evidence of widespread heterosexual transmission but as an important source of infection of the non-IVDA heterosexual middle class.

In fact, it was nothing of the sort. Indeed, the prostitution situation is something of a microcosm for the entire heterosexual AIDS debate.

As I noted earlier, prostitutes make handy scapegoats for men wishing to deny either homosexuality or drug abuse. If a man persists in his account, there is simply no way of telling whether he is speaking truthfully, since prostitutes are difficult to track down, especially if a man claims he has consorted with many. One way, however, of seeing whether prostitute-to-client transmission is occurring is to recruit men who have admitted to prostitute contact but are of undetermined sero-positivity. This is what Joyce Wallace and other doctors in New York City did by recruiting 340 men who denied both homosexual activity and drug abuse.* Of these, the average number of sexual exposures to prostitutes over the last ten years was 94, and the most common act was fellatio. They averaged one sexually transmitted disease a year; and while a third of them occasionally used condoms, one half never did. Of these 340 men, 6 tested positive. Three of these, upon requestioning, admitted to either drug use or homosexuality. Of the 3 remaining, they averaged 575 sexual exposures to prostitutes (six times the average number in the study group), and none had used condoms.[22] In other words, assuming these men had no other risk factors and were infected by prostitutes, they were exceptions because of exceptional behavior. They played the odds and lost. But just what were those odds? The entire group of men claimed a total of 31,960 partners between them. New York and New Jersey prostitutes have some of the highest infection rates in the country[23] (almost 60 percent were found to be infected in one New Jersey study[24]); but assuming for sake of argument that only 10 percent of these men's contacts were seropositive, that would mean 3,196 acts with infected partners. Well over half of these took place without a condom. If we assume that all 3 of the infected men had no other risk factors, that's over 1,000 acts with a seropositive prostitute per infected man, of whom over 500 were unprotected. Thus their being infected is hardly shocking. Further, considering the higher levels of STDs among New York and New Jersey prostitutes and the aforementioned role of STDs in facilitating transmission of HIV, these figures are very much in line with the Padian estimate of 1 infection per 1,000 contacts.†

The findings of other New York researchers have paralleled Wallace's. Recall that Rand Stoneburner noted that over 60 percent of the men diagnosed with AIDS, who originally claim prostitute contact as their only risk factor, will later, upon reinterview, admit to either IV drug use or homosexuality, and that it is suspected that most of the rest are lying as well.[25] This is the reason that New York, along with the CDC, does not place men claiming prostitute contact into the hetero-

---

*Because these men volunteered for this study, there can be no guarantee that they are truly representative of the clientele of New York prostitutes, but for our limited discussion purposes this should not be problematic.

†One mitigating factor is that many of the sexual contacts were probably oral (albeit some undoubtedly anal as well), but the number is not known.

sexual transmission category unless the prostitute is identified and tested. By no means, however, is this the case with every state. In New Jersey, if the man says that he believes the prostitute was an IVDA, the case is investigated no further; the patient's word is taken at face value.[26] In part because of this, New Jersey statistics showed 151 males infected through heterosexual contact[27] even while right across the border in New York City the total was seven.

Other than analyzing prostitutes' clients, there is also an indirect method of determining whether hookers are spreading the virus: that is, by determining whether prostitutes themselves are being infected by their clients. Considering evidence that HIV travels more efficiently from men to women, it would seem that if it were not going from clients to prostitutes, then it was not going from prostitutes to clients.

As noted, testing among prostitutes in one section of New Jersey has revealed almost 60 percent seropositives;[28] in South Florida, of 90 women tested, 41 percent proved seropositive.[29] Of 36 women tested in two cities in Italy, over a third were infected.[30] Such figures were to some proof positive not only of efficient heterosexual transmission and the dangers of multiple partners, but of the hazard to public health posed by prostitutes. After all, as high rates of syphilis and gonorrhea in prostitutes could have come only from their sex partners, from where else could the HIV infections have come? The simple answer is drug abuse. All of the areas (outside of Africa, which I shall discuss in detail later) where drug abuse was most prevalent also had the highest rates in prostitute infection with HIV. Newark, for example, is well known to be one of the worst areas in the nation for drug abuse. Miami, also, is notorious for drug abuse. Florida, with an estimated 41,000 IVDAs, is ranked in the top ten of states with drug abuse problems.[31] Thus, when intravenous drug abuse was specifically examined, it turned out to be the single most important risk factor for infection.[32] For example, the New Jersey study found that of 62 women who were seropositive, 76 percent had injected drugs.[33] In the Italian study, 59 percent of the drug users were infected, while none of the nonusers was.[34] Indeed, *none* of 50 prostitutes tested in a London STD clinic proved positive, nor did seropositives turn up among 56 prostitutes in Paris or 399 licensed prostitutes in Nuremberg.[35] (None of which, incidentally, kept German magazines from having a field day with articles on AIDS and prostitution, complete with photos of beautiful hookers wearing nothing but skimpy lingerie and a black bar over their eyes.) Likewise of 535 licensed prostitutes in Nevada's legal brothels, zero proved positive even while over 6 percent of incarcerated prostitutes in that state, of whom all had used IV drugs, proved positive.[36]

The authors of several of these studies drew conclusions, such as the Italians', that "female prostitutes and male prostitutes who are not homosexual are not at increased risk for AIDS while female and male prostitutes who are IVDA should be considered at risk for HIV infection."[37]

Yet that was not always the case. What about the other 24 percent, for example, in the New Jersey study where 76 percent of the prostitutes infected admitted to being IVDA? Of course, as with anybody, there may be a tendency on the part of prostitutes to lie about their risk behaviors and the source of their infection. One said to an inquiring Geraldo Rivera: "How'd I get the virus? I suppose it's from sexual intercourse with my dates and stuff."[38] And stuff. Thus, even the prostitutes themselves may have unwittingly contributed to their own status as the Typhoid Marys of heterosexual AIDS.

As to the remaining prostitutes who did not shoot up "stuff," the CDC's Dr. Darrow conducted a nationwide survey of 707 prostitutes with no evidence of IV drug abuse: that is, they denied use and they had no visible needle marks. Thirty-six of these women, or 5.1 percent, proved positive.[39] Nevertheless, of these 36 women, 24, or 66 percent, were from Miami, even though only 294, or 42 percent, of the total number of tested women had come from that city. The study concluded that "sexual activities with large numbers of clients . . . [was] *not* associated with HIV-I infection in our study"[40] (emphasis in original). "HIV infection in prostitutes with no evidence of IV-drug abuse was associated with [having been infected with] hepatitis B, recent infection with syphilis, and *sexual activities with nonpaying partners*"[41] (emphasis added). In fact, among the Miami prostitutes, these risk factors were far more prevalent, in addition to "sexual exposures with men from countries with a high-prevalence of AIDS."[42] (The importance of these factors will be discussed in chapter 10.)

Thus, while apparently some prostitutes are getting infected by sexual contact, it is not by their customers but through their pimps and boyfriends who themselves were infected through drug abuse. Instead of being the ultimate indictment of casual sex and the one-night stand, the evidence from prostitutes is a vindication of these practices. The reason goes back to the earlier discussion concerning the bugbear of the one-night stand. While a woman having sex with 1,500 men a year is probably at a significantly higher risk than our promiscuous college coed with 10 one-time partners a year, the odds of having sex with an infected customer, who probably tends to be middle-class and non-IVDA, is still probably quite low, and multiplying these odds by 1,500 doesn't much change this situation. Further, owing to the warnings against one-night stands, the rate of condom usage with prostitutes is reported to be extremely high.[43] On the other hand, the nonpaying partners of these women—be they pimps, boyfriends, or just friends—tend to have extremely high risk factors for infection, including drug use both IV and otherwise. About a third of Darrow's prostitute study group said their non-paying steady partners used IV drugs.[44] Further, barrier contraception is generally not used with steady sexual partners who may be seropositive[45]—again, probably because the focus of both the media and public health authorities has been casual, as opposed to long-term, sex.

Another factor that would tend to result in fewer prostitute infections through intercourse, and at the same time in fewer client infections from infected prostitutes, is that much, if not most, of the activities are not vaginal but oral, which is lower-risk. According to John French, chief of the office of data analysis and epidemiology for the New Jersey state health department, "for street prostitutes in the northern part of New Jersey, the general mode of sex is oral sex." He added, "There are not many brothels as might once have existed, so that a great deal of the sex is what they call 'working cars.' The vast majority of that—particularly with smaller cars today—is oral sex. And oral sex at this point appears to be a very inefficient means of spreading the infection."[46] Little do the Japanese know what they have done.

A final encouraging factor is that HIV seropositivity among prostitutes, as with positivity in other groups, has probably at least leveled off if, in fact, it is not dropping. Joyce Wallace has regularly tested prostitutes who work the streets in New York City, and found that while 19 percent were positive in 1985, only 9 percent were positive in 1986 and 6 percent in 1987. While her samples were probably too small (67 prostitutes in 1987) to extrapolate to all of the New York women working the street, they certainly do not indicate a raging increase in seropositivity and may indicate a decrease.[47] Likewise, HIV infection among licensed Greek prostitutes increased less than 1 percent in 1986 and not at all in 1987 and early 1988.[48] (Year-to-year comparisons for other countries are generally lacking.)

Carrying On a Tradition

The treatment of prostitutes during the AIDS crisis was but another example of a new disease being treated with old fears and prejudices. During the First World War, the medical historian Allan Brandt tells us in his authoritative social history of venereal disease since 1880, *No Magic Bullet,* prostitutes were portrayed as the enemy in the war against syphilis and thus as close allies of the Kaiser.[49] It was frequently said that 90 percent of these women were infected. "The prostitute," declared one writer, "is undoubtedly the most active single medium for the transmission of infection."[50] Thousands of women and girls, suspected of engaging in promiscuous sexual activities with soldiers during the war, were contacted. Though most were found to be first-time offenders and placed on probation, more than 18,000 women were committed to federally funded institutions between 1918 and 1920. Most, but by no means all, had venereal disease. In fact, the practice of releasing uninfected prostitutes became a source of criticism. Thus, notes Brandt, "the *possibility* of infection had become sufficient cause for incarceration."[51]

Prostitutes have certainly been treated better during the AIDS crisis, but the public attitude is the same: somebody has brought this horrible malady upon us, and somebody has to be punished. It was that way with the Black Death, when Jews were rounded up and accused of poisoning the wells;[52] it was that way with the Spanish flu pandemic of 1918–19, when agents carried by German U-boats were reported to have spread the disease in America.[53] Epidemics have always somehow been easier to endure if there were someone to blame for them, and it has never been hard to manufacture scapegoats. With syphilis (which wasn't even an epidemic when the scare hit; it was simply suddenly being given more attention), immigrants were blamed,[54] in addition to prostitutes. With AIDS the prostitutes' number came up again. IVDAs, conversely, responsible for the vast majority of heterosexual transmissions, were downplayed as carriers because so few of the white middle class have any contact with them. They would have made very poor scapegoats, indeed. Further, AIDS already having been identified as a disease of immoral behavior—specifically that involving baser physical pleasures—it was easy to extend this category to prostitutes.

Even if prostitutes were spreading HIV, cracking down on them in an effort to hinder or eliminate their trade is no way to deal with the problem. Whatever other merits there may be in outlawing the so-called world's oldest profession, preventing disease is not among them.

From Germany to Nevada to Greece, the lowest levels of HIV seropositivity are found in legal, licensed prostitutes. (It must be noted that even in places where prostitution is licensed, unlicensed prostitutes continue to work to some degree. Nevertheless, the men who patronize these women do so knowing they have higher levels of disease.) Thus, for those who saw AIDS as an opportunity to impose morality in the area of prostitution under the guise of AIDS, there was little fertile ground. Nevertheless, in 1986 a Nevada assemblywoman introduced a bill into the legislature to outlaw prostitution in the state; her stated reason: AIDS.[55]

While some used AIDS against prostitutes for moral reasons, in Nevada it was also used to restrain competition. The co-owner of the Chicken Ranch brothel near Pahrump urged Nevadans "to set an example for the rest of the world" by supporting a bill that would make prostitution while seropositive attempted murder.[56]

On the other extreme, one organization claimed that prostitutes could actually help staunch the epidemic:

> It's time to cast aside archaic moral judgements placed on prostitutes. We should endeavor to utilise the resources of our modern industrialised societies and promote AIDS Education. . . . Prostitutes, especially in less developed countries will acquire a broader base knowledge of the danger of contracting/transmitting the AIDS Virus. With their new found knowledge, the threat of death and safe sexual practice without exception, Prostitutes [sic] will ultimately pass on their knowledge of AIDS to their clients and others.[57]

As one might guess, this came from a prostitutes' organization, the Australian Prostitutes Collective. The view certainly is positive, though the wives and girlfriends of the prostitutes' clients might feel otherwise. Most prostitutes would probably have gladly eschewed a role as educator if only they could have gotten rid of their pariah status as well.

9

But What About Africa?

"AIDS in Africa," read the cover of *Newsweek* magazine in 1986.[1] "The Future is Now." This was to become one of the rallying cries of the alarmists. Any attempt to describe how meager a threat AIDS poses to non-IVDA American heterosexuals was met with the retort: "But what about Africa?"

Africa, all seemed to agree, was in a dire situation. ABC news reported that "an estimated ten percent of the healthy population [of Uganda] are infected with the AIDS virus."[2] A high Ugandan official stated in 1986 that within two years his country would be a desert.[3] One doctor, in a piece with the democratizing title of "We Must All Work Together Against AIDS," told the readers of his local newspaper that "at least 30 percent of the entire adult population of central Africa is infected with the AIDS virus."[4] *U.S. News & World Report*'s heterosexual scare cover piece, "AIDS: At the Dawn of Fear," also used the 30-percent figure.[5] The ubiquitous William Haseltine informed a Senate subcommittee that more than 10,000,000 natives in central Africa were infected.[6] Dr. Thomas Quinn estimated there are "possibly up to five million" infected in Africa.[7] The year after Quinn's statement, an ABC reporter on "Nightline" declared, "It's a virus that's infected ten million Africans so far, 20 million perhaps by next year—and by the year 2000, 50 million Africans may have died of AIDS."[8]* The typical newspaper headline ran "AIDS Epidemic Threatens to Depopulate Much of Africa."[9] And the question on Americans' minds was: Is this a preview for the United States?

Africans have not been happy, to say the least, about being depicted as the wellspring of the AIDS pandemic. Homosexuals have not liked

---

*Later in the show Ted Koppel challenged this figure.

the stigma associated with the disease, nor have minorities or Haitians. Nobody asked the drug abusers. But while these groups have been accused of spreading the virus, only Africa has been accused of *starting* its spread among humans. It is a tag Africans readily reject. Indeed, in Africa, AIDS is sometimes labeled the "American disease." (It is also called the "white disease"; but since white in Africa is also the color for death, it is not clear whether this description is a reference to race, to death, or perhaps to both.) One Ugandan health minister declared, "We don't have homosexuals and drug addicts. We don't have them. So this disease must be foreign."[10] A Kenyan newspaper writer seriously claimed that AIDS-infected foreign tourists were deliberately coming to Africa to spread the disease as part of an international conspiracy on the part of large drug companies seeking new markets for their drugs. Other Africans charged that AIDS was further evidence of how white supremacists try to thrust their own plagues onto hapless blacks.[11] For example, Dr. Ruhakana Rugunda, the health minister of Uganda, declared that "the AIDS problem has unmasked thinly veiled racism and fascism in some quarters where Africans are labeled the breeders of a scourge."[12]

Avoiding association with AIDS was not just a matter of pride. Tourism suffered in Haiti after the Centers for Disease Control declared Haitians to be a risk group. Tourism could be expected to decline in Africa as well. The 1987 *Fodor's Kenya* speculated that in some African countries the HIV infection rate may be 30 percent of the total population[13]—even though this statement had no scientific support, least of all in Kenya, where well-conducted studies of seroprevalence have shown much lower rates in the general population.[14]

The African Analogue

However the Africans may have thought of it, the alarmists readily pointed to the African experience as representing the future of the AIDS epidemic in the United States. There were many, many other allusions to this besides *Newsweek*'s, which concluded, "Already in much of Africa, no one is completely safe. Even allowing for the disparities between one culture and another, that may soon be true in much of the rest of the world too."[15]

An Associated Press dispatch, headlined "Spread in Africa Provides Glimpse into Future," warned: "Some scientists contend [AIDS] will soon spread into the general heterosexual population. If it does, it will be mimicking the course it has taken in Africa."[16] The *Reader's Digest* (in what was otherwise a sound article) entitled its exclusive report on Africa, "The Plague that Knows No Boundaries," and hinted that Africa's situation presaged that of the United States ("In Africa, the virus is transmitted primarily through heterosexual contact. . . . Already there are clear signs of accelerating heterosexual spread in the United States").[17] In early 1989, one could still buy magazines stating:

> It is already a near certainty that what we are seeing is only the beginning of something far more menacing: the transition of an epidemic now localized within a minority of the population into a pandemic affecting everyone. We have only to look at the course of events in parts of Africa, where whole settlements are now infected by AIDS. The virus is on the loose in Africa, and there is no reason to hope that it will not spread into the community at large in every other part of the world.[18]*

One proponent of the "Africa is America's future" theory was none other than the World Health Organization's director Jonathan Mann. In 1986, "Nightline"'s Ted Koppel asked him whether "it could happen in this country. That we could see over the years an equal spread among heterosexuals as we now see among homosexuals?" Mann replied:

> Well, it's actually already happening. In Europe, in the United States, the transmission of the disease from man to woman and woman to man is already a fact. So, it's begun. . . . I don't know if the United States and Europe will ever have a heterosexual AIDS problem similar to the problem in Africa, but the potential is clearly there.[20]

Other alarmist doctors were more adamant. Said Robert Redfield, "People say, oh that Africa, it's different. That's very colonialistic. The fact is, AIDS has moved. The infection has spread through Africa, like it's spreading through the U.S."[21] Dr. Haseltine put in his two cents, saying, "Many experts fear that, if the AIDS virus has gained a 'beach-head' in the heterosexual population of the United States, the experience of Africa could be repeated here."[22]

According to this theory, the alleged 90-percent heterosexual transmission rate in Africa is a portent of things to come in the United States. There are, however, two serious theoretical problems with this theory: first, it assumes that the African epidemic is more mature than ours; second, it assumes that Africa went through an epidemiological pattern similar to ours.

*Another diehard Africa citer, Shepherd Smith, president of Americans for a Sound AIDS Policy, states, "We have also felt that in time the African experience would be the most applicable model for America with this sexually transmitted disease [AIDS]."[19]

In fact, as noted in chapter 3, there is no evidence that AIDS cases began showing up there any earlier than in the United States; the epidemic was first recognized on both continents in 1981. The first blood-test–confirmed case of AIDS occurred not in Africa but in St. Louis, Missouri.[23] As Dr. Sebastian Lucas of the London School of Tropical Medicine has said, "Much of the evidence would suggest that it's virtually as recent an epidemic as it has been in America. . . . It would appear to have occurred fairly synchronously."[24] Dr. Luc Montagnier, co-discoverer of the AIDS virus, has also concluded, "The evidence does not support a conclusion that AIDS has its origin in Africa."[25] Even *Newsweek* admitted as much, conceding that "there is no proof that the AIDS epidemic began in Africa any earlier than in the United States."[26]

Furthermore, the evidence strongly weighs against the assumption that Africa went through an epidemiological pattern similar to ours. In the United States, AIDS has always been concentrated among homosexuals, IV drug users, receivers of blood products, and the sex partners of members of these groups. By contrast, even in areas of Africa such as Ghana, where the epidemic began comparatively recently, the epidemiological pattern of spread is similar to that in areas where it has raged for years.[27] One could as easily assert that America is Africa's future as the other way around; there is simply no evidence either way.

Hygiene (Blood and Needles)

What *is* going on in Africa? Why is it different from what's going on in America? Two possibilities that have been broached and dismissed concern the possibility of a more efficiently transmitted strain of HIV or of genetic predisposition. Genetic differences between Africans and Europeans and their descendants have been suggested, by several Indian and Caribbean investigators, to explain the level and extent of heterosexual transmission in Africa. But no genetic basis has been identified that is linked either with increased susceptibility to infection or with a greater capacity to disseminate HIV (as is discussed in greater detail in the next chapter). Nor have virological studies so far revealed any difference among any strains of HIV that would result in increased infectious capability.[28]

There was a time, probably up until mid-1987, when anyone who said he or she truly understood the AIDS situation in Africa should immediately have been dismissed as a liar. Yet information has been collected at an increasing rate, and far more is known than was the case just a couple of years ago.

In 1987, the Public Health Service issued a report which stated, "In Africa, over 90 percent of cases have occurred through heterosexual transmission."[29] In fact, the number of children with AIDS alone is probably enough to belie that statistic. At the Second International Symposium on AIDS in Africa in 1987, the central African nation of Rwanda reported that 35 percent of all its officially reported cases of AIDS are in children. Zaire and another central African country, Zambia, both reported that more than 20 percent of their AIDS cases involve children. The chief means of infection, according to a Zairian researcher, was either in the womb or at birth.[30] Writing in the *Lancet*, Johannesburg, South African virologists pointed out that 15 percent to 22 percent of AIDS cases there have occurred in children, either during pregnancy or from other causes having nothing to do with coitus.[31]

Additionally, a host of factors exist in Africa that do not exist here but that greatly facilitate the spread of HIV in nonsexual ways.

Because the cost of screening one blood donation in many African countries is more than the *entire* per-capita expenditure for medical expenses,[32] the process was virtually never performed until foreign AIDS assistance became available in the late 1980s. Until then, the blood supply was thoroughly contaminated. HIV prevalence in central and East Africa ranged from 2 percent to 18 percent;[33] although when CBS's "60 Minutes" observed testing at one hospital in Uganda, it found 28 percent of the blood donated that day was infected.[34] Since the average transfusion requires several pints of blood, receiving a transfusion in these areas was practically tantamount to being infected. "Don't have an accident [requiring a transfusion]," one doctor warned a visitor in Lusaka, Zambia. "Even if you survive the crash, you may not survive the treatment."[35] Some reports have stated that as many as 25 percent of central Africa's AIDS cases may have been caused by transfusions and injections,[36] a number that is borne out by several studies.[37]

When "60 Minutes" traveled to Uganda, its crew visited a hospital that had one of the country's five machines for screening blood to be used in transfusion, just a fraction of the number of such machines in New York City alone.

The day we were there, [said Diane Sawyer, the hospital] tested blood samples from donors, and the results were 28 percent positive. But when the donors who tested positive came to get their results, if they looked healthy, they weren't told they were carrying the virus. The doctors said there's no point in giving someone a possible death sentence when you have no counselors to help them deal with the news. Even if it means they spread the disease to others, the doctors say, one cruelty doesn't justify another. [One donor] saw ten doctors; no one told her the truth.[38]

From that statement alone, it should be readily discernible that the comparison between the spread of HIV in Africa and in the United States could not be more misleading.

Unsterilized needles used by untrained medical workers also greatly facilitate the spread of the virus. These needles are used in drawing blood for transfusions, for vaccinations, and for administering therapeutic drugs such as penicillin. In the United States they are simply discarded after use, but central and East African countries cannot afford to do this and may do nothing more to clean needles than run them under a faucet—a procedure useless for dislodging substances on the inside of a needle. The needles are simply used until they break.

Citizens of the Soviet republic of Kalmyk in 1988 learned a terrible lesson in AIDS hygiene when officials revealed that 27 children had become infected in a single hospital, most or all apparently through reuse of unsterilized needles. This was all the more shocking in a country that claimed to have only six persons suffering clinical symptoms of AIDS, with an additional 114 listed as being infected.[39] If one can imagine such an effect throughout an entire country, one can understand the potential for HIV spread in Africa through this practice alone.

One report noted that 80 percent of the AIDS patients in Kinshasa, the capital of Zaire, reported receiving medical injections before the onset of the syndrome; 29 percent went to traditional practitioners, who also provide injections; and 9 percent had received a blood transfusion in a three-year period before the onset of the illness.[40] A later report on hospital workers found that receiving medical injections and blood transfusions were significantly correlated with one's becoming infected.[41] While one study of Rwandese children showed no such correlation, it was pointed out that the Rwandese received far fewer injections than did the Ugandans.[42]

Native practices, such as ritual scarification of men and clitoridectomy of women, are also widespread. If a seropositive person is scarred with one of these instruments, it is possible that the virus will be passed along to someone scarred immediately thereafter. The extent to which such rituals contribute to the spread of HIV is, however, debatable. A letter to *Lancet* downplayed the importance of scarification, noting that, unlike hollow needles, razor blades allow quick drying of blood (and consequent destruction of HIV) and that treatment takes long enough that "by the time the razorblade is used again the retrovirus should be destroyed."[43] On the other hand, a doctor writing in *Science* stated, "It is noteworthy that the recent outbreaks of AIDS in Africa . . . correspond geographically to those regions in which female mutilation is still practiced."[44] Further, a recent report connected a case of HIV infection with acupuncture, a treatment that uses solid needles.[45] At any rate, the role of scarification should probably not be overplayed; the degree to which it may spread HIV is probably small.

All of these different modes of HIV transmission devastate the PHS's 90-percent figure, but the implications go far beyond. These numerous risk factors themselves contribute to the transmission of HIV through heterosexual intercourse in that they result in a much higher residual rate of infection than in America. In the United States, heterosexuals must worry about only IV drug abusers, bisexuals, and some hemophiliacs and transfusion recipients—a small percentage of the population. But in Africa, there is a vast number of conduits into the heterosexual population with a vast number of infected heterosexuals. (The importance of multiple conduits hearkens back to the discussion in chapter 2 on the various factors that may allow an expanding epidemic.) Put another way, if a heterosexual American goes to a singles bar in a northwest Chicago suburb, his chances of picking up an infected sexual partner could be less than 1 in 1,000. That same American visiting a bar in Kinshasa, Zaire, might find his odds increased to more than 1 in 10. Whatever other transmission factors are present, the bottom line is that one still cannot become infected sexually without an infected sexual partner, regardless of whether the source of the first infection was sexual or tainted blood or reused needles.

Sexual Practices

Nonetheless, it is fairly certain that the majority of AIDS cases in Africa arise from sexual transmission. The remaining questions, then, are what kind of sex, with whom, and with what complicating risk factors?

To refer to Africa as the "dark continent" nowadays is to be accused of racism and colonialist attitudes. Nevertheless, Africa's customs, habits, and mores are little known to Americans, and information about them is often difficult to come by. Again, it must be emphasized that the primary way—often the only way—a health worker can accurately determine the risk factors of an AIDS victim is through a personal interview. As difficult as such an interview may be with one New Yorker talking to another New Yorker, in Africa it is severely hampered by both language and cultural differences. Many Africans consider blunt, direct questions ill mannered and will not respond to them. Sexual vocabulary is always full of both euphemisms and slang (how many slang words for *penis* are in the English language?), but this is especially the case among Africans. *Vasectomy* may translate into *castration*, for example. The Swahili word for *plastic, elastic*, or *rubber* can mean a football or an inner tube as well as a diaphragm, an IUD, or a condom.[46]

Americans and Western Europeans are so open about sex that we find it hard to imagine a country where people still speak about it much as we did in Victorian times—when even table legs were often covered by the tablecloths so as not to seem suggestive. As in our Victorian era, it is not that taboo sexual acts don't take place in Africa, it is just that they are never spoken of. Imagine the feelings of an American or a European suffering from gonorrhea when a doctor pulls him aside and asks him how he got the disease. Say he got it through the last Western taboo—incest. Now, further suppose he is being asked by a foreign doctor who doesn't look like the patient, dress much like him, act like him, or talk like him. For all the patient knows, incest might be part of other cultures, but how compelled is he to confide in this doctor that, sure, he had sex with his daughter? On the other hand, it might be a native doctor who interviews him. In fact, the guy lives right down the block and the patient has known him all his life. How eager will the patient be to tell him that he's been having conjugal relations with a close relative?

In the same way, when a Western doctor asks about anal sex, an African says in alarm, "Oh no, we don't do that here!" The doctor marks it down. "Had any sex with men?" asks the doctor. "God forbid!" the African cries, knowing that God has indeed forbidden it. Thus, the doctor, used to hearing men in Los Angeles or San Francisco say, "Sure I use drugs" or "Sure, I'm homosexual," and finding that all of his African interviewees deny engaging in anal sex and bisexuality, simply takes the assertions as true.

As noted in chapter 2, a high level of partner switching is conducive to HIV spread. Many Africans go beyond denying homosexual practices and anal intercourse, to denying even promiscuity. The Ugandan ambassador to the United Nations told "60 Minutes," "I can tell you that I've lived in England the best part of seven years as a student and then 13 years as a solicitor—self-employed lawyer—there . . . and the extent of promiscuity is no different than it is in Africa."[47]

Some researchers seeking to discount African promiscuity will state, as one reporter put it, that "no research evidence exists showing that Africans are more promiscuous than Americans or Europeans."[48] But in respect to "research evidence," resistance on the part of both individuals and African governments would make it extremely difficult to collect such evidence outright.

Nevertheless, the observations of outsiders who have worked in Africa diverge sharply from the official government line. One British doctor who had worked extensively in Africa said, "There's no doubt there is a different attitude to sexual intercourse in many of these countries than we would have here. They are much less chaste than we are." He added that he was speaking not as a moralist but as a detached scientist, saying "I think to use the term 'promiscuous' is a bit derogatory—it's just a different way of life."[49]

An American gastroenterologist, who worked at Mulago Hospital in Kampala, declared, "There is profound promiscuity in Uganda, and a virus that takes advantage of it. The average Ugandan has sex with great frequency and with a great number of different partners."[50]

In some areas of Africa, in fact, promiscuity is practically institutionalized—as Edgar Gregerson in his *Sexual Practices* wrote:

> For a woman to have more than one husband has been described as almost nonexistent throughout Africa. But there are instances where a woman may have several recognized mates. What is clear is that in many societies—whatever the label given by the particular society itself to the arrangement—women are allowed to have many sexual partners.[51]

Gregerson went on to describe the Muslim Nupe tribe, "where married women are so free with their sexual favors that it has been described as bordering on prostitution." He further wrote that, in at least three societies, a widow must perform sexual intercourse ritually to remove her polluting status as a widow. The Twi of Ghana, for example, require that before a widow remarries, she must have sex with another man in order to cleanse her of the spirit of her dead husband.[52] (One newspaper article focused on an African man who was highly reluctant to cleanse his brother's widow: his brother had died of AIDS.)[53] It is probably fair to say, as NBC's science correspondent did after returning from Africa, that "sexual practices in Africa vary enormously from tribe to tribe, from country to country, from rural areas to cities. There can be no generalities, but in many parts of Africa and in other countries, it is traditional and accepted for people to have several sex partners."[54]

Anal Sex

Anal sex, by contrast, appears to be taboo virtually throughout Africa. In one of the most prominent early studies of prostitutes in Kenya, of 64 lower-class women and 26 women from higher socioeconomic status, absolutely none admitted to anal intercourse.[55] Dr. Thomas Quinn, widely considered one of America's foremost experts on AIDS in Africa, noted these denials and assumed their veracity. "Whereas anal receptive intercourse is a prominent sexual behavior that is associated with HIV infection among homosexuals in the U.S.," he told the President's AIDS commission, "this behavior does not appear to play any specific role in HIV transmission in Africa."[56]

But one British doctor who is a native of Africa returned to his native continent on a fact-finding tour and reported back:

> [I had] the privilege to interview 88 prostitutes in West, East, and central Africa as far down as Zimbabwe and there was no doubt that these girls divided all sexual intercourse into two categories only: *normal and abnormal.* Anything other than penovaginal was abnormal and they charged dearly for it because, as they put it, "it is very harmful." Some of their expatriate clients ask for anal intercourse, which the girls detest but which most accept "because of the double fee we charge."[57]

He noted further, "Even without anal intercourse, too-frequent normal penovaginal intercourse to which prostitutes subject themselves becomes *abnormal sex* because of the perintrauma involved." (The perineum is the area in front of the anus extending to the vulva in the female and to the scrotum in the male.) This doctor also stated, "In my Krobo tribe in West Africa, where prostitutes are the only people with AIDS (repatriated from neighboring Ivory Coast to die), the common feature in all the patients is perineal disintegration."[58]

Ann Guidici Fettner, whom no one can accuse of downplaying the risks of vaginal HIV transmission, nevertheless reported that an African doctor told her "anal sex in Africa is fairly common."[59]

Homosexuality and Bisexuality

The assumption that homosexuality in Africa is virtually nonexistent and hence not a factor in AIDS cases is—like many assumptions about AIDS—one that has become so commonly accepted and repeated that few have bothered to look at the evidence to see whether it is true. The assumption is based on the virtually universal propensity of seropositive Africans to deny homosexual contacts—a denial prompted by government laws against homosexuality and societal taboos. In fact, if a central or East African government has *not* passed a law against homosexual practices, it is probably because they are so taboo. As one Angolan diplomat put it, "the evil of homosexuality does not exist in our country, and it is consequently not mentioned in our legislation."[60] Doctors like Thomas Quinn have listened to the denials and accepted them as fact, then propagated them in turn.

Yet these denials do not stand up well to the evidence. First, it is fairly absurd to assume there is practically no homosexuality in Africa. Whether or not one buys into Dr. Kinsey's assertion that 4 percent of all males are "more or less exclusively homosexual throughout their lives,"[61] it cannot be denied that homosexuality is widespread in cultures with which we are familiar—those of North America and Western Europe, including blacks, whites, and Hispanics. Strictly on a theoretical basis, it is fairly absurd to assume that somehow this prevalence does not apply to Africa as well. On an empirical basis, there is indeed evidence that homosexual practices are engaged in in Africa and may even be widespread.

The aforementioned British doctor, who was native to Africa, noted, "The very first report on AIDS to come from Uganda (in a region the world press loved to describe as heterosexual) mentioned that traders who were found to be [seropositive] 'admitted to both heterosexual and homosexual casual contacts,' and one AIDS patient 'had a high recto-vaginal fistula of recent onset.' "[62] (A fistula is a narrow passage or duct formed by disease or injury, as one leading from an abscess to a free surface, or from one cavity to another; in this case, it indicates anal intercourse.)

Dr. Robert Gould, who taught sex education for the Family Life Division of Manhattan's Metropolitan Hospital, has written, "Year after year, the African nurses would confirm that homosexuality, although commonplace among their people, was not talked about or even acknowledged." Gould adds that it was

> not until the very end of the course did the nurses themselves begin to speak openly on the subject. So considering just how reluctant Africans are to talk about their homosexual practices even among themselves, I would question the information reported by African researchers and collected by western researchers regarding AIDS in the African heterosexual community.

Given my own experience, it is not farfetched to assume that the data may well reflect infection by homosexual activity (i.e., anal sex).[63]

The science writer John Langone has written, "There also seems little doubt that homosexuality is on the rise in major urban centers, both among the Western-educated middle classes and the rootless, detribalized masses who have moved in from the countryside";[64] and the late Dr. B. Frank Polk of Johns Hopkins University, after returning from a trip to central Africa, observed that "[homosexuality is] simply far more repressed, and most often is seen as bisexuality."[65]

Lest any doubt remain, a black writer for the homosexual newspaper the *New York Native* took a trip to Africa and had no trouble locating fellow homosexuals. In his article, "Inside Gay Africa," Cary Alan Johnson confirmed that the "vast majority of [African homosexuals] are married, affianced, have children, or are part of strong family units."[66] One contact he made while on his trip served as a microcosm for Polk's assertion. This man, while a homosexual, was also engaged. After the American reporter stayed with him, he was beaten by local authorities for allowing a visit by a known homosexual. Wrote Johnson, "Anyone who's spent a significant amount of time in the gay subculture of [Zaire] knows that no gay or bisexual Zairian would reveal himself to any investigator, local or foreign."[67] Unfortunately, that includes the American doctors who make short trips to Africa and come back parroting the African governments' "no-homosexuals" line, which is then picked up by the media.

While homosexual acts are clearly being practiced in Africa, it is true that homosexual communities like those in the United States and elsewhere in the West are nonexistent. Neither are there homosexual bathhouses, bars, bookstores, or other places where homosexual gatherings are socially acceptable. The effect of suppressing overt homosexuality is to eliminate it in open form and probably reduce its incidence over all. One aspect of this situation is, however, that those who in some other society might be purely homosexual adopt bisexuality instead. Instead of having sex with a stranger and going back home to a male lover, as a white homosexual might in the United States (American minorities present a different problem, as will be seen in the next chapter), an African homosexual is more likely to go back home and have relations with his wife or girlfriends. Thus, although in the United States female infection by a bisexual is comparatively infrequent, in Africa it could be a common route. In fact, Polk held that AIDS in Africa was best described as a heterosexual disease, but one that is mainly unidirectional—meaning that it travels most readily between men and then to women.[68]

One argument against widespread homosexual transmission in Africa is that, while in the United States the ratio of male AIDS cases to female ones has been about 12 to 1, in Africa the ratio is said to be about 1 to 1. In fact a 1-to-1 ratio by no means implies infection through heterosexual intercourse. Infections through needles and blood transfusions would both tend to leave ratios of 1 to 1. Widespread pure homosexuality would indeed tend to make the male side of the equation larger than the female, but that's not being addressed here; this is *bisexuality*. Writing in the *Journal of the American Medical Association,* Dr. Nancy Padian of Berkeley and Dr. John Pickering of the University of Georgia wrote, "If female-to-male transmission is rare in Africa, as it appears to be in the United States, then the low African ratio could be explained by a higher proportion of bisexual men in Africa than in the United States." In the extreme case, they said, "if few males are exclusively homosexual in Africa and if most homosexual behavior is among bisexual males, then bisexual males could be largely responsible for the sexual transmission of AIDS."[69] Nevertheless, because homosexual acts are so seldom admitted in Africa, Dr. Padian's theory will probably never be more than just that.

Sexually Transmitted Diseases

As noted in chapter 4, sexually transmitted diseases in either the HIV-infected person or that person's sex partner appear dramatically to increase the transmission efficiency of HIV. Most of these studies were conducted in Africa, one reason being that those areas of Africa struck hardest by AIDS are rife with STDs.

For example, one survey in the early 1970s showed rates of gonorrhea in Kampala, Uganda, and Nairobi, Kenya, to be more than ten times higher than in London and considerably greater than in Atlanta, Georgia. The syphilis rate in Kampala was seventy times that in London and almost seven times that in Atlanta.[70] Even the Atlanta figures were quite high compared with the United States as a whole, which in another study at about that time had a rate much closer to London's.[71]

According to the Panos Institute, "up to one in three people in some groups in Africa have had genital ulcers."[72] In fact, gonorrhea is so common that its symptoms are sometimes regarded as a sign of sexual awakening or potency.[73] According to researchers from the CDC and Family Health International, Africa has higher prevalence rates of traditional STD, such as gonorrhea and syphilis, higher proportions of antimicrobial-resistant organisms, and higher levels of complication, including pelvic inflammatory disease [PID], infertility, and adverse pregnancy outcomes. Between 20 and 40 percent of acute admissions to gynecology wards in Africa are related to PID. Infertility is as high as 50 percent in some areas; and as much as 80 percent of infertility is attributable to STD. . . . Gonococcal ophthalmia neonatorum, a severe gonorrheal inflammation of the eye in newborns, is over 50 times more common in Africa than in industrialized countries. Maternal syphilis seems to cause a fetal death or a syphilitic infant in five to eight percent of all pregnancies surviving past 12 weeks in many parts of Africa.[74]

The reason for such high STD rates in Africa is not just promiscuity; it's a lack of funds. In the United States, medical care is comparatively cheap, be it for diagnosis or actual treatment of STDs. In much of Africa, the cost of either a medical inspection or the treatment for an STD discovered by it can be more than the entire per-capita medical expenditures for that country.

Because of the STD co-factor problem, prostitutes in Africa constitute a permanent pool of infection. Thus, unlike in the United States, prostitutes appear to be a major HIV risk factor for men in Africa. In the United States, prostitutes can and do get treatment for their STDs. Since overall STD infection rates in the United States are so much lower than in Africa, the infection rate of American prostitutes' partners, too, is vastly lower than that of the prostitutes' clientele in central and East Africa.

Even if they don't transmit HIV to a customer, African prostitutes can still transmit the ulcerating STD that will make it easier for the man to get HIV from the next person with whom he has intercourse. Even for those who can afford to cure themselves, the STD rate among their clientele is so high and use of condoms so infrequent that, as one medical journal author put it, "the rate of reinfection observed among the prostitutes [in a sector in Nairobi] is astounding."[75] Among 52 women studied who were initially infected with gonorrhea, 28 became reinfected during the course of the study, taking an average of only 26 days after being cured to do so.[76] The result is that prostitutes in Africa, as opposed to those in the United States, are both receivers and transmitters of HIV. In major African cities, rates of HIV infection among prostitutes have been found from 27 percent to 88 percent,[77] with probably little if any of it attributable to IV-drug abuse,[78] which is, as noted earlier, the overwhelming risk factor for prostitutes in the United States.

A study in the *New England Journal of Medicine* found that 64 lower-class prostitutes in Nairobi, Kenya, averaged 963 partners a year at 50 cents apiece.[79] Of these, 55 percent tested currently had syphilis, 45 percent had gonorrhea, and 42 percent had genital ulcers.[80] Sixty-six percent of these also tested positive for HIV.[81] None of the prostitutes used condoms.[82] In a group of men seeking treatment for infections of the genitals and urinary tract at the Nairobi Special Treatment Clinic, of 40 tested for HIV, 58 percent had had intercourse with at least one prostitute. (Incidentally, they also averaged 17 partners in the previous year; and 1 of 3 testing positive admitted to being bisexual, neither of which lends support to those who insist that promiscuity is rare in Africa and homosexuality is not a factor.)[83] While it is improper to extrapolate from the patients at such a clinic to the sexually active population as a whole, other studies in Nairobi, Zaire, and Rwanda have implicated sexual contact with prostitutes as an important means of transmitting HIV.[84] While some African men claiming prostitute contact are probably disguising homosexual activities (as is often the case in the United States), it is easy to see how, considering the STD co-factor problem, prostitutes in Africa suffering from both HIV and other STDs could be a major means of infection of the population at large. The Nairobi study, in fact, was one of the earliest to theorize a link to STDs and HIV seropositivity; and lest one conclude that the relationship of these illnesses was coincidental rather than causal (that is, the more sex one has, the better one's chance of getting both genital sores and HIV), the study found no independent correlation between HIV infection and the number of sexual contacts;[85] nor did a later one in Nairobi.[86]

Circumcision

As early as 1986, Dr. Aaron Fink suggested that lack of circumcision could be a risk factor. In a letter to the *New England Journal of Medicine,* he wrote:

> It has been known for many years and has recently been documented again in studies in venereal disease clinics that both genital herpes and syphilis are more common in uncircumcised men. Since the infectious agents of both these diseases depend on a break or an abrasion in the skin to gain entry into the body, the likelihood that the cervical secretions of a woman infected with AIDS can be transferred by similar means is greater when the skin surface is delicate, easily abraded penile lining, such as the mucosal inner layer of the foreskin, than when the foreskin is absent.

The doctor said that he suspected that American men, in comparison
with those in Africa and some other places, have benefited from the
high rate of newborn circumcision in the United States—80 percent to
90 percent until recently, although the percentage has declined in the
last few years.[87]

Odd though it may seem to the layman, the question whether to
circumcise is extremely volatile among many doctors. This, combined
with the volatility of the debate over the etiology of AIDS, prompted
a couple of nasty replies to Dr. Fink's letter, including one that called
Fink's hypothesis "totally unfounded," and found it "unthinkable that
the prestigious *New England Journal of Medicine* would choose to
promulgate such irresponsible speculation."[88] Nevertheless, within six
months the first empirical evidence began rolling in to show that uncircumcised males indeed run a significantly higher chance of HIV infection. Several studies in both Africa and the United States have shown
that men who are uncircumcised have a far greater risk of contracting
HIV than those who have had the precupice of the penis removed. One
African study reported that lack of circumcision and genital ulceration
risk factors were found in 98 percent of all infections.[89] Another noted,
"Uncircumcised men reported a history of genital-ulcer disease more
frequently than circumcised men and they were also more frequently
seropositive for HIV," and "in uncircumcised men . . . the increased risk
of HIV was independent of the occurrence of genital-ulcer disease."[90]
Thus, being uncircumcised was a double whammy. First, it increased
a man's chances of developing ulceration, itself a risk factor. But even
aside from this, it still appeared to increase the transmission efficiency
of HIV. Indeed, according to one study, it increased a man's chances of
infection with HIV by a factor of from 5 to 10,[91] thus making the
difference between sex with circumcision and sex without on a par with
the difference between vaginal and anal intercourse.

Exactly why this is the case is not completely clear. Dr. Fink added
to his earlier explanation: "Circumcision . . . removes vulnerable mucosal lining . . . and allows the development of a protective stratum
corneum layer,"[92] meaning that the thickness of skin between vulnerable white blood cells and the outside world is greatly increased with the
buildup of tissue after circumcision. It is this increased thickness that
makes some men who were circumcised as adults claim that they have
reduced sensitivity during sex.

But for whatever exact reason, lack of circumcision clearly increases
a man's chances of seroconverting upon having sexual contact with an

infected woman. Epidemic areas of central and East Africa not only apparently have considerably higher levels of infected heterosexual women, they also have considerably higher levels of uncircumcised men than the United States. Although circumcision is widely practiced in the Moslem countries of northern Africa and in some other areas, this is not the case for the central region of what two researchers actually named the "circumcision line" where AIDS is most prevalent ("The majority of uncircumcised Kenyan men are native to areas bordering on regions of Uganda and Tanzania in which the prevalence of HIV is high").[93]

One final possible risk factor is a chronically agitated immune system. Like extremely sexually active homosexuals in the United States (especially in the pre-AIDS era), Africans in AIDS-affected areas of Africa often suffer from a wide variety of diseases, including cytomegalovirus, Epstein-Barr, hepatitis B, and herpes simplex virus, all of which are known to suppress the immune system. In addition, these Africans are exposed to malaria and other diseases that are also known to suppress immunity.[94] As one study noted, "individuals with prior immunologic alterations are possibly at greater risk of infection and disease progression."[95]

Is the African Situation Even as Bad as "The African Situation"?

As baseless as it is to say that the epidemic in America will become as bad as that in Africa, it must be said that even the epidemic in Africa is not as bad as it has been portrayed. In fact, all of the declarations of catastrophe with which this chapter began have proven grossly exaggerated. Uganda still suffers from AIDS; but far from having become a desert, its population continues to grow. By 1988, the director of project SIDA, the Zairian AIDS research program (regarded as the premier AIDS research program on the continent), was able to declare, "The epidemic now looks like it is beginning to level off. . . . There is no evidence of any increase" in levels of infections in the last several years.[96] The director, Robert W. Ryder, said, "The blood banks are as close as we can get to a survey of the general situation in the city. They come out at about six percent positive—we have done many studies over the past four years and it continues at six percent. It's just not going up."[97] One reason Ryder cited was saturation of the at-risk population. "Others leading traditional, middle-class African lives get infected at a lower rate," he said.[98] Ryder even suggested the possibility that not just infections but actually *cases* could be leveling off, or even dropping in some areas.

Notwithstanding earlier claims of 5,000,000, 10,000,000, and 20,000,-000 infected Africans, Jonathan Mann and the World Health Organization have since revised their estimate of seropositivity to state that there are perhaps 5,000,000 infections in the *world*, with two to three million of these in Africa.[99] The higher estimates were basically derived by sampling blood in the very worst of the areas and extrapolating to the rest of the country. Methodologically, this was as sound as sampling blood in New York's East Village and San Francisco's Castro section—areas with a heavy concentration of homosexuals—and extrapolating to the rest of the United States. But it made damned good headlines and, as the "social consciousness" theory goes, it went a long way toward focusing attention on a part of the planet that the rest of the world tends to ignore. In contrast to the alleged 2,000,000 to 3,000,000 infections in Africa, the deaths from which will be spread out over a number of years, *each year* in Africa an estimated:

- 10 million die of acute respiratory infections, 4,000,000 of them children.
- 1,000,000 die of malaria.
- 3,000,000 die of tuberculosis.
- 4,500,000 children die of diphtheria, neonatal tetanus, whooping cough, measles, and tuberculosis.
- 1,500,000 to 2,000,000 die of tropical diseases other than malaria.[100]

At a 1989 workshop in Lusaka, Zambia, sponsored by the African-American Institute of New York, African medical professionals expressed fear that the West might encourage distortions in Africa's health-care networks by placing excessive emphasis on AIDS research there. "We can get funding for AIDS projects with little delay," said one, "but you could talk until your hair falls out before you would get anything for malaria or diarrhea, which kill many more Africans every year than AIDS does."[101] Or will.

Writing in the *Lancet* in 1987, a year before researchers began to admit the African AIDS epidemic had been overplayed, Dr. Felix I. D. Konotey-Ahulu, an African-born doctor, discussed a tour he had taken of central Africa. After giving a laundry list of diseases he had seen kill patients in Ghana, he stated sardonically, "Today, because of AIDS, no one is allowed to die from these conditions any longer." Wrote the doctor, " 'Why do the world's media appear to have conspired with some scientists to become so gratuitously extravagant with the untruth?'—that was the question uppermost in the minds of intelligent Africans and Europeans I met on my tour. The answer is far from easy, but one thing is certain: this journalistic hyperbole has proved very expensive." In conclusion he wrote,

> It should not really have to fall to the lot of a black physician to write like this, because I know very many whites with a fund of goodwill for Africa who feel even more strongly than I do about the effect of the world's media on that continent. Perhaps they will now begin to speak up.[102]

As we now know, they did not.

And What about Haiti?

While it is closer in proximity to the United States, Haiti is more similar in many respects to Africa, whence its people trace their descent. There have been numerous bizarre theories why there is so much AIDS in Haiti. One doctor wrote to the *Journal of the American Medical Association:*

> Even now, many Haitians are voodoo serviteurs and partake in its rituals. Some . . . are suspected to use human blood itself in sacrificial worship. As [HIV] is known to be stable in aqueous solution at room temperature for at least a week, lay Haitian voodooists may be unsuspectingly infected with AIDS by ingestion, inhalation, or dermal contact with contaminated substances, as well as by sexual activity.[103]

As the CDC's chief epidemiologist Harold Jaffe says, you can't say that something will *never* be a method of transmission because there will always be someone out there to prove you wrong. Still, it would be amazing if more than one or two HIV infections came about this way. (One senses that the editors at the *Journal of the American Medical Association* felt the same way, as they entitled the letter "Night of the Living Dead II: Slow Virus Encephalopathies and AIDS: Do Necromantic Zombiists Transmit HTLV-III/LAV During Voodooistic Rituals?")[104]

But there *is* something unusual about Haiti. As noted earlier, Haitians AIDS victims originally confused American doctors by claiming they had no homosexual risk factors. This claim, however, quickly fell apart because it was fairly well known that Haiti was a favorite vacation spot for American homosexuals. Wrote the author David Black:

> On the main road from the Carrefour to the center of Port-au-Prince are the big whorehouses, like the Club Social Cabaret, which are surrounded by

massive walls. Inside are compounds with bars, shady groves, and little hovels
that the girls and boys use. In these "social clubs," for the price of [oral sex]
in Manhattan, $25 to $50, you can do anything with virtually anyone: male
and female, children and crones.

Such freedom offers not a test of sexual prowess but of the imagination.
What do you want? A thimblejob, an around-the-world, the rear-admiral, the
python dance, a rum-desire, the Macao sling—which involves two chickens
and some piano wire.[105]

According to Dr. Jean Pape, one of Haiti's leading AIDS researchers,
"the CDC never wondered why 88 percent of the early Haitian AIDS
cases in the United States occurred in males. In 1983 our group had
identified risk factors, bisexuality and blood transfusion, in 79 percent
of Haitian AIDS patients."[106] The reason for the CDC's befuddlement
was that its doctors asked Haitians if they were homosexuals, the Haitians said no, and that was the end of it. It turned out that while many
of them had engaged in regular sex with American homosexuals, they
weren't homosexual themselves because they didn't *enjoy* it. They did
it for money.[107] Of course, whether they enjoyed it or not was irrelevant
to its transmission efficiency. Again, it all comes back to: Ask the wrong
questions, get the wrong answers.

Alas, for this successful denial of risk factors, Haiti—already identified
by many Americans as primarily the land of zombies—was punished
with a tremendous dropoff in tourism and with discrimination against
its citizens abroad. Haitian community workers in the United States
reported that in some areas the unemployment rate for Haitians was
twice that of other black workers, a situation they felt was directly
attributable to AIDS. According to the AIDS Discrimination Unit of the
New York City Commission on Human Rights in 1987, "Haitian children have been beaten up and, in at least one case, shot in school.
Haitian families have been evicted from their homes."[108]

Ironically, HIV may have been brought to Haiti via its brothels by
U.S. citizens on vacation. Certainly there is no evidence that HIV was
present in the country before it was present in the United States.[109] As
it was, however, the Haitian AIDS epidemic appears to have begun in
the homosexual population. Notwithstanding its roots, it quickly fanned
out into the heterosexual population—so quickly, in fact, that it became
a major heterosexual problem before many American researchers even
realized it had originally started as a homosexual one. By 1985, the
demographics of AIDS in Haiti had changed so that women were making up a larger portion of the cases.[110]

But far from indicating that the United States, too, could go from a homosexual epidemic to heterosexual epidemic, Haiti was the exception that proved the rule. The alarmist author Chris Norwood wrote, "In 1983, only 22 percent of that nation's cases were heterosexually acquired. . . . Two years later 72 percent of the newly reported cases were men and women who had contracted the virus from heterosexual intercourse."[111] What this supposedly means for the United States is evident in the title of the chapter: "The Future of AIDS." But even as those words appeared in print, HIV had been in the American heterosexual population at least ten years. While HIV may survive in a fairly inhospitable atmosphere—as it apparently did for at least decades before causing sickness on a massive scale—it spreads rapidly when it finds a highly susceptible population; it doesn't spend a decade licking its chops before pouncing. HIV was allowed to shift in Haiti only because of factors present there and in Africa but far less so in the United States. As in Africa, blood contamination and needle reuse have been connected to seropositivity.[112] Hygiene in general is a nightmare. David Black wrote of his trip to Haiti:

> In 1975 I went to the Carrefour to research an article. I stayed with a *houn'gan,* a voodoo priest, whose powers had been studied at a parapsychology laboratory in the United States. By Carrefour standards this voodoo priest was a Rockefeller. He even had a gasoline-powered electric generator, which ran a tiny refrigerator in which he made ice—using water from the stream. [My host] took out a bottle of Coca-Cola, opened it, and poured an inch or so in our glasses—over ice that contained what looked like fecal matter. To refuse the drink would have been a mortal insult, so I gulped it as quickly as I could, before the ice had a chance to melt very much. Everyone in the family had bowel trouble. Now, so did I. At night, even though I was the third to get to the chamber pot (which was passed from room to room in a hierarchical order; to be third was also an honor, like being seated at a banquet above the salt), it was always full. Given my experience with Haitian hygiene, it didn't surprise me when Haitians were added to the list of AIDS risk groups.[113]

STDs are also a major problem in Haiti and have been linked in that country to HIV infection.[114] One study found that linking was the case independent of the number of partners, meaning the relationship between STDs and seropositivity could indeed be causal.[115]

One of the most important factors in the rapid spread of the virus to heterosexuals is that, again as in Africa, homosexuality means bisexuality. Dr. Warren D. Johnson, Jr., considered one of the top American experts on Haitian AIDS, said, "In Haiti, we see virtually no males who are exclusively homosexual. They're almost always bisexual."[116] Likewise, a *New York Native* reporter writing from Haiti said the doctors she spoke with stated, "We do not have homosexuals here, but we have men who are bisexual and promiscuous. In that sense we have a more serious problem than in the U.S."[117] Indeed. The severity of the problem is brought home when one hears Dr. Pape state that much Haitian homosexuality takes place for pay, and that after such intercourse the Haitian man would go to " 'cleanse' himself of his 'error' by having relations with a woman, a prostitute or otherwise."[118]

In sum, the African and Haitian epidemics are, in many areas, indeed devastating. But it was no more intelligent to deduce AIDS transmission patterns from these countries than to assume that because Africans suffer periodic famine, we will as well. With few exceptions, heterosexually transmitted AIDS is the problem—one among many—of Third World countries. It is a symptom of a society with underlying medical and hygienic problems. In a sense, just as AIDS destroys the immune system and allows opportunistic infections to grow, so does a society rife with genital disease and poor hygiene allow heterosexual AIDS the opportunity to proliferate. Most of the United States and most of Western Europe do not fall into that category—with one major exception. Indeed, the black and Hispanic ghettos of the nation are sometimes referred to as the "Third World" of the United States.

10

The Agony of the Underclass

"I enjoy sex," says the attractive woman on TV and in the magazine advertisements, "but I'm not ready to die for it."[1] The use of fear to sell condoms is hardly remarkable. Madison Avenue uses fear to advertise everything from mouthwash to dandruff shampoo to deodorant to seatbelt buckling. What should be remarkable is that the commercial's actress was a *white* woman. The condom manufacturers and, to a much greater extent, the media sold the nation on the idea that AIDS is of major concern not just to the heterosexual population, but specifically to the white, middle-class heterosexual population. Indeed, if one thing was clear from the media, it was that this was a disease of the white middle class. The film *Sex, Drugs, and AIDS*, originally made for the New York City Board of Education, was later distributed to and shown by high schools around the country. It featured one section with three girls talking about condom usage. All of them were white, even though it was made for a school system that was 80 percent black, Hispanic, and Asian.[2]

The heterosexual fear stories on the covers of the major newsmagazines have invariably pictured middle-class whites. The *Atlantic*'s heterosexual epidemic article portrayed illustrations of five people, all white and all dressed in yuppie garb; on the cover of the magazine were two more whites.[3] *Time*'s "The Big Chill" cover had two white heterosexuals on the cover,[4] as did *U.S. News*'s heterosexual scare cover, which featured a graph line depicting an exponential growth in AIDS cases over a man and woman's faces.[5] *People* magazine's "AIDS & the Single Woman" cover depicted the faces of ten women, eight of them white and none of them apparently anything less than middle-class.[6] The victims of AIDS on series television, in addition to being disproportionately heterosexual, were always white. When ABC's "Nightline"

ran a four-hour program on AIDS, it began the section on sexual transmission with a clip showing white, middle-class heterosexuals discussing
their fears of contracting AIDS. There was not a black or apparent
homosexual in sight, although a heterosexual Hispanic woman with
AIDS was finally shown later. Indeed, it seemed that practically the only
times the media chose to depict minorities was when they showed
someone who actually had the disease. As the ABC News commentator
Ted Koppel put it, "to use Ralph Ellison's old title, black people with
AIDS have become 'the invisible man' and the invisible woman again."[7]

To judge from the media, the typical profile of a victim of heterosexual AIDS transmission was either a white, upwardly mobile woman who
was infected after a one-night stand with a man who later proved to be
a bisexual, or a white, upwardly mobile man infected by a one-time
liaison with a woman who had had sex with a bisexual.[8] One couldn't
possibly guess that, in fact, the profile of the typical non-IVDA heterosexual AIDS victim was a lower-class black or Hispanic woman whose
regular sex partner was an IV drug user. White heterosexual transmission cases at the time of the media blitz on heterosexual AIDS (late 1986
to mid-1987) made up only about one-half of 1 percent of all AIDS
cases.* Only about 1 percent of white AIDS cases are attributable to
heterosexual transmission,[10] as opposed to 4 percent of Hispanic
cases,[11] 5 percent among blacks born in the United States (excluding
persons born in Africa and Haiti).[12] Of all native-born heterosexual
transmission cases, about 50 percent are black and 25 percent Hispanic.[13] In the Centers for Disease Control's heterosexual case category, which includes those born in Africa and Haiti, 65 percent of all
adult cases are black and 15 percent Hispanic.[14]

Even aside from heterosexual transmission, in every risk category
other than hemophilia,† blacks and Hispanics make up a disproportionately high percentage of AIDS cases.[16] Whereas blacks account for only
11.5 percent of the U.S. population, they represent about 25 percent of
all reported adult AIDS cases over all[17] and over 50 percent of all adult
women with AIDS.[18] Hispanics, at 6 percent of the population, represent 15 percent of adult U.S. AIDS cases[19] and 20 percent of all the
women's cases.[20] Thus minority women make up over 70 percent of all

---

*As of 7 September 1987, of 41,135 total cases reported, only 249 whites were listed
as being infected through heterosexual transmission.[9]

†Black men's lower risk of AIDS related to hemophilia suggests that this inherited
disorder may be less common in blacks than in whites, but demographic data on hemophiliacs are unavailable to substantiate this.[15]

female AIDS cases—a figure inversely proportional to the ratio displayed on the cover of *People* magazine.

Blood testing has shown similar disparities. Testing of civilian applicants to the Armed Forces from October 1985 to March 1988 showed that while only 8 of 10,000 white applicants were infected, with blacks it was 45 out of 10,000 and Hispanics had 23 seropositives per 10,000.[21] Among active-duty personnel, testing from January 1987 to 24 April 1988 showed 8 infected whites per 10,000 but 29 infected blacks and 20 infected Hispanics.[22]

Just as the media did its best to convince its audience that heterosexually transmitted AIDS was primarily a white, middle-class problem, it also disguised the reality that the great majority of children born with HIV were also black and Hispanic. *USA Today,*[23] *American Health,*[24] and other periodicals all used the pediatric figures without bothering to point out that the mothers were overwhelmingly black or Hispanic and poor. "Nightline" did an entire show on the subject without mentioning class or race.[25] The ads The American Foundation for Aids Research began showing in 1989 warning of perinatal transmission also showed a white baby. The CDC reported in late 1988 that AIDS had become the ninth leading cause of death among children age one to four and predicted at least 10,000 to 20,000 seropositive children by 1991. The *New York Times* printed an article on this in a prominent place (the back of the first section) but did not bother to mention race.[26] Yet less than 15 percent of seropositive babies are white, while over 60 percent are black.[27] Thus, black babies have a risk of neonatal infection over 35 times that of a white baby. Half of all white children infected became so through transfusion or hemophilia clotting factor,[28] neither of which are still major sources of infection since the blood supply was cleaned up in 1985.[29] But about 90 percent of black children and 80 percent of Hispanic ones are infected through the mother.[30] (Black and Hispanic children also have a higher risk of infection through transfusion than do white ones—probably due to their having a rate of low birth weight at least twice that of whites.)[31] As time progresses, then, blacks and Hispanics will constitute an ever greater majority of the pediatric category.

While fewer than 15 percent of white adults with AIDS are strictly heterosexual, 45 percent of black adults and 50 percent of Hispanics with AIDS fall into that category. The incidence of AIDS among black women is over 12 times the incidence among white women; in Hispanic women it is 8 times.[32]

As the media were wrong in portraying heterosexual AIDS as predominantly a white disease, they also were wrong in suggesting that it largely threatened the middle class. At least one study has found that even taking into account gender differences, race, sexual orientation, IV-drug use, and age, persons whose income was below the federal poverty level were significantly more likely to be seropositive than those above it.[33]

The "Color-Blind" Disease

The slogan used to appeal to blacks and Hispanics to beware of AIDS was the ubiquitous "AIDS doesn't discriminate." While this slogan was originally intended to draw attention away from the extraordinary percentage of AIDS victims who were homosexuals, those using it in their appeal to blacks and Hispanics wanted to signify that one need not be a white homosexual to get it. When the media finally did begin to write about AIDS and minorities, it used headlines like "AIDS and Minorities: Myths, Fear Shield Color-blind Killer"[34] and "AIDS Strikes Without Regard for Race."[35] In fact, in practice AIDS clearly did strike with regard for race. Even as the ads sought to convey the message that minorities are at equal risk for AIDS, it underplayed the truly scary fact that they are at significantly greater risk.

Again, this special selection was not simply the result of being black or Hispanic any more than it was of being homosexual. It's that these groupings are often associated with certain activities with other people engaged in certain activities, and these activities put them at higher risk. As the black AIDS researcher Dr. Wayne Greaves has stated, "The virus appears to be color-blind, though not culture blind."[36]

This in itself is nothing new: blacks suffer disproportionately from a wide variety of controllable diseases, as well as from cancer and homicide. "When Americans, as a whole, have a bad cold," said the Rev. Joseph E. Lowery, president of the Southern Christian Leadership Conference, "the black community has pneumonia."[37] Still, even by the usual standards, AIDS is striking a ferocious blow at minorities. Why? One obvious possibility is that they are genetically predispositioned. Indeed, some studies have indicated significant differences in the frequency of opportunistic infections that strike blacks, whites, and Hispanics, even when differences in drug use and homosexuality are taken into account.[38]* It has also been pointed out that blacks tend to live for

*For example, in one study, in non-IVDA homosexuals, Kaposi's sarcoma was 2.2 times as frequent in whites as in blacks. Again, among non-IVDA homosexuals, *Mycobacterium avium* infection was more common in blacks than in whites and Hispanics.[39]

a considerably shorter time after diagnosis than do whites;[40] but it may well be that blacks are being diagnosed later than whites, who tend to be more affluent and hence have better access to quality medical care.[41]*

At one time it was suggested that a protein found in blood and cell surfaces could be a key in determining whether some persons become infected, and that one of the three types of this protein was far more prevalent in persons who were infected. Further, this protein type was also far more prevalent in blacks than in caucasians.[43] "It attracted a lot of attention and a number of laboratories tried to repeat it, including us," Harold Jaffe of the CDC told me.[44] Finally the authors of the study retracted the conclusion, blaming laboratory error.[45]

It seems clear that the most important factor in higher rates of minority AIDS is intravenous drug abuse. About 7 percent of white adults with AIDS have been classified as nonhomosexual IVDA, with another 7 percent being homosexual IVDA. But among blacks, while homosexual IVDA is still only 7 percent, 38 percent of cases are in heterosexual IVDA. Among Hispanics, the IVDA categories are virtually identical to that of blacks.[46] These figures are hardly surprising, given the enormous drug problem in America's inner-city ghettos. Blacks appear to be no more likely to use drugs than are whites,† although it has been hypothesized that blacks are simply more likely to use *intravenous* drugs.[48] In any case, the most important determinant is not the use of intravenous drugs but the location and the frequency of sharing needles. This practice differs among the races. A study of 189 male inmates in a Worcester, Massachusetts, prison found that 27 percent of Hispanics, 17 percent of blacks, and only 4 percent of whites were seropositive. Despite this difference, a slightly higher proportion of whites shared needles than did blacks and Hispanics. But the Hispanics were almost twice as likely as whites to have used needles more than once a day, to have shared needles in a shooting gallery, or to have shared them in New York City. Frequency of needle use was similar for blacks and whites, but blacks were 2.6 times more likely to have shared needles in a shooting gallery and 3.3 times more likely to have shared needles in New York City than whites.[49] There are vast differences in seropositiv-

---

*Likewise, the feminist author Chris Norwood pointed out that while 57 percent of the men with AIDS had died, 63 percent of women had.[42] But, again, the difference—not much at any rate—is explained by most female AIDS victims being IVDAs while most male AIDS victims are homosexual.

†A 1985 national household survey on drug abusers found that persons admitting to illegal drug abuse were 82 percent white, 11 percent black.[47]

ity levels between East Coast IVDA and those on the West Coast and in the Midwest. In New York, testing consistently shows about 60 percent of IVDAs infected,[50] while a Los Angeles County study released in 1989 showed only 1.8 percent of tested IVDA in that area were infected.[51] This finding also indicates that HIV infection among IVDA is the result of culture or custom and by no means stems necessarily from the injecting of illegal drugs.*

The good news, then, is that to the extent people "have to" inject drugs, they don't have to get AIDS. The counteracting bad news stems from the fatalism that comes with being part of the worst of the drug subculture. As one IVDA prostitute put it, "If we're not worried about getting bad junk (heroin) that's going to kill us, or getting our throats slit by a weirdo customer, we're sure not going to worry about AIDS."[53] A social worker echoed this view. "Death has always been an alternative in addiction. So AIDS is just the same old problem, amplified."[54] Indeed, when researchers in Stockholm, Sweden, followed 270 seropositive IVDAs in that city who began becoming infected in 1983, they found that five years later 22 had died—but none of AIDS. Although many were showing immune dysfunction, only 4 percent had any major symptoms at all. The deaths came from other causes, such as overdose and suicide.[55] If this is the case in comparatively genteel Stockholm whose IVDAs tend to be middle class,[56] what's it like in New York City?

While drug abusers may be fairly intractable, those who work with them bitterly contest the assertion that they are utterly impervious to change. Indeed, almost half the IV-drug users in a San Francisco project reported using bleach that was distributed to sterilize needles, although it was not clear from the study design whether this slowed HIV spread.[57] Another study showed 87 percent of San Francisco users on the street using bleach.[58] "Addicts are educable. They are reachable," said the head of the AIDS office in Alameda County, in response to this news.[59] A needle-exchange program in New York City, in contrast, got off to a terrible start, with only 8 addicts signing up in the first four

---

*One national study found that while 99 percent of San Antonio addicts surveyed had shared a needle at least once, only 2 percent of the total were seropositive. In California, 97 percent had shared needles but only 1.5 percent had seroconverted. But in New York and Baltimore, where the shooting gallery is a part of the IVDA culture, rates were much higher. In Baltimore, 94 percent admitted to needle-sharing and 29 percent were seropositive; while in New York, only 70 percent of IVDAs admitted to needle sharing, but a tremendously high 61 percent were infected. Nor is the entire East Coast subject to the phenomenon. In Tampa, 72 percent of the IVDA admitted to needle sharing, but none were infected.[52]

days.[60] This is probably because the real problem is not so much a shortage of needles as a culture in which needle sharing with large numbers of persons is desired.[61] Even where needles cannot be legally dispensed without prescription (as is the case in most areas where IV-drug abuse is worst), a new needle and syringe are available on the street for $2 to $5 a set,[62] hardly a major occasional expense compared with the cost of a daily supply of heroin or cocaine. What is needed is to break the back of the needle-sharing culture.

Studies now show that seropositivity has clearly leveled off among IVDAs (as noted at 60 percent) in some of the worst areas in the New York city region.[63] Yet considering the high attrition in these ranks due to overdose, homicide, suicide, AIDS, and other diseases, a steady level of infection actually means many new infections from joiners to the ranks of the IVDA, a rate of about 7 percent a year in New York.[64]

Drug treatment programs in New York City have been shown to be effective in reducing the risk of HIV infection among IVDAs,[65] even though they often have high recidivism rates.[66] In most states, metha-done maintenance, although effective only with heroin addiction, has become the treatment of choice.[67] In 1987, New York had an estimated 225,000 IVDA and only 30,000 methadone maintenance slots available in 100 clinics throughout the city.[68] State drug-abuse officials said that the "word on the street" is that drug treatment programs are all filled and that few addicts try to join long waiting lists.[69] Yet the Reagan Administration effectively cut back spending on drug treatment, de-claring that it was primarily the job of state and local governments that would be administering the programs.[70] At the same time, the state and local governments wanted to stick the problem on the federal govern-ment, believing it had more money to spare.

This "not from my pocketbook" attitude was complemented by a "not in my backyard" attitude of communities toward having drug treatment centers in their vicinity. Everyone's arguments had some degree of merit; but while the arguing went on, the addicts were stay-ing addicted—risking their own infection and that of their fellow ad-dicts and sexual contacts.* For a nation that supposedly had declared a "war on drugs," it must have appeared to some that the white flag was being run up the mast with nary a shot fired.

---

*In the usual hyperbole that surrounds the issue of infectiousness, unnamed "experts" were cited as estimating that each infected addict would infect five other persons.[71] As late as 1987, this number was sheer nonsense: there simply were not enough uninfected addicts left for this to occur, even if each seropositive addict also infected a sexual partner.

Bisexuality

If needle sharing is at the root of most of black and Hispanic hetero-sexual AIDS cases, bisexuality also has played a major role—far more so than in the white population.

While bisexuals are to a great extent for whites just one more boogie-man for the media to dangle in front of terrified women, black and Hispanic women have much more to fear. Almost half of all cases in which a woman was infected through intercourse with a bisexual have occurred in blacks and Hispanics.[72] A black woman whose mate is a bisexual man has almost five times greater risk for AIDS than a white woman; a Hispanic woman almost four times the risk.[73] In part, the reason is that black and Hispanic male bisexuals are far more likely to be infected,[74] but also probably that black and Hispanic homosexuals are bisexual far more often than white homosexuals.[75]* For reasons that have nothing to do with Africa or Haiti geographically or racially, but everything to do with them socially, homosexuality among blacks, and to a great degree among Hispanics, appears to take the form of bisexual-ity much more than it does with whites.

Black civic leader after black civic leader has testified to the problem. "The black community is still deep into denial," said the founder of Lifelink, an interracial Washington, D.C.–based organization for AIDS victims. "The man who has a girlfriend or a wife and once a week has a sexual relationship with a man doesn't think of himself as gay."[77] Even among blacks who considered homosexuality in general as being ac-ceptable, black homosexuality is often disparaged. Lawrence A. Wash-ington, president of the (Washington) D.C. Coalition of Black Gay Men and Women said, "I've had [black politicians] tell me, 'I can understand white guys doing that, but the brothers, man, that's different.' "[78] In-deed, Washington's "coalition," despite being one of the best-known homosexual groups in the District of Columbia, had only 20 active members.[79]

Bisexuals in the Hispanic community are equally reticent about iden-tifying themselves. Often Hispanic men think that if they're the "macho man" in the homosexual relationship they're not homosexual.[80] Dr. George Samayoa, a physician from Guatemala who traveled around the United States trying to spread the AIDS message to the Latino community, told of having taken two male Hispanics with AIDS to

---

*Twenty-two percent of homosexual black males in one study reported heterosexual coitus in the past year, versus only 14 percent for white males. Hispanics in the study were classified as whites; hence, there is no separate data for them.[76]

community meetings in an effort to dramatize the reality of AIDS in the Hispanic population. "These men exposed themselves as homosexuals at these meetings and were humiliated in return," he said. "At the close of the meetings, people in the audience refused to shake their hands and treated them like dirt. Because of this, I had to stop taking them."[81]

The Crack Connection

By the mid-1980s there was a new burden for minority communities, and by 1988 it would become implicated in the spread of HIV. Cocaine in rock form, called crack, ingested through smoking, moved like a tidal wave into inner-city populations, again affecting minority populations disproportionately. Originally it was thought that crack use might actually help in controlling the spread of HIV, because it gives the user a "high" similar to that from injecting cocaine without the attendant needle usage and sharing.[82] But a study in New York City revealed that there appeared to be no "large-scale change" from injection to smoking cocaine.[83]

By 1988 reporters found a sexy new angle on the minority AIDS problem. Crack was reported to have an aphrodisiac effect. "What you have is marathon binges of cocaine use and sex," said Dr. Arnold Washton, executive director of the Washton Institute, a private addiction treatment clinic in Manhattan.[84] "Today's crack house may be comparable to the gay bathhouse of the late 1970s and early 1980s," said Dr. Willard Cates, Jr., director of the Division of Sexually Transmitted Diseases at the CDC.[85]

This is the same Willard Cates who three years earlier had stated, "Anyone who has the least ability to look into the future can already see the potential for this disease being much worse than anything mankind has seen before";[86] and comparing crackhouses to bathhouses was no doubt a similar exercise in rhetorical flourish. Yet, just as the direct effects of crack were one more cross for minority communities to bear, there were indeed ominous signs of a link between crack usage and increased seropositivity among minorities. According to clinicians who have treated cocaine smokers, both male and female users often experience heightened sexual desire and diminished inhibitions (including those that would prompt condom usage) while high.[87] In a population as syphilis-ridden as that in which crack is epidemic, and which already has comparatively high levels of HIV, this can only mean trouble. In fact, one CDC study in which 90 syphilis patients at STD centers in Philadelphia were interviewed showed that syphilis patients were at

least twice as likely as other patients to have used cocaine, to have
exchanged sex for drugs, or to have visited a crack house.[88]

Said the New York City Health Commissioner Stephen Joseph, "The
logical chain goes crack, syphilis, HIV."[89] Rand Stoneburner, an alarmist by nobody's measure, nevertheless told me that HIV testing in that
city is showing infections in blacks who appear to have no identified risk
factors; that "there very well may be an association with crack usage"
in these cases; and that this, in combination with high rates of syphilis,
could lead to tertiary transmission and "sub-pockets of epidemic in
some areas such as the South Bronx."[90]

The devastation caused by AIDS in some black populations has been
such that it is often compared to genocide. Sunny Rumsey, coordinator
of the community AIDS outreach program for the New York City Department of Health, explains this:

> Genocide by benign neglect. Clearly they believe that there has not been
> enough attention given to them on the issue of AIDS. If you had gone to the
> black community in New York four years ago or three years ago, . . . the only
> thing they had was posters in their communities that said this was germ
> warfare.[91]

Rumsey points out that the notion of a deliberate conspiracy against
blacks was lent credence by an experiment at the Tuskegee Institute
in Alabama in which 400 black men with syphilis were examined but
left untreated over a 40-year period, from 1932 until 1972, to observe
the effects of secondary and tertiary syphilis.[92] One black aide to the
then-mayor of Chicago Eugene Sawyer, in a lecture that eventually led
to his forced resignation, declared that the AIDS epidemic was "a result
of doctors, especially Jewish ones, who inject the AIDS virus in the
blacks."[93]

One clear illustration of Rumsey's "benign neglect" is the decreased
attention paid to syphilis over the last several years. Allan Brandt has
pointed out that the rise in syphilis incidence since its low point in 1950,
while attributed by many public health officials to the three "p's" of
permissiveness, promiscuity, and "the pill," also correlates with a substantial fall in funding for public venereal disease programs.[94] In the last
few years, the rate of syphilis infections among heterosexuals, especially
black and Hispanic ones, has gone up tremendously. In 1987, primary
and secondary syphilis rates increased 25 percent, the highest single-
year increase since 1960. While the rate increased somewhat for white

females, from 2.2 to 2.6 cases per 100,000 individuals, and actually dropped for white males (attributable to decreases among homosexuals), for black males the infection rate jumped from 106.2 to 144.9 per 100,000, for black females from 55.5 to 79.4, for Hispanic males from 66.0 to 70.7, and for Hispanic females from 17.8 to 22.[95] This notwithstanding a previous four-year decline in syphilis rates.[96]

Since it would be difficult to argue that in the age of AIDS minorities are having even more sex than before, the increase in STD rates is almost certainly linked to a decrease in resources used to counter their spread. Ironically, the reason funding syphilis and other STDs has declined is that a major portion of it is being siphoned off for AIDS. "When sexually transmitted disease clinics have fixed budgets, and 20 to 30 percent of those budgets suddenly has to go for AIDS control," something has to suffer, stated Dr. King Holmes, a Seattle health official and chairman of an advisory board to the CDC. "Funds for controlling those diseases have been deflected into AIDS efforts, and the other diseases have been getting worse," he said.[97]

Wendy Wertheimer, director of Public and Government Affairs of the American Social Health Association, the person most clearly associated with drawing attention to this problem, testified before the President's Commission on the HIV that, while funding for AIDS has shot up dramatically, funding for non-AIDS sexually transmitted diseases has only remained level. Yet, she says, even of this level funding, "millions of dollars . . . have been diverted to AIDS." Even more important,

> the brain drain has been severe and constant. In 1981, four [CDC] STD division members were assigned responsibility to review the literature and investigate the public health implications of AIDS. In 1982, eight members of the STD division were detailed to AIDS. In 1983, five headquarters staff and 10 field staff were reassigned to AIDS activities. In 1984, 3 headquarters staff and 20 field staff were reassigned to AIDS. In 1985, the Director of the Division of STDs was detailed to AIDS for part of the year, and 30 positions were diverted to AIDS. In 1986, 45 positions from the STD control program were diverted to AIDS programs; and in 1987 those 45 positions were *permanently* reassigned to AIDS activities.[98]

But it is even worse than that, testified Wertheimer. "A significant loss to the program does not show up on budget sheets" or in allocations:

> A recent study showed that only six of the more than 90 total STD staff actually devote all of their time to STD activities. Twenty-nine said they

spent up to 49 percent of their time on AIDS; 23 spent 50 to 70 percent of
their time on AIDS; and 38 members of the STD staff said they actually spent
between 70 and 100 percent of their time working on AIDS.[99]

Thus, just as AIDS would later begin to drain away the best and
brightest from research on cancer and other diseases, early on, despite
complaints from homosexual activists that the government virtually
ignored the disease until half a decade after it was discovered, AIDS had
already begun to drain off funds and personnel from other disease-
prevention programs. Thus, the Dr. Redfields of the world, who
claimed there were no risks in possibly overreacting to AIDS and that
"in the meantime we might have cut down on syphilis and other venereal diseases,"[100] were left choking on their words. One of the many
drawbacks of "erring on the side of caution" in overreacting to the
AIDS threat was to actually *increase* the threat to heterosexuals.

Let me qualify that. Studies around the country—from San Francisco
to Ohio to New York and points between—showed that, as the word got
out on AIDS, non-AIDS STD rates among homosexuals began to plummet.[101] STD rates among the white middle-class have not been much
affected. It's inner-city blacks and Hispanics who have suffered almost
exclusively from the money and brain drain from other STDs to AIDS.
Peter, already down on his luck, was robbed to pay Paul. And in the case
of middle-class white heterosexuals, Paul couldn't even use the money.

Behind the Media Whitewash: Bigotry or Just Bucks?

That the media were extremely reluctant to portray AIDS as a problem of blacks and Hispanics, and that Hollywood steadfastly refused to
depict minority AIDS victims, should not even be a matter of debate.
"The message," said an AIDS educator in the poor, predominantly
black Bayview–Hunter's Point area of San Francisco, "was that if you're
not gay, you're not white, you're not sleeping with anyone who's gay
or white, you're not at risk for the disease."[102]

The only real questions are, what was the effect of the "whitewash,"
and why did it occur? The *Village Voice* editor Richard Goldstein
emphasized one downside of what he calls the "color-blind" message:

> When race goes unremarked in an epidemic, nobody bothers to ask about
> the quality of care for minority patients. Nobody requires hospitals treating
> AIDS patients to hire bilingual staff. (At least one major treatment center, St.
> Luke's, has not a single Spanish-speaking doctor in its AIDS unit.) And no-
> body demands that minorities participate in making AIDS policy.[103]

An even greater danger (which Goldstein also alluded to) was that minorities would perceive their risks to be in proportion to the amount of attention they were getting in the media. Noting that "until very recently, the press has failed to report the overwhelming impact AIDS has had upon ethnic minority communities," Katherine Franke, an attorney with the AIDS and Employment project in San Francisco, wrote:

> This misinformation about the ethnic diversity of AIDS has had several dangerous results. First, a false sense of security has developed among many people of color that AIDS is not their issue. As a result, populations thought not to be at risk are reluctant to obtain the information they need. . . . This combination of misinformation and denial has had the effect of exacerbating the spread of the virus in ethnic minority communities.[104]

In one community survey in Detroit in the mid-1980s, only 13 percent of 62 black homosexual respondents correctly responded that the AIDS virus was transmitted through blood and semen, and only 19 percent were very worried that they might get AIDS (37 percent reported they were not worried about possible infection).[105] West Coast studies on high-risk behavior among blacks and Hispanics, released in 1987, also found that many Hispanics and especially blacks were neglecting to reduce their risk behavior.[106] The effect of the "whitewash" is clear: it was deadly.

Why did the media emphasis on whites occur? One possible answer is prejudice against blacks and Hispanics. Not an overt sort, as in a Stalinesque "One white death is a tragedy; a million minority deaths is but a statistic," but the sort that turns the New York strangling of Jennifer Levin, a white female debutante, by Robert Chambers, a white male yuppie, into a national event, while the daily murders of black persons in that city's ghettos barely make the local press. A white reporter or television producer, hearing of blacks or Hispanics being killed or threatened by AIDS, probably finds it more difficult to empathize with them than when the victims are white. A white person could have been a friend, a relative, even oneself. But a black addict, girlfriend of an addict, bisexual, or girlfriend of a bisexual is much more difficult for a white person to relate to. In America's ghettos, black families with a seropositive mother, father, and child are practically a dime a dozen. Rumsey told me,

> There is this kid Ryan White (a Caucasian youth in Indiana with hemophilia-caused AIDS). Now, he's doing a great job [of showing that AIDS

victims are normal human beings]. But isn't there a black or Hispanic Ryan White? White is middle America; it's the "Oh, poor baby" syndrome. We do send out a lot of messages that are either sexist or racist.[107]

Ryan White is a white, middle-class child whose initial infection came not from drug usage of his own or of a parent (read: guilty act) but from hemophilia clotting factor (read: innocent act). Sick blacks with no hope? What's new? Sick whites dying of an incurable transmissible disease? Now *that's* a tragedy.

It's probably this same, subtle sort of discrimination that accounted for the media's tendency to ignore AIDS in general before the alarmists succeeded in making it look like everyone's disease. That the media is probably as supportive of homosexuality as any institution in the country does not change the reality that homosexuals were still a "them," not an "us."

A second explanation is that some members of the media were bending over backward to avoid attributing such a stigmatized illness to minority groups. Clearly, middle-class blacks were very concerned with such stigmatization. "AIDS is one more crucifix on our back [*sic*]," said David Lampel, senior vice president of Inner City Broadcasting. "Now we're perceived as being carriers of a deadly disease, confirming the view that the world has of blacks as this beast entered from the cold."[108] Indeed, when the CDC tried to begin a national seroprevalence survey in Washington, D.C., the city with the highest ratio of minorities of any in the country, the public outrage and anxiety was such that the survey was scrapped,[109] despite support for the project from both the mayor and the public health commissioner.[110]

When I appeared with Stephen Joseph on a show hosted by the black columnist Tony Brown, much of the show consisted of Brown blasting Joseph for helping to portray AIDS as a disease of all blacks, not just those of the underclass. I explained that this was because the CDC broke figures down according to race, not class.[111] Yet even this was overly simplistic. Even a middle-class black is at increased risk of sexually transmitted AIDS, for the simple reason that middle-class blacks have a better chance of receiving the virus from a lower-class black than do whites from a lower-class white. My answer calmed things for the moment, but the very first question we took after the taping of the show was "Didn't the white man bring syphilis to Africa?" Obviously this audience of middle-class blacks, already branded to a great extent with the sins of their lower-class fellow blacks, were distressed to be painted as AIDS carriers merely because of the color of their skin. The fear of stigmatization has been so great, in fact, that the *Wall Street Journal* reported, "The black middle class also has been reluctant to offer support to people with AIDS, fearing the disease will be perceived as a black problem and thus increase racism."[112]

Another strong factor in the media's depicting of heterosexual AIDS as a disease of the white middle class was that that's who reads its magazines and watches its shows. Indeed, this explanation goes a long way toward explaining the heterosexual AIDS epidemic myth in general. Randy Shilts told me he confronted a television producer about why AIDS victims on TV were almost always heterosexual. "It won't make national TV unless it has a heterosexual in it," said the producer.[113]

"Erring on the Side of Caution" Revisited

The experience with black and Hispanic AIDS shows in a microcosm the problem with the "everyone's at risk approach" that characterized those who sought to "err on the side of caution." Instead of firing a narrow stream of information at those who needed it most, a shotgun approach was used that missed what should have been the target. Television shows that pretended to be public service messages ended up terrifying those not at risk and inducing complacency in those who were. The fluff pieces for magazines like *People, The Atlantic, Time, Newsweek,* and *U.S. News* had the same effect.

Unlike the media, the government did not actively avoid the black and Hispanic AIDS problem; it simply didn't pay it enough extra attention. As late as June 1988, the Office of Technology Assessment of the U.S. Congress could state: "Few educational programs have been targeted to homosexual and bisexual males who are black and Hispanic, who have low educational levels and low incomes, . . . and little is known about how to reach these groups."[114]

What did we gain from scaring the hell out of low-risk populations that made it worth inducing complacency in high-risk populations? The strategy of directing terror at low-risk populations with the hope that this would trickle down to the high-risk ones was nothing short of lose-lose. And the Africa situation, far from being a lesson in transmissibility for the U.S. heterosexual population as a whole, should provide a lesson that to the extent we allow African conditions to be imitated here, specifically in the presence of high rates of ulcerating disease, we can have African-type transmission. In all fairness to the alarmists, their tales of terror may have prevented a few cases of chlamydia or gonorrhea in white heterosexual college students, but at what price in terms of deprivation of funds and attention for minority AIDS?

In retrospect, the seemingly paranoid comparison between the treatment of blacks and Hispanics during the AIDS crisis and the Tuskegee experiment is not without merit; after all, the Tuskegee doctors didn't *give* syphilis to their charges, they simply allowed it to progress—an omission. Neither the media nor the government invented or spread AIDS. But to the extent they failed to give minorities much-needed extra attention, they left them in the back of the bus—or the back of a hearse.

11

The Liberal Democratizers

"AIDS is not a moral issue," says Ronald Reagan, Jr., in his video "AIDS: Changing the Rules": "You get AIDS because you're unlucky."[1] Declared ads for the American Foundation for AIDS Research (AmFAR), "AIDS is an equal opportunity destroyer." Dennis Weaver in television announcements stated, "AIDS is a terrible disease. . . . Anyone we know can get it." One would never know that these messages, labeled "public service announcements," were talking about a disease that can be transmitted only through blood products, shared needles, and sexual intercourse. Indeed, keeping the mind's eye away from visualizing these limited activities was the very idea.

These were the messages of the democratizers.

Those who spread the myth of the heterosexual AIDS epidemic did not necessarily have anything else in common. There was no conspiracy, because their actions were not concerted. Nor could it be said that there was a coalition. This said, I must also note that there were two factions with two distinct political impulses: the conservative moralists, whose agenda I will explore later; and the democratizers. The columnist George Will, in one of the earliest rejections of the myth of the heterosexual AIDS epidemic, wrote that "it is politically safe and socially soothing to pretend that AIDS is now a democratic, meaning universal, disease threatening us all equally."[2] Those who push this belief are the democratizers. Their object is not to sell papers or boost ratings. They are not seeking personal fame or fortune. Their intentions are to aid the plight of the homosexuals and, more than that, to assert their view on homosexuality and morality in general. The democratizers are basically politically liberal. They are probably strong supporters of affirmative action, of having women in combat roles in the military, of the doctrine of comparable pay (mandating, by government order, the paying of higher wages to traditionally female jobs).

To the extent that AIDS is perceived primarily as a "gay disease," the democratizers believe there would be two obnoxious effects. First, the heterosexual majority, feeling unthreatened, would not support massive funding for research into the prevention and cure of AIDS. Second, it would increase the stigma attached to homosexuality. To forestall both of these prospects, the democratizers have fought hard to characterize AIDS as a threat to the general heterosexual population.

"While at first it may seem almost foolish to speak of preventing a fatal venereal disease as a 'movement'—in the way that civil rights, feminism, and environmental protection have been 'movements,' " explained the alarmist Chris Norwood, "effective AIDS prevention undoubtedly has a similar strength. It is spurred by a committed moral energy that is totally different from life-denying 'just say no' slogans, an energy that reaffirms life through the human connection of personal and social responsibility."[3]

Some of the democratizers made the mistake of believing their own rhetoric and actually became convinced that a virus could not strike persons of one "sexual preference" more than another. Others knew better but maintained the rubric anyway. For the most part, given a choice between extending the epidemic or keeping it confined, they would have chosen the latter. But there was no need for such a choice, since, if they could extend the *perception* of the spread of the epidemic, they could accomplish exactly what an actual wider epidemic would accomplish.

Exaggerating the public's perception of the infectiousness of a disease to reduce stigma is hardly new. Allan Brandt notes in *No Magic Bullet* that some physicians claimed venereal infection could be caused by "whistles, pens, toilets, medical procedures, tattoos and toothbrushes, to name only a few."[4] Brandt went on to say:

> Since it is now known that syphilis and gonorrhea are almost never communicated in non-sexual ways, it seems that the frequent diagnosis of extragenital infections around the turn of the century reveals certain professional and public value-laden assumptions about sexuality and disease. Physicians he says pointed to these infections as a means of attempting to reduce the stigma of venereal disease, both for patients and for doctors. Until the "discovery" of these innocent infections, some members of the profession had refused to treat venereal diseases, and those who did held little professional stature.[5]

While much of the media's mishandling of AIDS is due to sheer ignorance or the crush of deadlines, part of it is influenced by intentional disinformation spread by democratizers. Perhaps the best example of a media democratizer is Ann Guidici Fettner. Fettner is an award-winning medical writer and co-author of *The Truth About AIDS: Evolution of an Epidemic,* who has also written about AIDS for *Redbook,* the *Village Voice,* and mostly the *New York Native,* where she was temporarily the science columnist.

In a 1984 interview, Fettner said, "The problem is that everybody says AIDS is a gay problem. Forget the hemophiliacs; what about the Africans, the women, the junkies? There is no central theory that explains all of these populations. . . . I don't think sex has a thing to do with it."[6] This a full three years after the sex connection was apparent enough to cause homosexual men to begin drastically curtailing their sexual practices. (Two years later, in a bitter denunciation of the Centers for Disease Control entitled "Is the CDC Dying of AIDS?" she would assert, somewhat inconsistently to say the least, "AIDS education should have been started the moment it was realized that the disease is sexually transmitted.")[7] But if denying the sex connection was a battle she could not win, Fettner made it clear she would do her damnedest to present AIDS as other than a "gay problem." AIDS might spread by insects, she told readers in several columns.[8] Time and again she attacked the assertion that AIDS is caused by HIV, and instead asserted that it may be caused by an African swine fever virus.[9]

Having made these arguments to the readers of the *New York Native,* Fettner then published articles in the lucrative women's magazine market, seeking in part to ease the very fears that she had helped create in the first place. Thus, after publishing at least two articles devoted to establishing that mosquitoes can spread the AIDS virus, she informed *Redbook* readers, "There is absolutely no evidence that AIDS can be transmitted this way," then proceeded to give all the excellent arguments against mosquito transmission she had ignored a year earlier.[10] After trying desperately to convince *Native* readers that AIDS is caused by practically anything *but* HIV, she told *Redbook* subscribers flatly that "the disease is caused by human immunodeficiency virus."[11] After blasting *Playboy* for declaring that deep kissing is almost certainly completely safe,[12] she gave *Redbook* readers an excellent rundown on evidence of how saliva may actually protect against HIV, and concluded, "The possibility of such infection [from deep kissing] is remote but probably not out of the question."[13]

A crucial part of the democratizers' game plan has been to keep up a pretense that there is basically nothing homosexuals do that heterosexuals do not. Thus, Dartmouth's "safer sex kits" contained instructions advising against "fisting," saying "Putting a hand or fist into someone's rectum or vagina is very dangerous." As the Dartmouth professor Jeffrey Hart observed, "There is every reason to doubt that heterosexual couples are 'fisting.' The word 'vagina' is present in the above sentence only in order to protect the gay practice."[14]

Dental dams, to prevent contact between the mouth and the orifice during oral-vaginal or oral-anal contact were also regularly included in such kits. Apart from the low risk of infection by this route, dental dams were a fairly silly idea at any rate. The whole idea of stimulating the vagina with the tongue is the sensitivity of the tongue to the receiver and the intimacy of touching the partner's genitals with one's tongue to the "giver." With a dental dam, both are lost. It recalls the scene in the comedy movie *Animal House* in which a woman masturbates her boyfriend in a car while wearing rubber gloves. Indeed, when one AIDS educator tried to introduce dental dams to a group of women in drug treatment, they found the whole idea so annoying and outlandish that they lost interest in the prevention lecture altogether.[15] It was perhaps testament to the obsessiveness of the "safe sex" educators that dental dams continued to be included in their kits. More important, however, dams are a democratizing device. Just as it is necessary to bring all sexually active heterosexuals under the "at risk" umbrella, along with all of their different methods of oral and genital contact, neither can lesbians be left out. Dental dams take care of the problem quite nicely.

A more sophisticated technique the democratizers have used to try to divert attention from the risk groups is to claim that it is wrong to classify individuals on the basis of what they considered artificial distinctions. "AIDS is not transmitted because of who you *are* but because of what you *do,*" an AIDS lobbyist told *Harper's* magazine,[16] in what was to become one of the most widespread AIDS epigrams. One witness before the U.S. Commission on Civil Rights complained of continuing to see the term "high-risk groups" which "feeds alarmist suggestions that AIDS is somehow a problem confined to social groups identifiable by certain characteristics or behaviors. The term fosters prejudice against those defined as high-risk people."[17] June Osborn, dean of the School of Public Health at the University of Michigan, stated, "People have to understand that getting AIDS has nothing to do with whether you're black, homosexual or Haitian . . . it's not who you are but what you do."[18]

The problem with these arguments is that, in the case of AIDS, what you are is often *defined by* what you do. Surgeon General Koop got in on the democratizers' act by telling the viewers of Home Box Office's *Everything You and Your Family Need to Know About AIDS*:

> Let's get rid of that word "high-risk group" because it's a misnomer. All kinds of people engage in high-risk *behavior* and so let's talk about the behavior. And those we consider to be practicing high-risk behavior are homosexual men, bisexual men, IV-drug abusers and heterosexual people who have multiple partners or who have sex habits which would get them into contact with other people who have high-risk behavior.[19]

Bingo! The high-risk groups are immediately brought back. If you have AIDS and have admitted to homosexual activity, you are classified in the homosexual/bisexual category. If you have admitted to needle sharing, you go into the IVDA category. The only classification not based on behavior was the Haitian one, which is why the CDC said in 1985 that it was dropping them from the groups at high risk, and commented that "the Haitians were the only risk group that were identified because of who they were rather than what they did."[20]

To support their thesis that AIDS is not a "gay plague," the democratizers pointed out that not all homosexuals are going to get AIDS. Benjamin Schatz, director of the AIDS Civil Rights Project of National Gay Rights Advocates, declared, "AIDS is not a 'gay disease.' According to current projections, the vast majority of gay and bisexual men will not develop AIDS."[21] The author of one self-help AIDS book wrote, "Remember that AIDS is not a gay (homosexual) disease. *All gay people are not infected with the AIDS virus*" (emphasis in original).[22] Applying this logic, sudden-infant-death syndrome (crib death) is not an infant's disease, black lung is not a coal miner's disease, and sickle cell anemia is not a disease of blacks; in fact, it's not even a disease of those with sickle-cell trait, since only a minority of those so afflicted will develop the anemia. One writer went even further, using pure semantics in pointing out that "very few female homosexuals (lesbians) have been infected with the virus through sexual contact. . . . This fact demonstrates conclusively that AIDS is *not* a 'homosexual' disease."[23] There now. Who could argue with that?

The central argument of the democratizers was expressed by Mathilde Krim when she declaimed, "Viruses do not discriminate on the basis of sexual preference."[24] Pop singer Madonna's 1989 "Like a Prayer" album contained a bulletin admonishing "AIDS is an equal opportunity disease."* Similarly, posters in Britain proclaimed, "AIDS Doesn't Discriminate"; and several American public health officials and homosexual rights advocates have parroted the nondiscrimination line with such slogans as, "We're all in this together."

The slogans have a nice ring to them, but quickly fall apart under scrutiny. Bullets and knives don't discriminate either, but you're far more likely to catch one walking through a dark South Bronx alley than strolling down a well-lit street on Manhattan's Upper East Side. What the nondiscrimination talk does—what it is presumably intended to do—is divert attention from the fact that it's not the *virus* that discriminates, but those who become infected with it. Most of these people are likely to have performed those acts that both cause contact with infected persons and allow the virus to be transmitted. To be sure, the purpose of these acts is not to transmit the virus. Those who choose to walk down a dark alley do not choose to be attacked. But they do choose to walk down the alley. It's not what you are; it's what you do. While we can perhaps argue that it's unfair that those walking down dark alleys be disproportionately attacked, or even that the government has an affirmative duty to prevent such attacks, it is hardly a sane policy to pretend that such attacks do not disproportionately occur simply because some of us feel that there's nothing morally wrong with walking down dark alleys.

Basic rules are just that. Exceptionless rules are something else. When we say that breast cancer is a woman's problem, are we assaulted by "experts" who insist that it isn't, because most women don't get it? Are those rare sufferers of male breast cancer trotted out, interviewed, displayed on the evening news—all for the purpose of proving that breast cancer is not a woman's disease? Do we aim breast cancer commercials at men instead of women because, after all, women already know they're at risk, therefore it's the men who think they're immune to breast cancer and therefore it's the men we have to warn?

The way cancer education works is that the risk of breast cancer for men is virtually ignored since their risk, while real, is so small. Instead,

*The Madonna album is of special interest in that it was a purely political reaction on the part of Warner records. Warner had earlier released an album by comedian Sam Kinison in which he joked about the connection between homosexuals and AIDS, declaring in so many words that it was "their" disease. After a coalition of West Coast groups voiced displeasure over Kinison's remarks, Warner offered its artists the option of including the bulletin, which also declared AIDS "affects men, women and children regardless of age, race, and sexual orientation."[25]

other male cancers such as prostate and testicular are emphasized to men. Even among women, the breast-cancer risk is differentiated. Young women with no history of breast cancer in the family are told to check themselves for lumps but that they have little to worry about. Older women are heavily targeted for education and often urged to get regular mammography screenings. Yet if the government ran a national breast-cancer campaign in the same way it does with AIDS, for every poster we saw warning of female breast cancer, there would be ten featuring male breast cancer. Movie stars would make commercial spots. "You know, I used to think only women could get breast cancer," macho Tony Danza would say. "Now I know that the disease of them is also the disease of us." Sixth-graders would be heavily dosed with information on breast cancer, some female, but mostly male. To the critics who pointed out that even among females, breast cancer in sixth-graders is virtually nonexistent, the answer would be that with such a big killer it's never too early to begin education. Indeed, some would advocate instruction for kindergarteners. Finally, we would see commercial spots of a hefty male construction worker saying, "I build skyscrapers for a living. And now I'm dying of breast cancer. If I can get breast cancer, so can you. Get the facts." Sound ridiculous? Would it sound more so or less so if one were to find out that, as rare as male breast cancer is,* more native-born American males are diagnosed with the disease *each year* than the total number who have contracted AIDS through heterosexual intercourse since the AIDS epidemic began?

The democratizers were boosted in their efforts by the Public Health Service. The same "Coolfont Report" that proved so instrumental in misleading the media stated, "It is clear that this virus does not discriminate by sex, age, race, ethnic group, or sexual orientation."[27] Yet in every single one of these categories there was a tremendously disparate impact by AIDS. Sex? AIDS cases are almost 90 percent male. Age? Transmission patterns for those under fifteen and over sixty are almost completely different from those of persons between those ages. (Between fifteen and sixty, transmission is primarily through coitus and needle sharing; outside this range, it is overwhelmingly perinatal or through transfusion or clotting factor.) Race and ethnic groups? Blacks and Hispanics with AIDS are twice their representative shares of the whole population; among heterosexuals alone, the disproportionate impact is far greater still. Asians, for their part, are significantly under-

---

*About 900 American males contract breast cancer each year, according to the National Cancer Institute.[26]

represented. Sexual orientation? At less than 5 percent of the population, homosexual males make up almost 75 percent of the total number of AIDS cases.

While it is not uncommon for epidemics to strike the older harder than the younger or the younger harder than the older or the poor more than the rich, it is rare when a disease breaks down so clearly along demographic lines as does AIDS.

But rather than note this and deal with it, the democratizers put the bulk of their efforts into denying it—even while accusing white heterosexuals of engaging in denial! Like the weatherman who predicts "sunny and clear for the next three days" even as the first drops begin to fall, like the general who declares victory is at hand even as all around his troops are throwing down their rifles and fleeing, the situation might be blackly humorous—if the stakes were not so high and the situation so tragic. If AIDS didn't discriminate, it would never have become politicized. If it didn't discriminate, the PHS wouldn't have rigged the numbers. If it didn't discriminate, there wouldn't have been marches and quilts and sit-ins. The "doesn't discriminate" language is Newspeak, nothing less. Susan Sontag points out, in *AIDS and Its Metaphors*, of the "The AIDS virus is an equal-opportunity destroyer" slogan: "Punning on 'equal-opportunity employer,' the phrase subliminally reaffirms what it means to deny: that AIDS is an illness that in this part of the world afflicts minorities, racial and sexual."[28]

Another popular democratizer shibboleth is "Someday we will all know someone who has died of AIDS."[29] The idea, of course, is that even if by the grace of God you personally escape the scourge, you cannot help but be personally touched. It was a halfway shibboleth, covering the ground between two other democratizer shibboleths: "Everyone is at risk," the most powerful statement but also the most clearly false; and "AIDS affects everyone," the most clearly true—allowing as it does for everything from changes in TV programming to changes in life style—but also the weakest statement. As a middle-strength expression, "Someday . . ." is also of middle truth. Certainly a lot more people know someone with AIDS than themselves have it, and this population will increase not only because there will be more AIDS victims but also because, as time goes on, people tend to meet more people, increasing the odds of meeting someone with AIDS. But the subtle message is that, even if you are not an AIDS victim, AIDS victims are really people just like you. You also probably don't have cancer or heart disease, it says, but you know people who have died of both, and you know that it's highly probable one of those diseases has your number or that of a close friend or relative. But, demographically speaking, this just isn't the case with AIDS. Thus, the CDC director of the Office of Public Affairs, Don Berreth, speaking at a conference on the media and AIDS, reported that "93 percent of Americans do not know anyone with AIDS,"[30] prompting the columnist Cal Thomas to suggest, "Perhaps this is because most Americans do not take drugs intravenously or engage in high-risk (that is, homosexual) conduct."[31] Truly, Brother Thomas was not filled with the spirit of democratization.

There was also more than just an element of democratization in the pronouncements of World Health Organization officials. Just as the American democratizers needed to bring heterosexuals into the risk group to get heterosexual funding, so too did WHO need to keep the United States and Europe interested in conditions in Africa. Thus, WHO's director Jonathan Mann proclaimed, "There is a global epidemic of AIDS that leaves no country untouched. We can't stop AIDS anywhere until we stop it everywhere."[32] *U.S. News & World Report* characterized Mann's declaration as "an international battle cry long overdue [as Mann] unveiled last week WHO's first blueprint for fighting a plague that threatens all people, white and black, rich and poor, Communist and non-Communist."[33]

It was the kind of language Churchill used to pull America deeper into his war against Nazi Germany. But whereas Churchill was almost certainly right about Germany's threat to America, Mann was on shaky grounds. While it's true that a pool of contagion in Africa might allow spread elsewhere, there are numerous diseases in Africa that kill tens of thousands, hundreds of thousands, even millions of Africans, but afflict very few North Americans or Western Europeans. Smallpox continued to kill Africans for thirty years after the last non-vaccine-related case in the United States was diagnosed.[34] Malaria was formerly a serious problem in parts of the United States. Today it causes about 1,000 cases a year in this country,[35] even while it kills a million a year in Africa.[36] There is simply no reason that AIDS could not become very well managed in the United States even while it continues at a considerably higher level in Africa or elsewhere. But for the sake of the worldwide struggle, neither Mann nor *U.S. News*'s editorializing writer could let it be so.

Mann's democratization of AIDS, however, crossed—as, indeed, it ultimately had to—from just comparing Africa and the United States to comparing heterosexuals and homosexuals. Thus, he told Jim Lehrer on the "MacNeil/Lehrer Newshour" that the reason AIDS was afflicting heterosexuals in Africa but primarily homosexuals in the United States

was that, "We think it may just be a historical accident that the virus
was principally introduced into this country, or began to appear in this
country, among male homosexuals and bisexuals. And that most of the
spread, therefore, occurred in that group, along with the spread among
intravenous drug users."[37] Mathilde Krim, likewise, has been quoted in
several places as saying "I think it's a fluke that AIDS emerged in the
gay community." A full-page advertisement in the *New York Times*
placed by the Ad Council declared, in huge print, "To start with, you
don't have to be gay or a drug user to get it. AIDS has hit these two
groups hardest because the AIDS virus hit them first." The ad was
placed in the waning days of 1988.[38]

"There but for the grace of God go you," one of the most popular
tactics of the democratizers, has been repeated over and over again.
The idea is that if only a heterosexual had been the first person in the
country with AIDS instead of a homosexual, it would be the homosexuals sitting back smugly watching the decimation of heterosexual society.
It is, of course, a fantastic notion, and one of many that assigns to AIDS
somehow superviral properties. At the same time as the democratizers
were saying that HIV could not possibly afflict primarily homosexuals
because a virus does not act at the behest of the Moral Majority, they
have tried to make us believe that the epidemiology of AIDS depends
on the flip of a coin. Either they don't see, or at least hope we won't see,
the inherent contradiction in saying, on the one hand, that the connections between the homosexual and the heterosexual populations are so
vast and close that what one suffers the other soon will, and, on the
other, that they are so disconnected that one can suffer terribly for years
even while the other remains relatively unaffected. Like many of the
alarmists' declarations, it is bad science and shallow thinking to boot.

Mathilde Krim—Waltzing with the Truth

Perhaps the best-known of the liberal democratizers is Mathilde
Krim, a founding chair of AmFAR. Krim has received numerous humanitarian awards and praiseful articles in *Ms.* and other women's
magazines, and been the subject of a Hollywood fete, featuring such
stars as Michael York, Faye Dunaway, Steve Martin, and Whoopi Gold-
berg. As Goldie Hawn handed her the AIDS Project Los Angeles Commitment to Life Award, she told Krim, "You are a gift from God."[39]

Krim is married to Arthur B. Krim, the chairman of Orion Pictures,
former finance chairman of the Democratic National Committee, and
advisor to presidents Kennedy, Johnson, and Carter. Mathilde Krim

began traveling in these political circles as well, and was appointed by President Johnson to the President's Committee on Mental Retardation.[40] Krim earned a doctorate in biology and became a cancer researcher, where she fell into researching interferon, a naturally occurring protein that seemed to hold some promise for combating cancer tumors. While other researchers remained skeptical, Krim promoted the substance and was in great part responsible for the spate of media stories to the effect that interferon could be the great cancer cure. As it turned out, it was found effective only in treating a rare form of leukemia[41] and genital warts. (Ironically, it was later approved for treatment of Kaposi's sarcoma, a cancer that often manifests in AIDS victims, though interferon was by no means miraculous here either.)[42] Sandra Panem, a former fellow at the Brookings Institution and author of *The AIDS Bureaucracy,* in an earlier book summed up the feeling of many cancer researchers saying, "One clear lesson of the interferon crusade is that rational biomedical policy cannot be based on hype."[43]

But it remained true that if interferon didn't work, the hype assuredly did; and Krim has used this same sort of promotion to raise funds for AIDS, campaigning, as the *New York Times* put it, "to persuade the public that we are all members of one large risk group."[44] That she does so out of sheer fund-raising cynicism is a charge she bitterly denies. Responding to Dr. Robert Gould (of *Cosmopolitan* fame) who said on "Nightline" that generalizing the risk of AIDS would increase research funding, Krim replied, "I find that statement deeply offensive to somebody like me, because my intent is not to fool the public, to raise money, it's really what I do and what I say done with great concern for the young generation. I want them to stop dying."[45]

When Krim was asked by an interviewer for the *New York Native* why she became interested in AIDS, she said, "I became interested because it was an intriguing scientific problem. But very early on I saw the implications and social repercussion of something like this."[46] A question later, she said, "Differences in sexual preference is an area we have not faced yet. So that aspect, the possible consequences of this disease, worries me a lot. And this is why I became involved more than in just research."[47] If that statement doesn't sound as if it has a whole lot to do with simply curing AIDS, it doesn't. In fact, as Krim candidly told *Newsweek,* "One of our [AmFAR's] main goals was to destigmatize the disease."[48]

As to the other goal, fund raising, nobody in the country can claim more expertise than Krim. In 1987, she staged a gala benefit at the Shubert Theater in New York. Rather than just dwell on the human devastation of the disease, according to *Newsweek,* "She told [the audience] that an unchecked epidemic 'could destroy the economy of New York City.' She told them AIDS could devastate the fashion, theater and restaurant trades and that the number of AIDS deaths could be extrapolated to horrendous figures. It was strong stuff."[49] Fashion, theater, restaurant—Krim knows how to hit a well-to-do audience where it hurts.

"It was an interesting ploy," said playwright Larry Kramer of the event. "She was trying to raise money from the straight community for AIDS as a straight problem. AmFAR distanced itself from the gay community."[50] While forecasting the decline of fashion and theater no doubt appeals to $150-a-plate guests in New York, it has limited use in appealing to the nation as a whole. Still, the reasoning would remain the same: If you want to raise money for AIDS, you don't talk about homosexuals, you talk about the audience. Thus for the national audience, Krim raised the specter of the ultimate loss—their lives.

Although Hollywood stars continue to gush over her, Krim has worn out the patience of even some of her liberal brethren. In an editorial in the *New York Native, Harper's* magazine publisher Lewis Lapham wrote:

> On a television program, I heard a doctor say, given the current doubling of cases every nine months . . . the entire population of the earth conceivably could perish within the next 60 years [actually it would be much less time than that]. Later in the program, again with what I took to be an air of unwarranted satisfaction, the doctor reported the disease making impressive gains within the heterosexual community. When it first appeared in 1981, it was thought to afflict only homosexuals, drug abusers, and Haitians.
>
> No longer, said the doctor. Carried across state lines and class lines by female prostitutes and bisexual men, the disease had begun to infiltrate the American mainstream.[51]

Sharon Churcher revealed, in the "Intelligencer" column of *New York* magazine, that this doctor was Mathilde Krim.[52] When *New York Native*'s publisher and editor, Charles Ortlieb, asked Krim to confirm this, he says she did.[53] Ortlieb went on to quote from a paper entitled "A Concise Statement on the AIDS Crisis in New York City," written by Krim: "AIDS is now on the loose and will soon threaten everyone. . . . If the spread of AIDS remains unchecked and the public remains uninformed about what risks are real and what is unfounded fear, much of the fabric of this city will come apart."[54] To which Ortlieb wrote, "I told Krim that I would blast her organization [AmFAR] if they set out to 'calm the public' in this manner."[55]

It is one of the great ironies of the AIDS crisis that the terrorists are often lauded as the heroes. Like the lad who invites his date onto the scariest ride in the carnival knowing she will throw her arms around him, the AIDS terrorists built up our fears and consequently put themselves in the positions of saviors. In its January 1986 issue, *Ms.* magazine gave Krim the "Woman of the Year Award" for "replacing fear with facts." An accompanying article declared that Krim "has been uniquely able to speak credibly *about* AIDS."[56] (Emphasis in original.)

Typical of the approach of Krim's AmFAR was its full-page magazine advertisement trumpeting in large letters the slogan Sontag referred to: "THE AIDS VIRUS IS AN EQUAL OPPORTUNITY DESTROYER." To illustrate the point, five persons were depicted illustrating a wide range of races, sexes, and socio-economic backgrounds. There were two women, casually dressed, in their late twenties; a strapping, perhaps somewhat paunched Latino man in his mid-thirties, again casually dressed; a white woman of perhaps fifty-five years in a sweater; and a white man with gray hair, in a business suit, looking to be in his late fifties. Absent were representatives of either of the highest-risk groups, male homosexuals or black male intravenous drug abusers. Granted that either of the two males could have been homosexuals and any of the five models could have been shooting drugs, this was not a subtle advertisement, and the copy was unambiguous: "AIDS is everyone's problem. To stop it, we must find a cure. But research takes money." It concluded in larger letters: "Please support AIDS research. It's everybody's problem."[57]

Other than promoting a misallocation of funds and fear, the greatest problem with the democratization of AIDS is that it conflicts with the message that AIDS is not casually contagious. On the one hand, the democratizers want to get everyone in on the act in order to destigmatize the disease and pump up research funds. But, on the other, they want to prevent outright panic and protect AIDS victims and homosexuals from discrimination and beatings by those who fear contracting AIDS by being breathed on or touched.

Logically, the democratizers are in an untenable position. Even if AIDS were as infectious as the most infectious of the sexually transmitted diseases, as many wanted us to believe, it would still not be true to say that "everyone is at risk" or "AIDS doesn't discriminate" or AIDS provides "equal opportunity" for death. Only a casually contagious

disease can put everyone at risk, and highly contagious STDs like gonorrhea and chlamydia still discriminate, because they virtually never affect those who do not engage in sexual intercourse.

Of course, the democratizers could extend the slogans to say that
"everyone is at risk who engages in ____" or "AIDS doesn't discriminate
among those who ____." But this is hardly satisfactory. For one, slogans
tend to lose their zip after a few words. Even more important, however,
the democratizers do not want anyone to feel exempt. *Nobody* is to be
able to opt out of the national risk group, any more than they could opt
out of being at risk for an Axis takeover in the Second World War. We
know what happens when the national will is splintered by those who
question the dire prophecies of a world occupied by the enemy; it's
called Vietnam. Nor is it enough for the democratizers to say, as I have,
that AIDS is everyone's problem—but only because we are all our
brother's keepers. Many of those Vietnam protestors had a very good
idea what would happen to South Vietnam if the North took over:
altruism did not stay their hands.

Consistency having proved impossible, the democratizers opted to
present an inconsistent message: everyone is at risk, but certain things
(casual transmission) don't put you at risk, and hence you might not be
at risk. The predictable result was confusion. Five years after the media,
the public health authorities, and the Mathilde Krims of the world
began a concerted effort to tell the public that AIDS is not casually
contagious, a good one fourth to one third of all Americans were telling
pollsters that they feared casual transmission.[58] While a little of this may
have been attributable to the efforts of some to assert that casual transmission was indeed a risk (covered in detail in chapter 13), much of it
was no doubt attributable to the democratizers' messages. Many of the
democratizers must have known that one by-product of their message
was terror of casual transmission. But as with the terror inflicted upon
low-risk sexually active heterosexuals, it was a price they were willing
to pay—or, more correctly, to let others pay.

Certainly the democratizers succeeded in their short-range goal of
driving up funding. AmFAR's budget grew fat, as did that for the Public
Health Service AIDS program. Mann's "we can't stop AIDS anywhere
until we stop it everywhere" approach contributed to converting
WHO's global AIDS coordinating office from a staff of one physician and
one secretary with a budget of $580,000 a year in November 1986 to
a full-time and part-time staff of almost 100 with a budget of $66 million
in 1988.[59] One could argue that no harm has been done by these efforts,
since in the joy over the declining epidemic, the dire predictions that

terrified us will all but be forgotten. But to the extent that people thought homosexuals deserved to die horribly, they probably still do, despite the best efforts of the liberal democratizers. As for Africa, the diseases whose fatalities have always dwarfed that of the AIDS epidemic will continue unabated.

What the democratizers have done is to apply a cynical solution in an increasingly cynical world. Instead of telling New York's social set that they were on the verge of losing their opera and ballet, Mathilde Krim could have tried appealing to their better sides, saying they have helped you enjoy your lives, now you should help them preserve theirs. Instead of telling Americans "Today Africa, tomorrow the world!" Jonathan Mann could have tried telling the truth and asked whether it wasn't about time that the world started giving a damn about Africa's health problems enough to do a little more than throwing spectacular but useless rock concerts. The democratizers' words were blunt and to the point *and only to the point.* Theirs is a message that will not carry even a day past that on which the risk of heterosexual AIDS is perceived to be gone. It may have been the only way, but one still ponders and mourns the lost opportunity.

12

Safe Sex and
the Condom Wars

It was called "condomania." Before the AIDS hysteria had quieted, the condom would become to this epidemic what mass seizures of wild dancing and general hysteria—known variously as "St. John's dance," "St. Vitus's dance," and "Tarantism"—were to the Black Death.[1] Surgeon General Koop defined *condomania* as "the activity on the part of some segments of the public to advertise, popularize, distribute, and otherwise focus attention on condoms as though that activity were the only thing that could prevent the spread of AIDS," adding, "I fault myself in no way for this phenomenon."[2] Many moralists, as shall be seen, disagreed with the last statement, but mania it truly was.

In 1987, New York City went on the offensive (perhaps in more ways than one) with a series of condom ads on TV created by a Madison Avenue agency and aimed at heterosexual women. The ads featured racially ambiguous actors and made no reference to homosexuals, a fact that drew the wrath of some homosexual activists.[3] The city also began to put up large numbers of condom-promoting posters, proclaiming such slogans as "Don't Die of Embarrassment" and "Don't Go Out Without your Rubbers."[4] A mother in a New York City commercial said to her son, "I hate the idea of you doing things you're not ready for, but listen, if you're doing anything, you use one of these, you understand?"

In late 1988, following New York City's lead, Surgeon General Koop unveiled the first national advertising campaign that would explicitly promote the use of condoms to prevent AIDS. The campaign, in English and Spanish, would feature four thirty-second TV commercials, three radio spots, and five print ads and placards for billboard and transit use, to be distributed through twenty thousand media outlets across the country. All three of the major networks agreed to air the ads. "I wish this wasn't necessary to talk about," said Koop, "but it is, and we can't let people die in ignorance."[5] He apparently honestly believed that, by the time the ads would start airing in 1989, there might still be somebody, somewhere in the country who hadn't yet heard about condoms and AIDS. Hollywood got in on the act, too. Justine Batemen of the "Family Ties" television series admonished: "Take the responsibility yourself. Buy a condom, carry it with you, make sure he wears it. It's still okay to think he's Mr. Wonderful. But there isn't a guy in the world with a body to die for."

Safe-sex valentines proliferated. One available at Long Beach State University in California featured a condom wrapped up as a gold coin ("Invest in our love") or as an Olympic medal ("Go for the gold!").[6]

In 1987, a Unitarian pastor, the Reverend Carl Thitchener, made national headlines by distributing condoms during services at his Amherst, New York, church. (He later wrote an article on the event for *The Humanist.*) After passing them out, he said, "Now that that's done, let's see if it worked. Let's all say the word correctly, 'Condom.' " The congregation replied, "Condom."[7] The condom distribution was primarily a publicity stunt, done on a single occasion and with a press photographer present. The idea was to emphasize the seriousness of AIDS and the propriety of condom usage. That message may have been a bit undermined when, a few weeks after the celebrated giveaway, it was discovered that the prophylactic-purveying pastor had been convicted five years earlier for parading naked in front of a troop of Brownies.[8] Before that, he had been charged with attempted rape and attempted burglary.[9]

When I was attending a federally sponsored conference on AIDS and minorities in 1988, I spotted a fairly attractive young woman with some of the strangest earrings I had seen. They were square, but there seemed to be something circular inside speckled with glittery sparkles. It wasn't until the second day of the conference that I realized the woman had glorified condom packages dangling from her ears.

Colleges became centers of condomania; and as so many trends do, condoms in dormitories began in California and spread eastward. At the University of California, Santa Cruz, condom-dispensing machines were installed in both men's and women's restrooms and in laundry rooms, next to AIDS-education brochures. Far West Vending Company installed machines at about twenty schools in the southwest.[10] Trustees of the San Jose/Evergreen Community College District voted unanimously to place between thirty and forty condom machines in men's and women's restrooms, earning the praise of the *San Francisco Chronicle* editorial board.[11] The president of the student senate at the University of Kansas agreed to spend student money on ten thousand condoms and distribute them on campus. The University of Virginia converted dozens of cigarette machines to condom dispensers. "I think from a health point of view, it's a wonderful statement," said Dr. Richard P. Keeling, the university's student health director.[12] A health educator at the University of New Hampshire, Durham, which had been holding out against the trend, declared, "If someone in a dorm in the middle of the night decides to have sex, they're not going to go to the health center or a drug store to buy condoms. They can get a quick fix from a Coca-Cola at two a.m.—why shouldn't they have access to safer sex?"[13]

On one occasion, the Mansfield University student newspaper enclosed a condom inside each of 2,500 copies on St. Valentine's Day. Mansfield's administrators supported the condom enclosure. In what one might consider a low threshold for responsibility, they declared, "We support any educational effort as long as it is sincere."[14]

On Safer Sex Awareness Day at the University of Wisconsin in Madison in 1988, an administrator dressed as a six-foot condom paraded down the middle of State Street, the main thoroughfare on campus. Called "Pat the Prophylactic," the mascot's job was to host the school's "Condom Olympics," a demonstration of the strength of some ten thousand condoms donated by a local company.

The condom craze was by no means limited to the American side of the Atlantic. In Norway, billboards depicted a huge erect penis, wearing a bowtie. The caption read: "Are you dressed to go out?"[15] Children were not to be spared the image. Danish television announced it would incorporate scenes depicting the dangers of catching the AIDS virus into four of Andersen's tales. To demonstrate the use of a condom to kids, the series would show a couple explicitly having intercourse.[16] Any guesses as to what the little match girl would be selling these days?

In Thailand, schoolchildren were taught to make a game of blowing up condoms like balloons. In Hong Kong and Mexico, clear plastic key rings encasing a condom—and reading, "In case of emergency, break glass!"—were distributed to teenagers. And in a Swedish government poster on AIDS, teenage males were encouraged to practice masturbating with a condom in place—no doubt the ultimate in safe sex.[17]

Condoms for adults, condoms for adolescents, condoms for teens: could condoms for children be far behind? In 1988, a small West Coast firm created a cartoon character known as "Calvin Condom," which, one newspaper reported, "the company hopes will become as widely used and well-known as Smokey the Bear."[18] The company sent a mass mailing to "every political leader in the United States" appealing for help in getting Calvin into the classrooms. "We feel that education regarding this devastating disease can never begin too early," said Calvin's promoters in a letter delivered to every member of Congress. A spokesman for the San Diego company said he hoped kids would learn to say to each other, "If Calvin's not with you, I'm not interested."[19]

Meanwhile, New York State's Board of Regents came within one vote of mandating that instruction for fourth-graders include the four "Rs"— reading, writing, 'rithmatic, and rubbers.[20]

Condom Counting

The Baltimore Health Department received a $25,000 grant from the Centers for Disease Control to count the number of condoms in city sewage to determine whether there was an increase in usage, and hence safe sex, over time. A *Washington Times* columnist, John Lofton—noting that an increase in condoms in sewage could simply mean that more people are having sex, or that more are flushing them rather than tossing them, and that therefore an increase in condom prevalence in sewage meant nothing—declared, "No more money should be appropriated [for AIDS research] until researchers misuse the money they already have."[21]

Geraldo Rivera introduced us to the condom cops. On one of his shows, he displayed a video clip of police confronting a man who had solicited sex with a police decoy:

"You ever been arrested before for anything?" they ask.
"No, I have never been arrested for anything," says the man.
"You wouldn't think to use a condom or anything?" asks an officer.
"Well, yeah."
Asks the officer, "Did you have one with you?"
"No, I didn't have one with me."
"So," says the officer, "you weren't too concerned about the fact that you could get AIDS?"
"I thought about it, yeah."[22]

The Birth Control Lobby

In short, America's obsession with AIDS became an obsession with condoms; and birth control advocates seized on the AIDS epidemic as a vehicle for promoting their chosen cause. Having tried for decades, with limited success, to get young people to use contraception to control births, they now sought to use fear of AIDS to get the recalcitrants to distribute or use condoms. The Maryland State Chapter of Planned Parenthood offered women a singular Valentine's Day gift for their sex partners: a heart-shaped box containing five condoms, a poem about them, and a pamphlet explaining their use.[23] The Center for Population Options in Washington, D.C., distributed a publication that suggested schools sponsor a Condom Couplet Contest, and that teenagers be given an optional homework assignment to purchase a packet of condoms.[24]

Nowhere was this linkage more apparent than in an episode of "Designing Women," "Killing All the Right People," when a debate takes place at a parent-teacher association meeting between one of the designing women, Mary Jo, and a prim-and-proper moralist. The caricatured moralist argues against birth control by claiming (correctly, by the way)[25] that the experience with free distribution of birth control at schools has resulted not in a decrease in pregnancies, but in an increase. She says that promoting chastity is the best way to prevent pregnancy. In rebuttal, Mary Jo agrees that pregnancy in teenagers is to be avoided, but adds, "I think I would be more concerned about my daughter getting something fatal." In consequence, she is dubbed the "Condom Queen."[26] Naturally, the show delighted the population control groups and sure enough, the Center for Population Options awarded the series its Nancy Susan Reynolds Award of the Center for Population Options for demonstrating sexual responsibility in the media for a comedy series.[27]

The exaggerated fear of heterosexual AIDS didn't exactly have condom manufacturers wearing mourning black. Condom sales rose slightly in 1986 and doubled during 1987 to almost $400 million. "Up until now," said one market analyst, "it was a business thought to be a mature if not dying market. There was not a lot left to get out of the market, until recently."[28] In 1985, stock in Carter-Wallace, the maker of Trojans condoms, sold anywhere from $19⅜ to $34½ dollars a share; by 1987, it was selling at $140 and climbing.[29] While neither the birth control organizations nor the condom companies could be accused of starting the heterosexual AIDS scare, both did far more than just ride the wave. The condom companies, for their part, began to throw "AIDS" into all their prophylactic ads, the vast majority of which were directed toward white, middle-class heterosexuals. The companies also took advantage of the hysteria to place their ads in media that would never have considered allowing them before.

The Taste Backlash

It was inevitable that there would be something of a backlash, if only on the grounds of taste alone. Such was the case when the Illinois governor, Jim Thompson, squelched a song called the "Condom Rag" that was to have been part of a state-sponsored anti-AIDS campaign. After telling listeners that "one size fits all," and that condoms come in various colors and textures, the song went on to say:

> And remember boys, don't be no dunce.
> Only use that condom once.
> See, it's easy and fun and it ain't a drag.
> Groovin' and doin' the condom rag.

Said the governor, "It's outrageous. Everyone will think we are lunatics." But a state health department official replied, "The use of condoms reduces the risk of AIDS. To deny that information to the public is to deny them information on a way to protect themselves."[30]

Another backlash occurred when *SPIN* magazine, a competitor of *Rolling Stone* published by the son of the *Penthouse* magnate Bob Guccione, distributed a free condom in its November 1988 issue. The giveaway was advertised in large letters on the cover. This proved too much for Safeway, A & P, Waldenbooks, 7-Eleven, and other chains, which instructed their stores not to sell the magazine that month. The junior Guccione said that sales for that issue were down 50 percent to 60 percent, but that it was worth it to show their "extensive editorial commitment to fighting AIDS."[31]

The Counterattack: Safe Sex Becomes Merely Safer

While AIDS was eventually to became universal, the word never has. In several languages it is *SIDA;* in Russian, *SPID.* In Great Britain, the acronym has turned into a full-fledged word: *Aids.* But the phrase *safe sex* has become universal. Say "please" or "help" on the European continent, and many will look at you askance. Say "safe sex," and they'll know exactly what you're talking about.

At times it seemed difficult to turn around without seeing those words. Madonna, in a concert tour, would flash a huge "SAFE SEX" on her background screen, while the crowd cheered.[32] The lyrics of another singer's tune, "Wild West," include the lines "Give me, give me wild west, give me, give me safe sex." The expression became so ubiquitous that it was ripe target for humor. Johnny Carson told the "Tonight Show" audience, "The surgeon general announced today that the earthquake we had today is the only safe sex left."[33]

Yet not long after the phrase appeared, it was attacked by a coalition of moralists and nonmoralist alarmists who thought the only "safe" odds against getting AIDS should be lower than those against a man metamorphosing into a giant insect. These were the anticondomites.

Since sex could not be made absolutely safe, declared the anticondomites, it must either be eschewed altogether or, at the very least, never be called anything stronger than "safer." Wrote the "Today Show" 's physician, Art Ulene, in his *Safe Sex in a Dangerous World,* "Truly 'safe sex' is an all-or-nothing thing"; and, "Sex is either 100 percent safe or it's not, even when it's 'almost safe.' "[34] It was as if it had never occurred to the anticondomites that, in any field, safety devices cannot always be completely protective. Did they think that since safety belts cannot always prevent injury, they should therefore be called "safer belts"? Shouldn't safety pins be called "safer pins"? Safes for valuables, "safers"? No, but in the hysteria surrounding AIDS, nothing was to be judged by any other standard than an absolute one. Thus, "safe sex" was quickly replaced by "safer sex," because, after all, one can never be 100-percent sure that one's partner is uninfected, or 100 percent sure that a condom will be an effective barrier. The term *Russian roulette* was popularized. A booklet circulated by Education Department staffers, and co-authored by none other than Robert Redfield, warned in full capitals:

DON'T ENGAGE IN INTIMATE CONTACT AT ALL. IF YOU HAVE HAD THAT KIND OF CONTACT IN THE PAST, STOP NOW. THAT IS THE ONLY "SAFE SEX." IF YOU ENGAGE IN CLOSE SEXUAL CONDUCT, YOU ARE PLAYING RUSSIAN ROULETTE WITH YOUR LIFE.[35]

About one half of the time—mostly in side collisions—seat belts do not prevent loss of life.[36] If the anticondomite logic were to be applied here, seat belts would be blasted as "horribly unsafe." No matter that seat belts tremendously increase one's odds of survival: if they aren't completely foolproof, they're no good.

Why this disproportion? Simply this: the moralists saw utility in driving a car; they saw none (presumably) in illicit coitus. Thus, even the act of driving to the store to buy a candy bar and the latest issue of the *Star* had some utility and hence was worth the relatively tiny possibility of an accident. But no act of coitus outside of a monogamous relationship could possibly have any utility. Therefore, any risk was too great.

As another risk-reducing measure, some, including Ulene, have advocated blood tests to ensure against infection.[37] (Recall the five *Playboy* Playmates in chapter 1.) Blood tests used as a risk-reducing measure can be very effective, yet they can also be extremely infringing. There is such a long delay in getting back results (sometimes several weeks) that the test is useless to a person determined to have sex on short notice. The test also requires a comparatively high expenditure in money and some expense in pain. Most women demanding a blood test cannot offer a man the kind of incentive a *Playboy* Playmate does. The upshot is that precoital blood testing among comparatively low-risk populations will probably be comparatively rare. Further, if absolute safety is demanded, blood tests do not offer this any more than do condoms or anything else short of abstinence, a point Ulene concedes.[38] Blood tests can allow a false negative due to an extremely recent infection. Further, a negative test by no means ensures that a sex partner won't become infected *after* the test is performed. None of which implies that blood testing isn't an effective way to screen a potential sex partner, but it simply cannot reduce the risk to zero.

The Moralists

No doubt what traumatized many of the anticondomites was not that condoms sometimes fail, but that for the most part they do not. In *No Magic Bullet,* Allan Brandt writes that, during the syphilis scare at the turn of the nineteenth century, moralists were infuriated by attempts to regulate prostitution to allow only uninfected hookers to stay in business, not because they (the moralists) thought such a procedure might fail to reduce the incidence of venereal disease, but precisely because they feared it would. While the moralists then made some meritorious arguments, Brandt notes that the

basic assumption lurking behind the attacks on [regulation] was that venereal disease among prostitutes served as an effective discouragement to immorality. Fear of venereal disease, according to these reformers, contributed
to sexual morality and therefore should not in all cases be removed as a
threat. . . . In this light, venereal disease was seen as *serving* the sexual order
by deterring "immoral" behavior.[39]

The syphilis moralists were at no loss for arguments against cleaning
up the same prostitute trade they so viciously attacked as the prime
spreader of disease. But the 1909 announcement of Salvarsan as the first
effective treatment for syphilis sent them scraping for arguments about
why abstinence and monogamy within marriage were still the only safe
means of syphilis prevention. "It . . . does not cure syphilis, although it
has remarkable effects in suppressing certain manifestations," said
Prince Albert Morrow, a dermatologist and a leader of the "social hygiene" movement, of the Salvarsan treatment. "Unfortunately, they
always come back, and often with a train of disagreeable symptoms that
were not present at first."[40] The statement had a shade of truth. If
Salvarsan treatment were begun but not completed, as often was the
case, the disease would not be cured and symptoms would return.[41] But
Morrow gave away his fear of effective treatment when he concluded,
"So, for the present at least, men and women cannot sin with impunity."[42] Howard Kelly of Johns Hopkins University offered similar senti-
ments, noting the valuable role that venereal disease played in curbing
sensuality: "I believe that if we could in an instant eradicate the diseases, we would also forget at once the moral side of the question, and
would then, in one short generation, fall wholly under the domination
of animal passions, becoming grossly and universally immoral."[43]* During the syphilis era, says Brandt, "The question was thus boldly posed:
Which was the greater threat to society, venereal disease or immorality?"[45] The question would be posed again with AIDS; and again, many
moralists would throw their lot in with the latter.

During the syphilis epidemic, condoms also came under direct attack,
even though their usefulness in preventing transmission had been
clearly recognized. The military bent over backward to avoid using
them, instead establishing a series of prophylactic stations where a
soldier could take a disinfective treatment after sex, which included a

---

*Also very much along these lines was the view expressed by the military physician,
Dr. Glantz, in William Styron's play about venereal disease in the Second World War:
"Won't [penicillin] open up the floodgates of vice? For if a libertine knows he can indulge
himself with impunity, he will throw all caution to the winds. What universal debauchery
this might portend for our nation!"[44]

painful injection into the urethra. Not taking the treatment and subsequently developing syphilis was a court-marital offense.[46] Thus, sex
necessarily meant pain, and many a young man learned the meaning
of the words *love hurts.* The "problem" then—that condoms were, if
not particularly desirable, a nevertheless painless alternative to remaining chaste—was as irritating to the moralists in 1918 as it was to them
in the 1980s.*

Representative of the anticondom AIDS moralists was a statement in
the *HLI (Human Life International) Reports* of Gaithersburg, Maryland. Drawing its own interpretation of a redraft of the Roman Catholic
bishops' document on AIDS,[48] the newsletter stated, "The now [*sic*]
document is expected to be clearer, stating unambiguously that the use
of condoms protects the user neither from hell nor from AIDS."[49] The
John Birch Society organ *The New American* stated, "In the name of
fighting AIDS, millions of children are being indoctrinated in amorality
and immorality, which will result in many of them losing their souls as
well as their lives. It is time for the truth, difficult as that may be for
many to accept: 'Safe sex' is moral sex—the kind that takes place within
a monogamous, heterosexual marriage."[50]

Having seized upon AIDS as the savior in the losing fight against
promiscuity, moralists were infuriated at the surgeon general's decision
to promote condom use as a method of prevention. Paul Cameron,
chairman of the Family Research Foundation, practically became apo-
plectic after the surgeon general told a preselected young audience on
"Good Morning America" that "for many young people [abstinence] is
a very viable way to live, but for adults it isn't viable," and proceeded
to discuss the proper use of condoms.[51] Wrote Cameron in his "Family
Research" newsletter:

> "REAL MEN HAVE TO, KIDS DON'T" asserts the Surgeon General! He
> *dared* these boys and millions viewing to become *adults.* REAL MEN DO,
> says Dr. Koop, AND THEY SHOULD USE CONDOMS! Better this bumbler
> preach "eat your spinach to grow strong." Instead he intones "want to *STAY*
> *A KID?* That's nice don't have sex. Want to *BE ADULT?* HAVE *CONDO-*
> *MIZED* SEX"! MILLIONS of normal American adults manage to live without
> sex. Our public health officials have been imbibing at the Gay Task Force well
> of wisdom much too long. [All emphasis in the original][52]

---

*When smallpox was associated with immoral behavior, the treatments were often
repugnant as well: one treatment, for example, consisted of a drink made from sheep's
dung, the idea being that medicine would drive out evil influence only if its repugnance
was in proportion to the sin.[47]

Preventing Decadence Versus Preventing AIDS

On another occasion, Koop said, "Of course you speak of abstinence, of course you speak of monogamous marriage, but you also speak of condoms. . . . This conservative antagonism to the truth is ridiculous."[53] Perhaps, but it is important to understand that to many people the condom is something far beyond a rubber sheath to prevent contact between genitalia. Whatever its disease-preventing faculties, the condom clearly means one thing: somebody is having sex purely for the sake of pleasure. This many conservatives continue to view as the ultimate symbol of debauchery and national and cultural moral decay.

Condoms are always used in sex for pleasure: hence, condoms are always bad. If this sounds like puritanism, so it is. As a staffer for Gary Bauer in the White House Office of Policy Development, James Warner, a staunch conservative, worked with many leaders who fought against condom use. "These people are truly characteristic of what Mencken said about those who are afraid that somebody, somewhere might be having fun," Warner told me. "They are strange. Thoughts about sex play a very strong role in their lives."[54]

Sometimes the puritans inadvertently showed their hands even to persons outside their workplace. In the material the Education Department regularly sent out during Secretary William J. Bennett's tenure, a *Los Angeles Times* piece, which was just another in a long litany of "AIDS Has Ended the Sexual Revolution" articles, was marked by Education officials for categorization purposes under "VICE (Perversion/ AIDS)."

Having already come up with their conclusion, the moralists were left only to decide on their arguments. While some used a forthright approach, saying that mortal preservation wasn't worth moral compromise, others sought to combine the two. But the most cynical of the moralists realized the inherent dangers of preaching morality to what they considered to be at best amoral rabble. And so, disguising their moral indignation behind the shield of practicality, moralists sought to impeach the value of the condom in the prevention of AIDS.

Thus did those who saw any sex outside marriage as evil—the moralists—combine under the anticondomite umbrella with the nonmoralist hysterics who saw virtually any sex as incredibly risky. One of these supposedly scientific arguments ran as follows:

> Condom use pregnancy prevention failure rates of between 10 and 30 percent are reported and that involves a peak ovulation "window" of only

about 12 to 24 hours or so between each menstrual cycle. AIDS, on the other hand, never sleeps—so its carriers are always ready to transfer a potentially infectious dosage of AIDS virus no matter what time of month it is.[55]

This is a mixture of nonscience and nonsense. First, a peak is just that: A woman is susceptible to pregnancy half of the time.[56] Second, regardless of ovulation cycles and peaks, it is far easier for a fertile man to impregnate a fertile woman than it is for him to infect her if he's carrying HIV. Recall that over a period of several years, only 10 percent to 20 percent of seropositive male hemophiliacs and transfusion recipients managed to infect their wives. If the fertility rate weren't considerably higher than that, the human race would quickly die out. Finally, the vast majority of heterosexual men are fertile, but they are not infectious.

There was also a good deal of confusion over the meaning of the "failure rate" of condoms. Thus it was popular to use the 10-percent condom-failure rate in preventing pregnancy from a well-publicized Planned Parenthood study[57] as if this rate somehow meant that one out of ten condoms failed. Secretary Bennett's booklet on AIDS warned, "When condoms are used for contraceptive measures, *they* fail about ten percent of the time" (emphasis added).[58] The booklet went on to cite a study by Margaret Fischl.[59] Claimed Bennett's chief of staff, John Walters, "Condoms have a particularly high failure rate when used by young people,"[60] as if condoms somehow popped more leaks when young people were using them.

In fact, as Surgeon General Koop points out well, it's not that simple:

> Let's say that a surveyor approaches a couple and says, "What method of birth control do you use?" [And they say,] "Well, we use condoms." "Have you ever had a failure?" "Yes, we had a child we didn't expect." So that gets checked off as a failure of condoms. However, you go back and talk to that couple and say, "Tell me exactly how you used your condoms?" "Well, you see we really practice [the] rhythm [method] unless my wife thinks she's fertile." Well, that is not the condoms, that is again human unreliability. So one has to be very careful about using statistics that are taken from surveys.[61]

A distinction the condom opponents were loath to make was between equipment failure and user failure. The first, referring to an actual problem with the condom itself, poses by far the least difficulty. The second refers to the failure to use condoms properly. The Fischl study that Bennett's booklet cited, for example, stated, "Only three spouses used barrier contraceptives regularly during a two-to-five year period prior to enrollment [in the study]; all three were seronegative for

[HIV]."[62] The problem of condoms versus some prophylactics, such as the Pill or the IUD, is that since the condom can be used only once, a special effort must be made each time one wishes to have intercourse. The problem with condoms versus even other one-time contraceptives is that the former can be put on only immediately prior to intercourse. Female barrier contraceptives—sponges, foams, jellies, diaphragms— can all be applied several minutes to several hours prior to intercourse. Thus, condoms are the form of birth control least conducive to spontaneity.

One month after New York City unveiled its slick condom campaign, Mayor Edward Koch suddenly came out against promoting prophylactics as the first line of defense in favor of promoting abstinence. "Flip-Flop Ed" read the *Post* headline, although the mayor said he still completely favored the condom ads.[63] Koch's reasoning was simple: Condoms are "Russian roulette." Said the mayor, "There are six bullets in a revolver." Since "leakage" is found in about 17 percent of condoms, "it's roughly the same kind of odds."[64] The reference was, of course, to the Fischl study, and the "leakage" statement was fatuous. The study had nothing to do with measuring the permeability of condoms. All it measured was seroprevalence rates of those who claimed to use condoms as opposed to those who did not make such a claim. Studies that have measured leakage have essentially found nothing to measure. As *Consumer Reports* stated, based on its own study and those of others, "Intact latex condoms won't let even the smallest microbe through."[65]* It stated also, "In principle, latex condoms can be close to 100 percent effective."[66]

Thus—at the risk of sounding like a National Rifle Association slogan—condoms don't usually fail, people do. Telling a couple that using condoms leaves a 10-percent or 17-percent chance of HIV transmission, if one is seropositive, is as fallacious as telling a thirty-year-old college-educated woman—who may be ravishing, charming, and intelligent— that, based on Census Bureau statistics, her probability of marriage is only 20 percent. People decide their own risks. A couple using condoms correctly and consistently incurs little chance of transmitting HIV or anything else.†

*A study done by Dr. Marcus Conant of the University of California, San Francisco demonstrated that twelve varieties of latex condoms proved inpenetrable to HIV, herpes-virus one and two, and cytomegalovirus, another STD which especially plagues homosexual men. There was, however, occasional leakage in the natural membrane condoms.
†Studies among prostitutes in Kenya and Zaire found that those who insisted that their clients use condoms had a much lower rate of seropositivity than those whose partners did not use condoms. The authors of the Kenyan study reported, "There is a striking

The Condomites

By the same token, those who supported the widespread distribution of condoms were equally prone to hyperbole and misinformation. They probably did not know, and might not have cared if they did, that different studies have shown that distribution of free condoms at sexually transmitted disease clinics, even in combination with special counseling, have had no effect in reducing STD reinfection.[69]

The problem the condomites had was the proverbial problem with the horse: you can bring him to water, but you can't make him drink. Couples fail to use condoms not because they lack access to them, but because they don't *want* to.

The reasons for their reticence are twofold. First, condom sensitivity is inverse to safety. Noted one study in the *British Medical Journal,* "In general, the stiffest condoms seemed to be safer than the others, but they were also the least liked and therefore unacceptable to the participants."[70] Second, in the case of heterosexual intercourse, the persons most at risk are least likely to be bothered by the lack of sensitivity, and vice versa. In other words, because a man in the United States or Europe is far more likely to be infected than a woman, a woman is at greater risk for infection; yet because the nerve endings on the inside of the vagina are not especially sensitive, she is less likely to complain about use of a prophylactic. Men, on the other hand, are far more likely to complain that coitus with a condom is like "taking a shower with a raincoat on"; or, to use an expression popular in Britain, "You can't taste a sweet with the wrapper on." This discrepancy created a tension for which there was no easy answer. One possibility was to try to persuade men that while they were at less risk than women, they were still at great risk. Many of the condomites did just that, revealing themselves to be just as willing to engage in deception as the anticondomites. Even so, many men refused and continued to be more willing to take risks than women seemed to be. Prostitutes often report great difficulties in getting their clients to wear condoms. If men don't want to wear prophylactics with women who are perceived to be highly likely to harbor

reduction in risk of seroconversion with increasing levels of condom use." Although only one woman in the entire study of 595 prostitutes claimed to use condoms 100 percent of the time, "*Any* condom use resulted in a three-fold reduction in risk of seroconversion" (emphasis added).[67] The Zairian study also found a more or less direct correlation between frequency of usage and seroconversion rates.[68] If condoms will protect women in Africa with large numbers of infected partners who often have ulcerating STDs to boot, they'll protect lower-risk Americans just as well.

and transmit HIV, it's obviously an uphill battle to get men to wear them with "nice girls."

Thus, the condomites had to wage a two-front war. First, they had to establish that condoms were effective. Second, they had to convince sexually active heterosexuals, especially men, that condoms would not significantly interfere with the enjoyment of the sex act. The second front proved to be far more difficult, primarily because they were not telling the truth. So desperate attempts were made to convince people that sex with condoms was every bit as good as sex without—even better. Some manufacturers tried using a "macho" approach. For example, in Great Britain the advertising slogan of a brand of condom called Jiffi was "Real men come in a Jiffi."[71] (Presumably these ads were always visual; *heard,* the pitch might sound like a promotion for premature ejaculation.)

Others tried to make condoms to sex what strawberries are to cheesecake. Wrote the feminist AIDS author Diane Richardson:

> Condoms make sex safer; they can also make sex more exciting.... For men who have difficulties maintaining an erection, a condom which fits tightly will tend to make erections harder and orgasms more intense. Condoms also cut down on friction, especially the lubricated kind. This can aid women who experience vaginal dryness and find intercourse uncomfortable. . . . Some men who climax too quickly find that wearing a condom can delay this and give them and their partner more satisfaction.[72]

The Condom Irony

The irony of condoms would prove to be that they were of greatest efficiency to those who needed them least—anyone engaging in oral sex and heterosexuals engaging in vaginal sex—and of least efficiency to those who needed them most—homosexuals engaging in anal intercourse. But while ironic, this isn't especially mysterious. Anal sex is the most dangerous form of intercourse in part because it allows the most friction with the least lubrication. The same factors that cause mucous membrane tearing in the anus can and will cause such tearing in the membrane of a condom as well. Asked if condoms were a good protection during anal sex, Surgeon General Koop replied:

> That's entirely different. The rectum was not made for intercourse. It's at the wrong angle, it's the wrong size, it doesn't have the same kind of tough lining that the vagina does. It has its blood supply directly under the mucosa. Therefore, you would expect a great many more failures of condoms in rectal

intercourse than you would in vaginal intercourse, and it's important to know that.[73]

While many homosexuals might consider such a statement to be "homophobic," the case against relying on condoms for protection during anal intercourse is strong. An Australian study, reported in the July 1987 *American Journal of Public Health,* showed that 27 percent of homosexuals using condoms reported "a few" or "many" breaks, with an additional 4 percent indicating "other problems" with condom strength.[74] By 1988, homosexual groups were also warning against relying on condoms during anal sex.[75]

Sorting It Out: How Valuable Are Condoms?

The practical effect of all this is that it is foolhardy to tell a man that he has little to worry about if he engages in receptive anal intercourse and uses a condom, and that it is equally foolish to tell a college woman that she should not trust a condom to protect her either. On the other hand, it must be stated that if a man insists on engaging in anal intercourse, a condom will still, with all its risks, substantially reduce his risk; while the college coed is already at such low risk that in practical terms a condom won't make any difference to her one way or the other.

Brandt notes that the military, having learned its lesson from its emphasis on chastity and pain in the First World War, decided in the Second that troops must be equipped with condoms to prevent infection. The military program, which combined a massive education program, prophylaxis, and rapid treatment without punitive measures, proved highly successful as rates of disease were controlled, even prior to the introduction of penicillin.[76]

By contrast, condoms are still of limited use in combating the AIDS epidemic. "Instead of putting up condom posters on subway walls, we need to use teams of ex-addicts to attack drug addiction in the streets," said Manhattan's borough president, David N. Dinkins.[77] But distributing free condoms or putting up educational posters on condoms—or posters in general, for that matter—is an easy, cheap way of pretending to be doing something important. It makes expensive solutions, like putting more addicts into treatment programs, seem less necessary.

At any rate, for some the efficacy point was moot. One strong element of the "safe sex/safer sex" mania was that old stand-by, social consciousness. Noting that condom giveaways appear to have little correlation with condom usage, what was the purpose of such distribution, be it in

Spin magazine, the Mansfield student newspaper, or the Dartmouth Safe Sex kits? What was the purpose in Madonna's flashing "SAFE SEX" on the view screen at her concerts or for a popular group to sing "Give me, give me wild west; give me, give me safe sex"? The answer is that the Eighties were characterized by high-profile events which resulted in very low impact. Remember Farm AID? Farm AID II? Hands Across America? How many people know where the money they raised went? How many care? For participants and promoters alike, the importance of these events was that they were consciousness-raisers. Condom giveaways, like holding hands with a stranger, accomplished virtually nothing, but they were a cheap, easy way of saying: "Hey! Look at me! I'm socially conscious!" Or, as Robert Guccione, Jr. put it, "I'm proud to be part of a magazine that said something."[78] *What* was said doesn't seem to be of as much importance. What was important was *feeling good.* When one rents a car from Budget on the east coast, one finds that affixed to the back bumper is a square sticker with the word "hunger" in a circle with a slash through it. Now everyone in the world will know that both the driver and Budget oppose hunger. It's a courageous stand, but somebody had to make it. When the background video at Madonna's concerts flashed "SAFE SEX," perhaps it didn't accomplish anything toward stemming the tide of AIDS, but who cares? It made the audience feel good for a moment, whereupon they turned their attention back to Madonna who was sensuously squirming all over the stage singing, "Like a virgin (ooh!), touched for the very first time . . ."

A Pox on Both Houses

A joke making the rounds:

> FIRST DRUG ADDICT: Hey! Don't shoot up with that dirty needle; you could get AIDS!
> SECOND DRUG ADDICT: Don't worry, I'm wearing a condom!

Harold Jaffe puts it more seriously: "You just can't tell people it's all right to do whatever you want so long as you wear a condom. It's just too dangerous a disease to say that."[79]

Clearly, condoms are no talisman. One can't hang them around one's neck and expect them to be protective. Just saying one uses them doesn't protect one; and to the extent one uses them but does so irregularly or incorrectly, their efficacy is reduced. Furthermore, the moralists are also absolutely right when they say condoms can't make sinful sex safe, as in safe for the soul.

But used properly, condoms can substantially reduce the odds of transmitting HIV, along with any number of less dangerous diseases. That they can thus facilitate immorality is hardly an unimportant point; but it is a point that does not alter their ability to prevent disease.

Nevertheless, those who urged a strategy of letting a million condoms bloom* were just as far off the target. Condoms in the right hands, which is to say the hands of persons sufficiently motivated to obtain them and to learn how to use them properly, can be virtually 100-percent foolproof. But tossed at people like party favors, the vast majority of prophylactics probably ended up in the trash or in the backs of drawers. Further, since willingness to use a condom is closely tied to perception of one's risk, condomites had a natural incentive to overplay the risks of heterosexual-HIV transmission. Indeed, to the extent that it was was aimed at the general population, condom distribution was *ipso facto* spreading the fear of heterosexual AIDS.

Finally, the foisting of condoms onto children, the effort to accustom teenagers to their use, and treatment of condoms generally that bordered on the ancient Roman worship of phalluses, is difficult to construe as anything less than decadent. One need not be a certified moralist, a conservative, or a Christian to be horrified at what the condomites passed off as responsible behavior in time of crisis.

As with any religious war, the excesses of the zealots on both sides were stomach turning. But here the carnage was even more pitiful. For here the excesses—the profligate prevarication of the anticondomites and the deific adoration of a tube of rubber on the part of the condomites—were both committed in the name of a single god, and that god was a false one. This Lord of the Flies was the epidemic of heterosexual AIDS.

---

*In his remarks before the House Select Committee on Narcotics Abuse and Control, on 27 July 1987, New York's mayor Edward I. Koch told of plans to distribute 1,000,000 condoms.[80]

13

The Conservative Alarmists

In the AIDS epidemic, some conservatives believe they have found a shiny weapon with which to recapture their vision of a better world—one where homosexuality is pushed back into the closet (or further); where chastity, monogamy, and sexual morality are revered; and where sexual behavior is once again within the domain of law. But as with all the other groups who have sought to gain from AIDS, the conservatives have been forced to distort the true nature of the epidemic—to shape it to fit their wishes. Unlike most of these other groups, however, their efforts have ultimately done little to further their particular agenda.

At the root of the conservative alarmist confusion over AIDS policy is confusion over the transmissibility of the AIDS virus, using any combination of three theories. Theory 1 assumes that in addition to being blood-borne, the contagion can be transmitted casually: that is, that a person can through mere proximity transmit the virus; and that while sexual intercourse may facilitate transmission, it is not necessary. Theory 2 assumes that HIV, in addition to being blood-borne, is transmitted efficiently through sexual intercourse, both homosexual and heterosexual. Theory 3, the correct one, is that because HIV is blood-borne, it will continue to be spread through anal sex and shared needles, but will pose far less of a threat to the general heterosexual population.

As a matter of logic, all three of these theories cannot be right. Either it is "a fluke of fate that AIDS landed in the gay community," as Mathilde Krim says;[1] or it is confined by its very nature primarily to homosexuals (and drug users). Similarly, either AIDS is casually transmitted and hence no more a behavioral contagion than tuberculosis or influenza, or it is not. Yet conservative alarmists frequently combine all three, depending on their state of confusion and, perhaps more important, on their agenda.

Because few people enjoy operating in the dark, writers and some doctors have sought an analogy to another sexually transmitted disease, although HIV is epidemiologically unique. While hepatitis B would be the most logical choice, many have instead seized upon syphilis. Neither analogy is complete, but syphilis is by far the worse choice. Syphilis is a spirochete, rather than a virus, and readily infects the penile, vaginal, and rectal mucous membranes by boring right into intact skin. In fact, syphilis is so infectious that you can get it on the back of your hand.[2] The infection rate of this microbe during coitus is thought to be about 20 percent per contact, although no per-contact study has been done.[3] HIV, as noted previously, has an infection rate of less than one tenth of 1 percent from male to female. Thus, combating HIV spread as if it were syphilis makes as much sense as would treating syphilis as if it were tuberculosis or using anti-aircraft weapons to shoot at tanks. Yet the syphilis model seized the imagination of many conservative writers and leaders.

The most immediate and visible consequence of this analogy was that officials of the Reagan administration insisted upon using their influence to fight AIDS by the methods of the pre-penicillin campaign to control syphilis. Both President Reagan's secretary of education, William J. Bennett, and his chief of domestic policy, Gary Bauer, urged states to require routine HIV testing for marriage licenses. President Reagan supported expanding mandatory blood testing beyond blood banks and the military, as to some extent did all four of the original conservative Republican presidential contenders in the 1988 presidential race—Jack Kemp, Pierre du Pont, Alexander Haig, and Pat Robertson.[4] Senator Jesse Helms (Republican, of North Carolina), normally a fierce champion of federalism, introduced legislation in the Senate that would penalize states that refuse to mandate premarital testing.[5] Representative William Dannemeyer (Republican, of California), another normally staunch federalist, introduced similar legislation in the House of Representatives.[6] The conservative weekly *Human Events* did a cover story urging that the syphilis strategy be used against HIV.[7]

The conservative AIDS alarmists fancied themselves inheritors of Thomas Parran's ideas. The young bucks in William J. Bennett's Department of Education circulated memos to each other—subsequently made public through regular mailings to interested parties—which included sections of Parran's book on syphilis, *Shadow on the Land.* They also circulated memos calling for a variety of testing schemes ostensibly mimicking Parran's mass-testing programs, including one under which all 125,000,000 Americans, from age fifteen to forty-nine, would be tested.[8]*

In fact, these men had about as much claim to descending from Parran as Mussolini did to descending from the Roman Empire. For one thing, virtually all of them emphasized moral restraint as a corollary to mandatory testing; yet Parran was a strong critic of relying on moralism to combat venereal disease.[10] "Greater progress," he wrote, "will be made by concentration of effort on the medical aspect of control rather than through continued scattering of effort in an attempt to carry out the 'ideal program' . . . for moral prophylaxis."[11] Indeed, with syphilis, the moralists eventually lost out to those who prescribed amoral medical preventatives.[12] More important, when Parran's testing began, syphilis was treatable with Salvarsan and had been for decades. With AIDS antibody testing, there was no cure—indeed, no effective treatment of any kind—for the afflicted. Thus, while Parran had proposed identifying targets for cure, his would-be imitators proposed identifying them for the sheer sake of identification—along with the hope that identification would somehow substitute for cure.

Finally, as Dr. Allan Brandt points out about Parran's mandatory testing for syphilis, "so few cases were found this way—less than one percent at a cost of about $250,000 per case—that even this wasn't cost effective."[13] What the "let's test for AIDS like we do for syphilis" crowd never pointed out was that, in fact, twenty-two states have *repealed* their premarital blood-test requirements since 1980 alone.[14] If syphilis premarital testing was virtually useless, such testing for HIV is completely so—because couples preparing for marriage are, by virtue of that fact, in an extremely low-risk group for HIV infection. Some may be drug abusers or bisexuals, but few are pure homosexuals. In Illinois, during the first year of testing, of 150,000 applicants tested in the first eleven months since it became mandatory, only 23 positives were identified. Since test costs ranged from $25 to $125 a person, a spokesperson for the State Department of Health said that using a "conservative" average of $35 a test, the cost of finding each of the 23 seropositives was more than $228,000.[15] Louisiana, the only other state in the country to implement mandatory premarital testing, got similar results and dropped the test requirement within a few months.[16] Nevertheless, the conservative Illinois state representative Penny Pullen, who had been a member of President Reagan's AIDS Commission, declared that re-

---

*This aping was such that Dr. Redfield and his superior officer, Donald Burke, even entitled a paper of theirs on AIDS, "Shadow on the Land."[9]

pealing the testing law would send a message that Illinois no longer regarded AIDS as a serious problem—an analysis the legislatures in forty-nine other states might disagree with. Said Pullen, "This program is giving thousands of Illinois couples the good news that they are not infected." What she was saying is that, having terrified persons into thinking they might be suffering a silent but fatal, horrible illness, these persons are now benefited by being able to rejoice at being absolved of that fate. Betraying her moralistic perspective, she added, "[In] this society, with its current mores, that can be very good news indeed."[17]

For all the money spent in Illinois, there is no evidence that a single case of AIDS was prevented.* Surely that money could have been spent more efficiently to reduce HIV transmission where it was really occurring, or perhaps to combat some other life-threatening malady.[18]

Casual Contagion and the Conspiracy Theory

As unfounded as the syphilis model is, the casual contagion one is nothing short of bizarre. And, unlike the syphilis theory, it appears to be almost solely in the domain of the right. By 1987, if not sooner, no doctor working for the U.S. Public Health Service or for the public health departments of any major U.S. city would give credence to the possibility that AIDS is casually transmitted. Further, as poor as the media's track record has been in exaggerating the threat of AIDS to heterosexuals, they have been fairly consistent in their efforts to inform the public that AIDS cannot be transmitted by coughing, food handling, or sharing drinking glasses.

Because responsible public officials and reporters will not credit the casual contagion model, its proponents tend to articulate a conspiracy theory. To those persons, AIDS has become the new fluoride. The guru of the casual contagion theory is John Seale, a British venerealogist who has declared that "the genetic information contained in [HIV's] tiny strip of RNA has all that is needed to render the human race extinct within fifty years."[19] Seale submitted to the House of Commons, in May 1987, a report that admitted—indeed, trumpeted—that the material in it was completely in conflict with the reports reproduced in British and

*Education Department and White House staffers made absolutely no effort to show how by diagnosing HIV in one person, who was now beyond help, they could prevent any cases of AIDS. Many couples, upon finding out that one member is seropositive, continue to have sex anyway. Add to that couples where the first partner has already infected the second, and those where the second partner would have remained among the majority who did not become infected anyway, and it is clear that premarital testing was a foolish way of preventing new AIDS cases or saving money.

American medical journals.[20] Among Seale's assertions totally in conflict with accepted understanding of HIV transmissibility was that,
"Male homosexual contact of the finger, penis, or tongue with the rectal
wall of another man transmits the virus very easily." According to Dr.
Seale:

> Moderately efficient means of transmission include mouth-to-mouth and
> genital contact [and] oral salivary contact between small children. . . . Finally,
> highly inefficient "contacts" which occur very frequently indeed, such as
> coughing and sneezing in public, and being bitten by insects, will infect many
> people as millions of infected persons interact with the non-infected, and
> saturation of the entire British population becomes inevitable.[21]

Lest we wonder why these verities have gone unmentioned by the
media, Dr. Seale tells us that "journalists and media editors have been
frightened to contradict the conventional wisdom being put across.
. . . There has been no serious attempt at investigative journalism into
the wealth of scientific scandals surrounding AIDS." Politicians fear that
"taking AIDS seriously would gain them few votes"; homosexual leaders "actively [obstruct] the publication, in the scientific or general press,
of facts and conclusions which they want suppressed."[22]

Virtually the only people taking Dr. Seale seriously, at least on this
side of the Atlantic, were conservative writers and publishers. Reed
Irvine's "Accuracy in Media" newsletter and its sister publication, the
Washington Inquirer, have both used Seale's material to accuse the
scientific journals and the media of "downplaying evidence that AIDS
is being transmitted in ways other than sexual contact, IV needles and
blood transfusion."[23] (Almost as an afterthought, they threw in the
caveat that "Seale contends that the AIDS virus is man-made, and
accidentally released during scientific experiments.")[24]

Some conservatives have been less honest about their sensationalist
source. In a scathing critique of "The Surgeon General's Report on
AIDS" in National Review, Wayne Lutton, a writer who specializes in
extolling the evils of immigration, made no mention of Seale's quirks in
quoting him as saying AIDS has "the molecular biological equivalent of
the nuclear bomb," and in repeating the assertion that the human race
could become extinct as a result of the virus.[25] In December 1987, the
presidential candidate Pat Robertson, in an interview with the editorial
board of New Hampshire's Concord Monitor, declared that medical
authorities have not been honest in asserting that the virus has limited
ways of being spread. "If, say, we're in a room with 25 people with AIDS
and they're breathing various things into the atmosphere, the chance

of somebody catching it has become quite strong," the *Monitor* quoted Robertson as saying. Robertson's source, according to a spokesman, was Dr. John Seale.[26]

Some conservatives, such as then nationally syndicated columnist Gregory Fossedal, did not even feel the need to cite a physician or a theorist like Dr. Seale to push the casual transmission line. Wrote Fossedal in one column:

> Polls show that a majority of Americans think they are being lied to about the disease, and they're right as the provocative book *The AIDS Cover-up?* suggests. They can tell that doctors are telling the truth but not the whole truth when they say there's no evidence AIDS can be spread through casual contact. (There's nothing proving it can't, and common sense suggests erring on caution's side.)[27]

Fossedal was merely stating the logical proposition that one cannot prove a negative. That AIDS is not casually transmitted is demonstrated in the same way so many other negatives we accept are demonstrated— by lack of evidence on the other side. AIDS has been recognized as an epidemic for nine years now. During that time, there has yet to be a single verified case of casual transmission. Numerous studies done in the United States have shown no higher incidence of HIV in households of HIV-positive individuals except as a result of a sexual relationship. Further, sheer intuition tells one that casual transmission is not taking place. If it were, there would not just be an isolated case here or there, any more than there is with the flu, which strikes tens of millions in this country each season. Why some of our most brilliant conservative writers and publishers have been so willing to suspend that intuition is certainly a mystery.

Conservatives pushing the casual transmission line pointed to the "undetermined" section of the CDC statistics as providing evidence. As Representative Dannemeyer put it in 1986, "Of the 21,000 cases that CDC tells us about nationally, there's about six percent or 1,200 where they can't establish how that person got AIDS. No one can say for certain that AIDS may not be transmitted socially."[28] A year later he was still at it: "The fact of the matter," he told "Nightline"'s "Town Meeting on AIDS" audience, "is that three or four percent of the 35 [*sic*] cases reported by CDC of AIDS in America, CDC can't tell us how they got it. . . . I'm not suggesting that proves social transmissibility, but I don't believe we should exclude it."[29] It didn't matter how many times it was explained that this category consisted primarily of those who had not yet been interviewed, died before interview, or refused interview.

Further, the ages and other demographic characteristics of the victims closely correspond to the ages in the sexually transmitted and IV-drug cases.[30] Why would HIV be casually transmitted only to those in the age groups most likely to use drugs and have sex? But the Dannemeyers of the world simply could not be satisfied.

Likewise, Paul Cameron's group grasped so hard for proof of casual transmission that it took a report from the *American Medical News* that genital herpes could be transmitted despite a lack of symptoms in the infectious, and said it vindicated parents who were afraid of casual transmission of herpes in school. This piece of "information" was slapped in a newsletter below an article entitled, "Casual Spread of AIDS a Possibility?"[31]

The AIDS Cover-up?

The book cited by Fossedal, and used as the title of the *Washington Inquirer* article citing Seale, was written by Gene Antonio, a heretofore-unknown former minister, and published by the conservative Catholic Ignatius Press. *The AIDS Cover-up?* became a cult classic, with over 300,000 copies sold, according to its author. It is a terrifying book. "I got a copy of it from my dentist," one friend told me, after which she, a virgin until her marriage a year earlier, almost decided to have her blood tested for HIV. *The AIDS Cover-up?* has been offered as a primary selection of the Conservative Book Club. Copies of the text are displayed prominently on conservatives' bookshelves and desks throughout Washington; and to be a conservative journalist who writes about AIDS is to be plagued with the question "Have you read Gene Antonio's book?" Antonio has written updates which are circulated by the Department of Education, and speaks often at church gatherings, meetings of Phyllis Schafly's Eagle Forum, and the like.

The AIDS Cover-up? relies heavily on Seale's pronouncements, citing him thirteen times. Another doctor who figures heavily in Antonio's book is William Haseltine, whose contribution to the heterosexual AIDS panic I noted earlier. Antonio is fully capable of his own apocalyptics, predicting that as many as 8,000,000 Americans would be infected by the end of 1987 and 64,000,000 by the end of 1990. (His calculations are examined in greater detail in chapter 21.) In the near future, according to Antonio, "the entire population will shudder as the anguished cries of the demented and dying rise in a ghastly crescendo. Unless drastic measures are taken . . . AIDS may well become *everyone's* Final Epidemic."[32]

Antonio presents an entire chapter on casual transmission, although most of the casual transmission about which he writes is not of the AIDS virus at all, but of secondary illnesses such as tuberculosis which frequently plagues AIDS victims and can be casually transmitted (although even with this disease extended contact is usually required). Antonio's prime arguments for casual transmission of HIV appears to be: (1) HIV is a lentivirus; (2) there is a lentivirus that affects sheep; (3) the sheep virus is casually transmitted; and therefore, (4) the AIDS virus may be capable of casual transmission. "Lentivirus in sheep involves a means of spread consonant with casual transmission in man," writes Antonio. "Simply put, the lentivirus which causes lethal pneumonia in sheep is spread by coughing."[33] But a virus's mode of transmission has absolutely nothing to do with the manifestation of symptoms caused by the virus. While both the common cold and pulmonary plague are spread by coughing, the first is never fatal in a previously healthy individual, whereas the latter was almost always fatal during the plague epidemics.[34]

As with virtually every published article, good or bad, on AIDS, most of what Antonio presents is true. But it is the untruths that have gained the book its notoriety and made it the AIDS bible of conspiracy-minded conservatives.

One source quoted in *The AIDS Cover-up?* probably constitutes the most egregious AIDS scare article printed in the conservative press. The March 1986 *American Spectator* featured on its cover a man and woman taking apples from a tree consisting of a human skeleton. The article provides the somewhat questionable estimate that 30 percent of all men patronize prostitutes,[35] suggests that cow's milk could transmit the virus (how it would get into cow's milk, since cows don't carry HIV, we are not told),[36] and uses the same fallacy that Antonio does in assuming that since the sheep lentivirus can be transmitted by coughing, so can HIV.[37] After summarizing the various categories of persons at risk, the article concluded ominously, "who will be left?"[38] To which the apparent answer is "nobody."

The article ran after heated internal debate at the magazine, debate that exploded into print when next the *Spectator* ran an AIDS scare piece. This article, written by a former special adviser to Margaret Thatcher, called for compulsory universal testing with enforced isolation for seropositives. In a published letter to the editor, the assistant managing editor, Andrew Ferguson, called the article an "insult and an embarrassment to all associated with *The American Spectator.*"[39] Explained the managing editor, Wladyslaw Pleszczynski, to me later, "At the time information was still quite sketchy, and we thought it prudent to go ahead with a warning article."[40] Pleszczynski was more skeptical half a year later, when the authors offered to do a follow-up after three health-care workers were reported to have contracted HIV after being splashed with infected blood. The *Spectator* declined.

Nevertheless, the loss of one forum did not stop one of the co-authors, A. D. J. Robertson, from continuing to spread his message. He continued to be called upon by Gary Bauer in the White House for advice. Nor were other conservative publications quick to follow the *Spectator*'s lead in accepting that AIDS was not the risk to the general population once thought. The *Wall Street Journal*, with the most prestigious conservative op-ed page in the country, has run many pieces pushing the heterosexual AIDS breakout theme. One was the prostitution piece, discussed in chapter 8, in which the author claimed, without citing any source, that "between 1000 and 10,000 men will become infected with the AIDS virus this year by having sex with female prostitutes."[41] The *Journal* also ran two rather strange AIDS op-eds, one by Katie Leishman, pushing her "AIDS is syphilis" theory;[42]* and another by two doctors, asserting that AIDS is caused by immune overload†—a popular theory early on, but the *Journal* ran the piece well *after* the discovery of HIV. In its own editorial, the *Journal* stated, "An African-style epidemic is certainly possible, especially with a mutation of the virus."[45] (In fact, as noted earlier, such a mutation would be without precedent.) The *Journal* attempts to show its diversity by running a regular column by the far-left Alexander Cockburn; but when it came to AIDS, no diversity was to be tolerated. At least two writers' attempts to publish pieces downplaying the heterosexual threat, or the scope of the AIDS epidemic in general, were repeatedly rebuffed, the result of which was that the *Journal*'s op-ed page—open to heterosexual alarmists and bi-

---

*When I first made this assertion about Leishman and syphilis in the pages of the *New Republic*, Leishman replied: "Fumento's statement in his article . . . that my op-ed piece in the *Wall Street Journal* 'pushes the theory that AIDS is really syphilis' is incorrect. My article pointed out that heterodox theories about the nature of AIDS, such as those proposed by Professor Peter Duesberg . . . , were not being given a fair hearing. Mr. Duesberg does not in fact believe that AIDS is really syphilis."[43] All fine perhaps, except that the quote she excerpted from my article does not mention Duesberg; it says *she* pushed the theory. In my reply I reprinted the section of her op-ed that indicated her support for the AIDS-syphilis theory, and further noted that she had written a massive piece called "AIDS and Syphilis" for the *Atlantic* (see Katie Leishman, "AIDS and Syphilis," *Atlantic Monthly* 261, no. 1, January 1988, p. 17), whose thesis was clearly spelled out in the title.

†The writers stated, "It appears that AIDS patients have not been healthy people who got AIDS simply because they had sex with the wrong person. Rather, they seem to have been people who already were sick in the sense of having a damaged immune system."[44]

zarre theorists—never published a piece challenging the heterosexual epidemic myth.

Prudery as Policy

The major thrust of the conservative position on AIDS was to discourage heterosexuals from engaging in illicit relations. They had an ally in the *Soho Weekly News,* which explained, "Perhaps it's current sexual practice that is the real epidemic and the rash of sexually transmitted diseases raging through the city simply a symptom."[46] One newsletter sprang up, whose sole policy was to terrify heterosexuals into chastity. Featuring a logo representing a family, and with the ironic motto "Reliable information has life-sustaining power," the "AIDS Protection" monthly is chock full of stories that serve its point. Take the one about the virginal co-ed who goes down to Florida for spring break, whereupon a female friend talks her into giving up her virginity, and she allows herself to be taken by four lusty young males. A few weeks later, she falls ill, takes the AIDS virus test, and, sure enough, she's positive.[47] A life shot to hell for a few moments of passion. The problem is that, like the boogeyman story to which it compares, this one seems to have little basis in fact. A request for information on this case was refused by the newsletter's editor, H. Edward Rowe (who, like Antonio, has his degrees in theology). He cited confidentiality in refusing so much as to provide the name of the health department that interviewed the girl.[48] Thus, a newsletter that tells its readers not to trust condoms, and to look upon Public Health Service missives with a jaundiced eye, nevertheless wants those readers to put blind faith in its own veracity.

Such apocryphal stories are by no means new when it comes to sexually transmitted diseases. One turn-of-the-century lecturer told the grim story of a football squad who celebrated a big victory by "breaking training" in a nearby city. Seven of the eleven developed venereal infections. "Three of them are now six feet under the sod," the lecturer said solemnly, "dead with the most loathsome of diseases, syphilis."[49]

It is probably not surprising that the honorary national chairman of the AIDS Prevention Institute is Pat Boone, who is to premarital sex what Anita Bryant is to homosexuals. The newsletter prints blocked-off, oversized fillers which blare such admonitions as: "Save sex for marriage! You owe it to your future children!" Authorities such as Miss America 1988 are cited as calling for mandatory testing.[50] One story in the newsletter relates the story of a heterosexually promiscuous young man who, with no other symptoms than glands that remained swollen for more than a week, sweats through an AIDS test that after an agonizing wait comes back negative. "Never again!" proclaims the prodigal youth.[51] It's the old perpetual motion machine of fear. The newsletter terrifies heterosexuals into thinking they may be infected, then uses accounts of those needlessly terrified heterosexuals to terrify more heterosexuals.

AIDS-induced chastity has also gone high-tech. Goodday Video, a Texas producer, says it has sold to schools more than one thousand copies of its video "AIDS: Suddenly Sex Has Become Very Dangerous"—a large number considering that a school need buy only one copy. In one of the five original vignettes, a young woman is shown trying on her wedding dress when she receives a call from her doctor telling her she has AIDS. The video warns that the only truly safe way to avoid such calls is to avoid sex. The video makes no mention of homosexuality, but does warn sternly against deep kissing.[52]

Theodore A. Leslie, a director at Goodday Video, is undaunted by the astronomical odds of acquiring HIV through intercourse with other drug-free heterosexuals. "If there is one chance in ten million that a kid will catch AIDS, he shouldn't take it."[53] What Leslie is saying in effect is that, to him, extramarital sex has zero utility. Unfortunately, he doesn't have the honesty to come out and say so. It is dishonesty that underlies the entire moralistic scheme to exaggerate the heterosexual AIDS problem. Frustrated with the reaction to their admonition that "Sex will cost you your soul," the moralists have cynically exchanged it for "Sex will cost you your life." Moral suasion is replaced with mortal terror.

The Problems of Chastity at Gunpoint

The idea of disease as a morality modifier is old. "The fear of disease is a happy restraint to men," declared the preacher Edmund Massed in Holborn, England, on 2 July 1722. "If men were more healthy, 'tis a great chance they would be less righteous."[54]

The syphilis moralists were much more willing than the AIDS moralists to admit to using fear to promote morals. Only a well-developed awe of infection, suggested Dr. Abraham Wolbarst in 1910, could control the sexual drive in men. "The sexual instinct is imperative and will only listen to fear," he noted. "Ninety-nine out of one hundred persons could be frightened into being good by the fear of evil consequences."[55]

But can they?

The problem with pragmatic arguments against premarital sex is that they can nearly always be overcome by pragmatic means. Pregnancy? Take birth control, and if that fails, get an abortion. Sexually transmitted disease? Use a condom or get a dose of antibiotics. Even herpes is treatable. The only argument against premarital sex that cannot be overcome is one that isn't pragmatic but moral: that the act is wrong, and preventing the physical consequences cannot forestall the spiritual ones. In real life, people often "get away" with immoral behavior. To believe that adverse temporal consequences must follow immoral behavior is bad theology and will ultimately undermine itself.

Second, the virtue that comes from abstinence can come about only if that abstinence results from morally praiseworthy motives. If John finds Fred's wife sexually attractive but refuses her advances out of a sense of morality, John has acted virtuously. If, conversely, he resists her advances because Fred is a hot-tempered, suspicious NFL linebacker, then John is merely acting expediently. In either case, John's abstinence from sex with his neighbor is the proper action, but in only one case was it done for the morally correct reason. People can be forced through fear to behave correctly, but virtue must be chosen of free will: it cannot be enforced at the end of a bullwhip or through the services of a boogeyman with a scarlet "A" tattooed on his chest. Yet such an approach is fraught with danger. At some point, sexually active heterosexuals are going to wake up and find they're still alive. And the ant, who so fastidiously practiced celibacy while the apparently foolish grasshopper fiddled away, will find he's been duped.*

Eventually there will be a vaccine, or a treatment bordering on a cure. What then? If the moral position is abandoned for the pragmatic one, how can the moral one be reclaimed once the reason for pragmatism is gone? Whatever short-term gains the moralists make through use of the AIDS threat will be lost once the falsely induced hysteria inevitably abates.

But all of these arguments were probably lost on the AIDS moralists, who seemed to have little conception of morality as being something chosen of free will. Illicit sex to them was something to be prevented at all costs. It is hardly surprising, then, that their most strident—and inconsistent—rhetoric about AIDS was directed against homosexuals.

One moralist was willing to change the etiology of HIV because it suited his homosexual-bashing purposes better. In a speech delivered at

---

*Indeed, it's already happening. One youth, "Marc T.," a seventeen-year-old from a middle-class family in Washington, told a reporter, "A lot of my friends feel that everybody's using the AIDS thing to scare kids into not having sex. It's not going to work. I don't know of one person my age who has died of AIDS."[56]

Valley Christian University and reprinted in *Vital Speeches*, Melvin Anchell makes no reference whatever to anal-genital intercourse, instead claiming that his "forty years of critical, clinical observations" leads him to believe that the primary, if not only, risk factor is mouth contact with the anus, which explains why the body structures most frequently infected by the AIDS virus are the eye, the brain, and the intestinal tract.[57] (In fact, in terms of severity, it would be the lungs— *pneumocystis* pneumonia—and skin—Kaposi's sarcoma; and in frequency, it would be the mouth and throat—oral thrush—and lymph glands—lymphadenopathy.)

One moralist group that employs a dual agenda, urging both chastity and homosexual bashing, is the Family Research Foundation, run by Paul Cameron. Cameron clearly qualifies as the single person most reviled by homosexuals. When he appears at conferences, they seek to terrorize him by spitting at him, since he asserts that the AIDS virus can be transmitted this way. Just as clearly, he hates homosexuals. Cameron has co-authored books with the aforementioned Wayne Lutton.

A good portrait of Cameron's agenda is revealed in a listing of measures advocated to control HIV spread as presented in the "Family Research" newsletter, written entirely by Cameron. Stating that the "assumptions undergirding these proposals include: (1) homosexuality, not AIDS, is the world's #1 public health problem," Cameron urges mass screening with infected adults to be "semipermanently [whatever this means] tattooed on their right cheek. . . . Hiding the mark would be a banishable offense. . . . Molokai, breeding ground of the hammerhead shark, might be suitable [as a location for banishment]." Writes Cameron, "New hires [*sic*] would have to swear that since 1977 they had not engaged in homosexuality, prostitution or drug abuse." Making the apparent assumption that pornography encourages illicit and HIV-transmitted sex, Cameron urges, "Books or magazines for sale having photographs of the human genitalia to be locally taxed" either with a generalized $10 tax per item or with a $1 stamp affixed directly to the photograph itself. "The state should reward virtue as well as punish malefactors," he says. "Those who: (1) remain chaste until marriage, (2) remain in longevous marriages, and/or (3) rear children in intact homes should be rewarded with suitable grants or tax credits."[58]

To make all of his points, Cameron simultaneously adopts all three—mutually contradictory—epidemiological theories of HIV transmission. The "gay plague" model serves his purpose of illustrating the vile homosexual life style he constantly and graphically seeks to expose. The generalized STD model serves to urge heterosexuals to remain chaste and to bash homosexuals for spreading the disease to good and decent folk. The casual contagion model serves to illustrate the Grand Conspiracy.

One media fallacy, however, was that those advocating Christian beliefs were vicious "I told you so-ers." As time went on, more Christian groups began to disavow the "God's wrath" theory. In the October 1988 issue of *Moody Monthly,* published by the fundamentalist Moody Bible Institute in Chicago, there appeared a 12-page section on AIDS patients and ways that Christians can minister to them. Included was a piece by a hospital chaplain relating his change of heart after meeting a man dying of AIDS and after asking himself why, if AIDS were God's judgment for homosexuality, lesbians didn't get it even while babies and transfusion recipients did.[59] An organization called AIDS Crisis and Christians Today was organized by a Nashville singer and songwriter in collusion with an evangelical writer and lecturer. One attested that he was "ashamed of what my attitude used to be" toward AIDS sufferers, and that Christians "need to be leading the way on AIDS because Jesus went to the lepers."[60]

A University of Virginia sociologist, Jeffrey Hadden, in a presentation before the 1988 World Congress of Political Science, stated that the widespread perception that Christian evangelicals believe AIDS to be God's plague on homosexuals had been created by the media but is inaccurate. After a broad survey of evangelical literature, Hadden concluded "that these general perceptions people have about 'fundamentalists' do not match the evidence very well."

He said that, to the degree that evangelicals have distorted the AIDS crisis, it has been in the unequivocal claim that only chastity and monogamous marriage can stem the epidemic, but added "It is inconceivable to me that they could take any other position."[61]

Ignoring the Drug Connection

Conservatives in power positions have to a great extent ignored the IV-drug aspect of AIDS, presumably because IV-drug abuse has nothing to do with syphilis or chastity. Given the overemphasis on heterosexual AIDS cases, this obliviousness is rather amazing. Over 80 percent of native-born American heterosexually transmitted cases occur in the partners of IV-drug abusers;[62] while close to 100 percent of males infected through heterosexual intercourse were the partners of IV-drug abusers, since the only other ways they can get it is through tertiary transmission (which, as noted earlier, is extremely rare) or intercourse with one of the tiny number of female transfusion victims. Yet at this writing, no conservative member of Congress has introduced legislation dealing directly with the AIDS/IV-drug connection.

Mention of the AIDS/IV-drug abuse connection was almost absent from the speeches of Secretary Bennett and Gary Bauer. Bennett's booklet, "AIDS and the Education of our Children," was put out in October 1987—some assert in response to the surgeon general's report, which many conservatives felt overemphasized condoms and under-emphasized moral restraint. Almost two million copies have been printed. A count of lines directly relating to sex and drugs in the intro-duction and body of the booklet reveals that fifteen sentences concern drugs only, thirteen concern both sex and drugs, three sentences con-cern exclusively homosexual intercourse, and two sentences exclusively heterosexual intercourse. By contrast, a whooping seventy-nine sen-tences make reference to sex in general, without mentioning drugs and without differentiating between homosexual and heterosexual inter-course. (Of these, eighteen were devoted to disparaging condom usage.) Nowhere is anal sex mentioned. What can be said of a man who objects to the surgeon general's report as being incomplete because it does not mention condom failure, whose own report fails to mention that anal sex is responsible for the overwhelming percentage of sexual transmis-sions of HIV? Nowhere is the reader told that cases of AIDS in men whose partners did not inject drugs are virtually nonexistent. This si-lence was all the more amazing given the Reagan administration's usual policy of inveighing against drug use at any possible opportunity. And the irony was fully brought home when the Bush administration later named Bennett as its so-called "drug czar."

By concentrating on virtually nonexistent heterosexual tertiary trans-mission, while ignoring the drug connection, chastity-pushing conser-vatives (along with their condom-pushing counterparts) ignored the opportunity to pass laws that could have had a serious impact on needle-transmitted AIDS and consequently heterosexually transmitted AIDS. Penalties could have been increased for the sale and possession of in-jectable drugs. Methadone programs could have been funded out of AIDS-earmarked monies so that everyone seeking treatment could get it immediately. But since none of these are suggested by the etiology of syphilis and have nothing to do with promoting chastity, they were ignored by Bennett and Bauer as well as by conservatives in Congress. The concentration on the tiny percentage of AIDS cases that were heterosexually transmitted was an enormous distraction of attention and funds from where the problems really lay. While conservative alarmists continued to pour water on a smoldering sapling, the forest fire continued to rage.

That Bennett was not about to let veracity get in the way of his booklet's chastity message is shown by what occurred at a meeting between White House officials and CDC officials on 16 September 1987. Bennett confronted the CDC's director, James Mason. Bennett said, "You mean this thing is not exploding into the heterosexual community?" Dr. Mason replied, "No, it's not." Whereupon Bennett said, "Well, why have you been telling everyone that it is?"[63] Why indeed? But why did Bennett then proceed with the mailing of his booklet, with a reprinting several months later?

Bauer had his own little problem with expertise contrary to his message when his staffer, James Warner, prepared a paper indicating that not only had the threat to heterosexuals been vastly overstated, but also the overall seropositivity estimates of the CDC were far too high.[64] So Bauer brought one of Bennett's staffers into his shop, a devotee of Robert Redfield associated with Americans for a Sound AIDS Policy. Warner was quickly pushed out of his AIDS position. Problem solved.

Warner says, however, that Bauer's deception probably applied to himself as well. "To my knowledge, he never really knew what was going on," Warner told me. In fact, "he didn't understand AIDS at all. All he knew was what was going on with evangelical groups, and things that were causing them discomfort he would kill and things they liked he would push and that was the total extent of his interest in AIDS."[65] When Bauer left the White House he became the chairman of the Family Research Council, an evangelical group.

Spoiled Chances

Despite their best efforts, whatever impact the conservative alarmists had, it probably paled in comparison with that of their liberal counterparts. Control of the White House was nothing compared with control of the media, and nobody on the conservative side had the punch of a liberal like Mathilde Krim. But conservatives as a whole, alarmist and non-alarmist, were also a distant second in taking advantage of a bad situation to effect long-term changes. For example, by successfully desensitizing the public to condoms, the long-term goal of liberals to provide greater access to and emphasis on birth control was clearly realized. Even more significant, sex education became universally accepted. But the conservatives who eagerly latched onto the heterosexual AIDS myth, in order to promote chastity or stigmatize homosexuals, played right into the hands of their opponents. By agreeing that the homosexual scourge had now become the heterosexual scourge, they lent credibility to the liberal democratizers and homosexuals who insisted there were no fundamental differences between homosexual sexual habits and heterosexual ones, save choice of orifice.

A few conservatives were able to resist becoming strange bedfellows with their liberal counterparts. The publisher and columnist Norman Podhoretz was able to take advantage of the disease to emphasize what he and his fellow conservatives regard as the degradation of the moral life style.[66] The columnist and director of media communications in the Reagan White House, Patrick J. Buchanan, did likewise. Buchanan's exhortation to "the poor homosexuals—they have declared war upon nature and now nature is exacting an awful retribution"[67] became one of the classic lines of the AIDS era. It cut so deeply into homosexuals' worst fears (both of Buchanan being right and of others thinking he was right) that, on the literary scene at least, he would become Enemy Number 1. (Ironically, a homosexual, Randy Shilts, would do a far more effective job of villifying homosexual sexual excesses, if only because he was a veteran of them.)[68] The *Washington Times,* second only to the *Wall Street Journal* in conservative influence, took the opposite tack of that paper, going on record denouncing what it called the "heterosexual AIDS myth."[69] The columnists George Will,[70] James J. Kilpatrick,[71] and the neoconservative Charles Krauthammer[72] applied traditional conservative skepticism to come to the conclusion that the threat to heterosexuals was being exaggerated. Buchanan, in fact, became the first nationally syndicated columnist to assert that the scope of the entire epidemic had been overstated;[73] and on a television show he co-hosts, "Crossfire," he found himself arguing against a homosexual who was asserting that heterosexuals would be the next to go.[74]

Another victory scored by conservatives was in shedding light on the policies of the Food and Drug Administration that result in holding up new drugs for years while Americans die of the diseases the drugs are supposed to treat. The *Wall Street Journal* fired salvo after salvo at the FDA[75] and was joined by the *National Review,*[76] the Competitive Enterprise Institute, and the Heritage Foundation.[77] This FDA policy had long been a sore spot with conservatives; AIDS provided the perfect opportunity to form a coalition with the left to attack it.

Yet these successes were few and far between. By tossing in their lot with the casual contagion kooks and the Bennett-Bauer axis of moralists, conservatives tossed away most of their chances. Most important, they shrugged off their responsibility to act *conservatively.* The father of modern conservatism is Edmund Burke, a British statesman best known for his inveighing against the excesses of the French Revolution long before they would become generally acknowledged. If conservatism means anything, it should mean restraint in the face of hysteria. This was exactly the view of Andrew Ferguson's dissent at the *American Spectator,* which, long after it no longer applied to that magazine, continued to apply to the conservative alarmists. Wrote Ferguson:

> This grotesque but recently voguish hysteria is ludicrous on its face, or anyway it should seem so to someone who prizes the principles on which this magazine is supposed to be based—limited government, prudence, and individual responsibility, to name a few. It is simply the latest version of the totalitarian flim-flam that is forever drawing believers from the ranks of the weak-minded and the perpetually alarmed.[78]

Conservatives, with their traditional skepticism of fads and their more modern distrust of the media, should have led the fight against the alarmists, instead of seeking to lead them. And when the federal AIDS budget began to strip away funds and researchers from other diseases, as I shall describe in detail in chapter 22, it should have been conservatives, with their traditional skepticism of government spending, who began to question whether this area of spending were not going out of control and being wasted. But having thrown in their lot with those predicting millions or tens of millions or hundreds of millions of deaths, the conservative alarmists had succeeded only in hamstringing themselves and their principles. Their real enemy here was not the liberals; it was the person who looked back at them from the shaving mirror.

14

The Homosexual Lobby

Nineteen sixty-nine was to prove a watershed year for homosexuals. In that year occurred two disparate events: one would lead to the homosexual population's great triumph; the other, to their greatest tragedy.

The first occurred in a bar in New York's Greenwich Village, the section of the city most heavily populated by open homosexuals. For years, police had routinely harassed the transvestite patrons of the Stonewall Inn; but that June the "drag queens" fought back, violently. The Stonewall riot sparked the gay liberation movement. Homosexuals, especially those in the big cities, fought for rights they felt had been denied since before the Old Testament proscribed death for their "abomination."[1]

Within the homosexual population, liberation meant many things to many different people. To some, it meant living without the fear of being fired or thrown out of one's apartment because of the public discovery of one's life style. To others, it meant migration to beautiful, liberal San Francisco, where they were able to elect leaders who were sympathetic to demands going far beyond merely being left alone, all the way to establishing quotas for homosexuals on the police force. To still others, liberation meant sexual liberation: being able to have sex with as many men as possible in as many ways as possible. "Whenever I threw my legs in the air," one AIDS victim remarked, "I thought I was doing my bit for gay liberation."[2] Bathhouses and bars with darkened back rooms began to proliferate, and sexually transmitted disease rates began to soar.* The incessant sexual activity prompted one doctor to

*In *AIDS in the Mind of America,* homosexual author Dennis Altman writes, "Large-scale luxurious pleasure palaces where everyone is potentially an immediate sexual partner are a common sexual fantasy; only for gay men they are a commonplace reality."[3] He goes on to say: "Men in bathhouses rarely talk much, and it is quite common for sex to take place without words, let alone names, being exchanged. . . . The willingness to have remark in 1980 that "if something new gets loose here, we're going to have hell to pay."[6]

In 1969 as well, fifteen hundred miles away from the Stonewall, a black youth in his early teens, called Robert R. by his doctors, died in a St. Louis hospital. He had been gradually wasting away and suffered from a case of chlamydia that his immune system seemed unable to combat. At autopsy, it was revealed that he had also suffered from Kaposi's sarcoma, a disease that sometimes struck elderly men of Mediterranean descent, but simply was not seen in persons of that young age. The doctors suspected the youth might have been a male prostitute, but had no reason to suspect that his malady had been the result of sexual transmission. Indeed, they had no idea what the underlying disease was, let alone how he'd gotten it. A battery of tests on his blood and tissue nearly two decades later revealed he had died of AIDS.[7]

The rest of the story is well known. What it is difficult for the average heterosexual fully to understand is how it felt for a homosexual to go from the heady days of "Gay Liberation" to the days of "Gay Related Immune Deficiency," or "GRID" as AIDS was first called, and finally to the days when it was expected that a few communities—Greenwich Village, the Castro in San Francisco, West Hollywood—would see death percentages higher than some European cities saw during the Black Death.

As if the death of vast numbers of one's friends, the destruction of one's community and life style, and the mortal terror for one's own life were not enough, there is still another factor to add to the agony of homosexuals. For their medieval counterparts suffering the scythe of the bubonic plague, at least death was more or less an equal opportunity employer. No country or town was left untouched. The rich, with their ability to retain doctors and perhaps flee town ahead of the crowd, fared better than the poor, but not by much.[8] But with the exception of IV-drug abusers—another class traditionally loathed by society—homosexuals are going it virtually alone.

The stigma associated with AIDS is horrific. Perhaps no disease in history, other than leprosy, has been so identified with uncleanliness as AIDS. In part, this attitude is probably because it is the only contagious disease that is always, or virtually always, fatal. It may also be because

---

sex immediately, promiscuously, with people about whom one knows nothing and from whom one demands only physical contact, can be seen as a sort of Whitmanesque democracy."[4] But, lest one think Altman necessarily disapproved, as late as 1982 he was defending bathhouses and the fast-lane homosexual culture in general.[5]

the symptoms of AIDS are particularly terrible. As opposed to, say, tuberculosis, which eats at the body from the inside, AIDS appears to eat away from the outside. The victims become emaciated and often are covered with lesions of Kaposi's sarcoma or herpes zoster (shingles). Death visibly announces its advent with repulsive symptoms.[9]

Particularly frustrating to homosexuals is the characterization of nonhomosexual, non–drug-abusing sufferers of AIDS as innocent victims. Wrote the *Village Voice*'s editor Richard Goldstein, "In AIDS we see our fate writ large, as the inchoate rage and revulsion that underlies homophobia resurfaces as concern for the 'innocent.' As if I am not innocent."[10] In addition to levying guilt on homosexuals for their own disease, the labeling of only those who get AIDS from donated blood or plasma as victims implies that they were victims of a culprit; since the vast majority of tainted blood has undoubtedly been from homosexuals, it is not paranoid for homosexuals to feel themselves blamed.

Given these circumstances, it is easy to see why so many homosexuals have been eager to promote the thesis of a general heterosexual breakout. They have been motivated by two major factors: denial, and the need for research funds.

Denial

Denial was a major feature of homosexual reaction to AIDS. For years the homosexual newspaper the *New York Native* attempted to persuade its readers that HIV was not the cause of AIDS. Articles abounded about AIDS victims who survived several years; and indeed these survivors, like self-proclaimed Kaposi's sarcoma "poster boy" Bobbi Campbell, were celebrated.[11]* When researchers began to express their belief that HIV infection might eventually prove fatal to virtually all seropositives, homosexuals reacted bitterly, just as they earlier railed against the term *AIDS test,* because it implied that all seropositives had or would have AIDS.[13] They even tried (and with many journalists and others succeeded) to alter the terminology of AIDS, insisting that "AIDS victim" or "AIDS sufferer" be changed to the more neutral-sounding "people with AIDS." This appellation was eventually modified to "people *living* with AIDS," in an attempt to

---

*The long-term survivor Michael Callen complains bitterly, "The unthinking repetition of the notion that everyone dies from AIDS denies both the reality of—but more importantly the possibility of—our survival."[12]

make a positive statement against the assumption that AIDS is a death sentence.[14]*

The executive director of the People with AIDS Coalition even went so far as to protest the obituary of the coalition's co-founder, Kenneth Meeks, telling the *New York Times* in a letter that, "the labeling of People with AIDS as 'victims' in [the] obit was incorrect and more so in light of Ken's extensive work to end such practices. We are greatly disappointed in such practices." The news editor of the *Times* wrote back that the term was not pejorative: "Along with most of society, we have long written about 'stroke victims,' 'heart attack victims,' and 'cancer victims.' The logic is equally applicable to AIDS, and I am uncomfortable about drying idiom [*sic*] for any cause, no matter how meritorious."[16]

The homosexual author Dennis Altman wrote in his acclaimed *AIDS in the Mind of America:* "From available evidence it appears that the Administration, particularly the White House, has collaborated in fostering the idea that AIDS should be seen as a gay issue rather than a health emergency which should transcend the characteristics of those involved."[17] Altman argued that "AIDS is American and homosexual only in the sense that the first group in which the disease was discovered was American homosexuals,"[18] and later asserted, "AIDS is intrinsically no more gay or American than Legionnaires's disease is an illness of ex-soldiers or than rubella (German measles) is inherently German."[19] The comparison is hardly fair: Germans do not account for 73 percent of all rubella victims, as did homosexuals of AIDS victims, at the time of Altman's writing; nor have the tens of thousands of American homosexuals who contracted AIDS all just happened to be in the wrong hotel at the wrong time. Altman is a highly intelligent writer, and *AIDS in the Mind of America* stands out as one of the few well-researched, generally worthwhile books written on AIDS. That even such a work stooped to fatuous reasoning to de-homosexualize the disease is telling evidence of the pervasiveness of denial.

---

*The "Statement of Purpose" of the National Association of People with AIDS states: "We do not see ourselves as victims. We will not be victimized. We have the right to be treated with respect, dignity, compassion, and understanding. We have the right to live fulfilling, productive lives—to live and die with dignity and compassion. . . . We are born of and inextricably bound to the historical struggle for rights—civil, feminist, disability, lesbian and gay, and human. We will not be denied our rights!"[15]

Research

"The plain fact of it is that this society wants homosexual people to die."[20] So stated one *Native* writer in explanation of why, seven years into the AIDS epidemic, the only antiviral drug approved for AIDS, AZT, was not only not especially effective but was itself potentially harmful and even lethal.

The belief that many heterosexuals did not see them as having equal worth prompted many homosexuals to assume early on that if AIDS continued to be perceived as strictly a problem of homosexuals and equally undesirable drug abusers, the funds needed to combat the disease would never materialize. That belief was by no means groundless. Dr. Joel Weisman, a Los Angeles private practitioner, told one writer, "I remember calling a person [in infectious diseases] to describe what was occurring. He said—and this was a theme very early on—'I don't know what you're making such a big deal of it for. If it kills a few of them off, it will make society a better place.' "[21] Members of the Ku Klux Klan paraded with signs declaring, "Praise God for AIDS."[22]

The homosexual activist and playwright Larry Kramer stated, "There is no question that if this epidemic were happening to the straight, white, non-intravenous drug using middle-class, that money would have been into use almost two years ago."[23]

The same view was held by Representative Henry Waxman (Democrat, of California), who chaired a subcommittee with oversight over the Public Health Service. Speaking in 1982, he said, "There is no doubt in my mind that if the same disease had appeared among Americans of Norwegian descent, or among tennis players, rather than among gay males, the response of both the government and the medical community would have been different."[24]

Randy Shilts makes a compelling argument that AIDS was initially severely underfunded despite the recommendations of some very knowledgeable health officials,[25] although it would seem he falls short of establishing that this underfunding was a direct result of antihomosexuality as opposed to the usual bureaucratic bungling and the fact that crises are usually mishandled. The scope of the AIDS epidemic was underestimated in the early 1980s just as Shilts maintains that with regard to non–drug-using heterosexuals it is now overstated.

In a statement that played right into the hands of those seeking drastic action (such as quarantine) against HIV carriers or homosexuals in general, the former president of the Texas Human Rights Foundation, dying of AIDS, proclaimed, "There has come the idea that if research money is not forthcoming at a certain level by a certain date, all gay males should give blood. . . . Whatever action is required to get national attention is valid. If that includes blood terrorism, so be it."[26]*

"A lot of gay people in AIDS organizations have spent years watching friends and lovers die," Shilts told me, and are convinced that research money has been slow in coming because AIDS is not perceived as a general threat. Hence, he says, the "concerted effort" to create heterosexual panic that is being made by "gays, public-health officials, and scientists who want research dollars."[28]

Shifting Blame

A common reaction to infectious diseases is the desire to blame them on somebody else. Thus, syphilis was the "French pox" to the English, *morbus Germanicus* to the Parisians, the "Naples sickness" to the Florentines, and the "Chinese disease" to the Japanese.[29] Italians called it the "French pox," which proved to be its most popular name; but the French called it the "Italian pox." The English also called it the "Spanish pox"; Poles called it the "German pox"; and Russians called it the "Polish pox,"[30] which was okay, because the Poles called it the disease of the Russians. The Persians labeled it the disease of the Turks; and the Japanese, when they weren't blaming the Chinese, also called it the disease of the Portuguese.[31] Of course, it remains a persistent belief that Columbus brought it back from America in 1492, thereby making it the disease of the Indians.

For homosexuals in the 1980s, pinning the blame on someone else meant sticking it to the intravenous-drug abusers, the Haitians, or the Africans. Thus, one writer countered a controversial antihomosexuality AIDS piece in the *Claremont Review of Books*[32] by declaring that "at least 79 percent of AIDS patients, gay and non-gay, have abused drugs"; thus, he conveniently blurred the distinction between intravenous drugs, which spread HIV, and non-intravenous drugs, which do not. He also cited a *Los Angeles Times* article describing a Harvard study that supposedly "traces AIDS in America to intravenous drug use, not to homosexuality."[33] In fact, the article quotes New York researcher Don Des Jarlais as saying that "the spread [is believed to be] from gays to drug users rather than vice versa."[34]

Writing in the *New York Native,* Dr. George E. Dematrakopoulos

*The Reverend Jerry Falwell would later, in a direct-mail letter to members of the Moral Majority, write that homosexuals "have expressed the attitude that 'they know they are going to die—and they are going to take as many people with them as they can.' "[27]

noted that there were 62 cases of AIDS per 100,000 Haitian immigrants in the United States and then stated:

> In view of the fact that approximately 17 to 22 million Americans pursue bisexual or homosexual lifestyles, while the adult Haitian immigrants in this country number well below 100,000, the incidence of AIDS in these two populations shows that the relative risk for contracting the syndrome is 5 per 100,000 for a bisexual and homosexual male. This fact alone indicates that if we are searching for an AIDS "causative agent" we'll have a much better chance of finding it among Haitian immigrants.
>
> Additionally, it has become known that occasional cases . . . began appearing in the United States as early as 1976 . . . a year or so after the 1975 influx of 20,000 "raft-boat" Haitian immigrants. . . . This may indicate that [AIDS was] indeed imported into the United States, which would, of course, mean that sexual lifestyles cannot be held responsible for the appearance of this agent.[35]

The calculations were a mess, including putting lesbians in the denominator in order to lower the homosexual ratio. Further, we now know that many of those Haitian cases were in men who had sex with men. But Dr. Dematrakopoulos's reasoning was typical of the effort to divert attention from the obvious.[36]

Homosexuals also sought to blame Africans. Wrote Arthur Frederick Ide in *AIDS Hysteria,* "When ministers get up to speak, they preach a message of depression and misinformation, lamenting the genesis of AIDS as a 'gay disease'—even though medical evidence . . . specifically proves that AIDS began among *heterosexuals* in Africa."[37] Ide is a member of the Dallas Gay Alliance and author of such works as *Gomorrah and the Rise of Homophobia*[38] and *City of Sodom and Homosexuality in Western Religious Thought to 603 CE.*[39]

Dennis Altman likewise complained:

> Thus a *Newsweek* story at the end of 1984 remarked that "even such remote countries as Rwanda and Zaire in Black Africa have reported AIDS cases," with no acknowledgment of the extent of the disease in these countries or of the theories that central Africa was the place where AIDS most likely originated. It is my experience that otherwise well-informed people have managed to ignore the reports from Africa that do exist, and that throw severe doubt on the whole concept of AIDS as a "gay disease."[40]

The Heterosexual Epidemic

Making other groups responsible for the origin of the disease was psychologically important for many homosexuals, but their primary goal was still to come up with facts, figures, and theories showing that AIDS was now exploding into the heterosexual population as well. One convoluted and ultimately self-defeating version of this argument was proposed by an antidiscrimination lawyer in the *Native*. Lee Oliver, in "AIDS and the Heterosexual Myth: The Scapegoating of the Gay Male Population," declared that even if AIDS were a homosexual disease, it would still affect a tremendous portion of the heterosexual population, because so many so-called heterosexuals engage in homosexual practices. Oliver said that the Kinsey data indicated, "Only 50 percent of all men are exclusively heterosexual throughout their adult lives. One of every two men you meet have sexual responses to men and 37 percent have sexual relations with men during the course of their lives."[41] He added, "we have never been told that more than a third of the *adult* American male population is at risk for AIDS, even if AIDS only struck men who have sex with men."[42]

In fact, the Kinsey bisexuality figures are the most controversial in his book, in part because he recruited participants out of prison where one might expect more homosexual contacts either through lack of women or through rape. (A more recent survey by the Kinsey Institute, published in *Science* magazine in January 1989, found the number of men with at least one homosexual experience to be only 20 percent.)[43] In any case, it hardly follows that a man who engaged in one act of insertive oral intercourse with a man some thirty years earlier now threatens his wife with AIDS. Yet it is this man and his fellows who allow the Kinsey figures to expand all the way up to 37 percent. And although Oliver's argument is intended to disprove the link between AIDS and homosexuality, in fact he ends up stating that even a single homosexual experience puts one at substantial risk for AIDS,[44] and thereby defeats his entire purpose.

While it was rare for a homosexual or a homosexual ally to come right out and say in public that it's good to exaggerate the threat of heterosexual AIDS in order to generate research funds, a column by George Will, saying the threat to heterosexuals had been greatly overstated,[45] elicited just such a response from a physician named Neil Ravin, who stated, "There is now the likelihood that the heterosexual majority will be less keen to support research for a disease that is confined to a rather unpopular minority."[46]

Indeed, while many of the nonhomosexual alarmists cheerfully set about calling press conferences, writing books, and sending out newsletters to spread the myth of the heterosexual epidemic, had homosexuals tried to do the same it would surely have been looked upon with a suspicious eye. Thus, many of them, like Neil Ravin, reserved their disinformation for making rebuttals against those who claimed the disease was remaining confined to the old risk groups. After the columnist James J. Kilpatrick's column "Aren't We Overreacting to AIDS?" appeared in the *Washington Post*, homosexuals (or their supporters; most homosexuals don't identify themselves as such in letters) poured out of the woodwork to challenge his assertion that a disease limited to a small proportion of the population deserved only a concomitant share of attention and resources. One homosexual declared, "AIDS is *contagious* and is spreading very rapidly in the United States, with decreasing discrimination." (An odd choice of words: to say that it is discriminating less is to admit that it nonetheless discriminates.) Another declared that 1.5 million Americans were infected, "a rapidly growing figure," after the Centers for Disease Control had already *lowered* its top-end estimate from 1.5 million to 1.4 million. Another stated, "This type of article does no one any good. . . . It is simply a way to say (quite ignorantly) that white, upper-middle-class, heterosexual Americans should not have to worry about or pay for AIDS."[47]

One homosexual activist who wages an active campaign of disinformation is Robert Kunst, a tireless self-promoter who takes personal credit for "throwing Anita Bryant out of Dade County and the State of Florida."[48] Kunst directs a group called Cure AIDS Now in the Miami area, and claims to have "participated in 1,500 radio, television, conference, and lecture forums in 1987."[49] Puffery, to be sure, but he is not without influence. Kunst in his newsletter talks about the infections of "600,000 Americans doubling annually," with "millions of carriers who don't know it."[50] Kunst also related that there were 100 million persons infected in the world "doubling annually."[51] Some of his material had grains of truth; some was simply made up. He attributed a figure of "100 to 160 million infections around the world in the next five years"[52] to the U.S. Government Accounting Office, which, in its only publication dealing with the world AIDS problem, merely repeated the WHO estimate of as many as 100,000,000 infections by 1991.[53] He has also quoted the 1 February 1987 *New England Journal of Medicine* as stating, "It is estimated that in the United States, for every one individual diagnosed with the disease, another 300 individuals may be infected."[54] There was no issue of this journal with that date. Kunst also throws the word *heterosexual* around whenever possible, continually noting that "40 percent of our caseload [in Florida] is heterosexual,"[55] or that Florida has a "40 percent heterosexual factor,"[56] both of which simply mean that since, like New York and New Jersey, Florida has a terrible drug problem, its percentage of heterosexual IVDA cases is exceptionally high. Not incidentally, Kunst believes his figures strongly support substantial increases for AIDS research funding. His declarations of doom are regularly accompanied by calls for $5 billion in AIDS research spending a year.[57]

Obviously Kunst has credibility problems, but this has not stopped the media from treating him as an authority on epidemiology. Thus, a UPI story stated, "Kunst said state statistics show 40,000 Florida residents have AIDS-related complex, or 'pre-AIDS,' with at least 500,000 to one million infected with the AIDS virus without showing symptoms."[58] Had UPI's reporter bothered to call state authorities, he would have found that Florida keeps no figures on AIDS-related complex or on asymptomatic seropositives. It should also have occurred to the reporter that Florida would probably not have up to two thirds of the AIDS infections in the entire nation. But as was so often their wont, the media relied on the figures of a highly partial advocate, at least when those figures made good copy.

Defending the Kinsey Myth

In July 1988, the *New York Times* ran an article[59] that quoted community leaders' responses to the news that AIDS researchers were coming to a consensus that almost all seropositives, of which New York had an estimated 400,000, would eventually fall ill.[60] Said the chairman of New York State's AIDS Advisory Council, "I shudder to think what happens if we try to put 400,000 people into the system without better preparation than we have shown to date."[61] A spokesman for the Gay Men's Health Crisis, a major private agency, said the projection was "numbing, absolutely numbing."[62] Mathilde Krim rounded the New York City Department of Health figure up to half a million *and* accelerated the incubation rate by assuming they would all die within a decade: "Half a million people are going to die here in the next 10 years."[63]

No one quoted by the article noted that the 400,000 figure was completely at odds with the CDC estimate of 1,000,000 to 1,400,000 infections in the nation and with the Department of Health's estimate that 15 percent of those cases would be New Yorkers.[64] The resulting figure would be 142,000 to 210,000—half the New York figure.* Nor did

---

*New Yorkers currently make up one fifth of all AIDS cases. But their proportion to the nation's cases continues to drop. Because of the time lag between initial infection and full-blown AIDS, we may infer that New York has fewer than one fifth of the nation's HIV

anyone quoted by the article note that the 400,000 figure was incompatible with the peaking of new AIDS cases in the city at less than 20,000, as will be discussed in chapter 21.

Thus, it came as a shock when the following week the New York City Department of Health released new figures slicing the old estimate in half. The adjustment was necessitated by the reduction of the estimate of infected New York homosexuals in the city from 250,000 to 50,000. According to the director of the Department of Health, Stephen Joseph, "Our previous estimates were based upon extrapolation from data published by Kinsey several decades ago, estimating that one out of ten men engaged in homosexual behavior."[65] The new estimate, he explained, was based on more refined estimates of the number of homosexuals in San Francisco, which a telephone poll in 1984 indicated to be about 56,000, including bisexuals.

> For some time . . . Health Department researchers have noted a disparity between the ratio of AIDS cases to the estimated number of gay men in New York City versus San Francisco: New York City, with a total population ten times that of San Francisco, has been estimated to have a population of gay men several times larger than San Francisco's, yet its AIDS caseload of homosexual men is less than twice that.[66]

On the assumption that the ratio of seropositive homosexual men with AIDS to the total number of homosexual men is about the same in the two cities, "that would produce," said Joseph, "an estimate of 50,000 HIV-infected gay men in New York City, rather than the previously estimated 200,000 to 250,000."[67]

With the 400,000 figure generating such dread, one might think that the revised, lower estimate would cause an outpouring of relief and joy. Not a chance. Members of a homosexual activist group called the AIDS Coalition to Unleash Power (ACT-UP), which concentrates primarily on promoting the curing and patient care of those now suffering from the HIV, besieged Joseph. They heckled him at public appearances, disrupted his private meetings, and demanded his resignation. Joseph says he has also received hostile phone calls at home and at work.[68] Twelve ACT-UP members were arrested at a sit-in outside his office.[69] The *New York Native*, the city's primary homosexual newspaper, later depicted Joseph on its cover with a Cheshire-cat grin, spouting mumbo-jumbo about the number of seropositives in the city.[70] "It's the statistical cure

---

infections. Yet one fifth of even CDC's top-end figure of 1,400,000 would still only be 280,000.

of AIDS," said Dr. Barry Leibowitz, president of the Doctors Council, a union representing physicians on the Health Department staff and at several hospitals. He said he feared damage from the new estimate "being used to give us less when we desperately need more" funds and services to treat current as well as future patients.[71]

But the lowered estimate was a cure for nothing except an earlier faulty estimate, and Joseph and his staff were quick to point out that the estimates upon which the city planned its medical services were not based on the estimate of seropositivity. Instead, they were calculated from the projected caseload for the next three years, a mathematical extrapolation from the present caseload trend.

The bitter reaction of the New York homosexual population to the new figure was a natural response to a double whammy. First, homosexuals worried that the reduced estimate might reduce the impetus to find a cure. But, second, any dramatic reduction of the size of the homosexual population seriously threatens their own power base. Could the long-assumed Kinsey "10 percent" be just a myth?

According to lore, Alfred Kinsey, in his landmark 1948 study, found that 10 percent of all Americans are homosexual.[72] The importance of this 40-year-old statistical assumption to the cause of the acceptance of homosexuality in our society simply cannot be overstated. "We are everywhere!" was one of the rallying cries of the Gay Liberation Movement. The 10-percent figure is also regularly employed as a lobbying tool by such groups as the National Gay and Lesbian Task Force (NGLTF), which claims to represent "20 million gay and lesbian persons"[73] (presumably children are excluded), and by the Human Rights Campaign Fund, a homosexual political action committee which, in an AIDS lobbying effort, declared "there are 12 million registered gay voters."[74]

But the fact is that Kinsey never gave any such 10-percent figure. What he said was that 10 percent of males are "more or less exclusively homosexual for at least three years between the ages of 16 and 55."[75] Dropping the "more or less," and the "three years" reduces to 4 percent the figure that Kinsey says applies to men who are exclusively homosexual throughout their lives.[76] A new Kinsey Institute report, conducted in 1970 but just released in 1989, found this number to be substantially lower at only 1.4 percent, providing support for those who have long argued that Alfred Kinsey's methodology tended to exaggerate the level of male homosexuality in the population.* Further, the

*In their conclusion the authors note, "it is estimated that 1.4 percent of men had adult homosexual contacts (for example, at age 20 years and older) whose frequency was characterized as being fairly often (at some point in time). An additional 1.9 percent of

Kinsey studies indicated that there are far fewer lesbians than male homosexuals.*

Whether for purposes of deciding who is represented by the NGLTF or who has HIV, the 10-percent figure hardly seems a good indicator. Nevertheless, it is the 10-percent figure that New York had used for its 400,000 figure. (The CDC, by contrast, uses the 4-percent figure in its calculations.)[79]

Buffeted by AIDS, by the public scrutiny the epidemic has brought to the homosexual population and its sexual practices, and by the inherent stigma in being identified with a particularly hideous disease, the last thing homosexual activists wanted to hear was that they are far rarer than had been popularly believed. Indeed, at least one conservative columnist, Patrick Buchanan, picked up on the New York figures and used them to assert just that.[80]

Such was the outcry at the new figures that New York City quickly came up with yet another estimate. This time it covered itself in two ways. First, it took a hint from the CDC and set a *range* of seropositivity—from 149,000 to 229,000—effectively allowing its estimate to go even lower. Next, it denied that its lower estimate necessarily meant that there were fewer homosexuals in the city than previously believed. "A number of commentators have inferred that our new estimate of infection strongly implies that the male gay/bisexual population . . . is much smaller than the 250,000–500,000 commonly asserted," said the report.[81] Instead, it stated that the lowered number of infected homosexuals could simply mean that the percentage of homosexuals infected was much smaller than previously believed.[82]

It indeed is possible that seropositivity levels are much lower than previously believed. Estimates of seropositivity in New York are based

---

men had adult experiences whose frequency was characterized as occasionally. Taken together, these two groups made up 3.3 percent of the adult male population, . . . Overall, these numbers appear similar to the 1948 Kinsey estimate used by the Public Health Service in its projections (that is, that 4 percent of the U.S. men are 'exclusively homosexual' throughout their lives). In fact, the interpretation of our estimates is different. Most of the men included in our 3.3 percent estimate could not be classified as exclusively homosexual throughout their lives. Thus . . . men who are currently or were previously married (who are a much larger segment of the total population) account for the majority of men who would be included in our estimate that 3.3 percent of adult men in 1970 had same-gender sexual contacts during adulthood whose frequency (at their peak) was characterized as 'fairly often' (1.4 percent) or 'occasional' (1.9 percent)."[77]

*"The incidence and frequencies of homosexual responses and contacts, and consequently the incidence of the homosexual ratings, were much lower among the females in our sample than they were among the males on whom we have previously reported [citing *Sexual Behavior in the Human Male*]"—a conclusion they say is confirmed by three other authors.[78]

on sampling at STD clinics which might well be unrepresentative of most homosexuals. But this rationale clearly contradicts Joseph's earlier statements. There can be no other conclusion but that Joseph was saying New York had little more than twice as many homosexuals as San Francisco's 56,000, and that therefore New York's homosexual population is far below the alleged Kinsey 10 percent. Further, the explanation that it might not be that there are fewer homosexuals, just fewer infected individuals, is an implicit rejection of the validity of San Francisco's seropositivity studies, occurring in the New York City explanatory report just pages after the phrase, "San Francisco has been able to develop a *reliable* estimate of the size of its gay/bisexual population *and its seroprevalence"* (emphasis added).[83] In order to keep the homosexual level in New York at 250,000, the seropositivity level would have to be reduced from 50 percent to about 20 percent. San Francisco's seropositivity studies all indicate that about 50 percent of that city's homosexuals are infected.

Nevertheless, as convoluted and inconsistent as this new explanation was, it helped get New York City off the hook with angry homosexuals. Joseph also used the new explanation to blast columnist Buchanan, accusing him of advancing "an agenda of bigotry and divisiveness,"[84] notwithstanding that the *New York Times* had come to the same obvious conclusion that Buchanan had, stating "the methodology suggests that the homosexual and bisexual population . . . is only 100,000."[85]

As to the true level of seropositivity among homosexuals, the explanation for the lack of infected homosexuals is probably a combination of both fewer homosexuals and lowered levels of seropositivity. Kinsey properly rated homosexuals on a continuum instead of making a flat calculation. Similar caution should prevent us from offering a flat figure for the number of homosexuals who are seropositive. If one regards any man who has ever engaged in a sex act with another man as a homosexual, then the degree of seropositivity among homosexuals is probably quite low. If one regards this category as comprising only those who engage in a fairly active homosexual life style (what most of us regard as being homosexual), open or closeted, then the seropositive rate is probably quite high. In any case, the myth of the Kinsey 10 percent could prove to be yet another casualty of the AIDS epidemic.

Having viewed the political pitfalls New York City encountered with its estimates, the New York State Department of Health stuck its fingers into the political winds and was much more circumspect. It announced that it would not rely upon the new New York seropositivity estimate;[86] and in December 1988, completely ignoring the plateauing or near-plateauing of actual cases in the city, New York State health officials extended their projections to show an unabated increase in cases for the next five years.[87]

On another occasion, ACT-UP showed its willingness to take to the streets to fight the assertion that AIDS would remain essentially confined to homosexuals and drug abusers. This occurred after *Cosmopolitan* published Dr. Gould's January 1988 article, "Reassuring News About AIDS."[88] One hundred fifty ACT-UP members picketed the magazine's headquarters in New York chanting, among other things, "For every *Cosmo* lie, more women die."[89] But Gould, a long-time supporter of homosexual rights, told me that at least part of this action was due to their fear that portraying most heterosexuals as being safe from the disease would increase homophobia and hurt their efforts to generate more research funds.

The Intellectual Dissent

If exaggerating the heterosexual threat of AIDS was the basic rule among homosexual spokespersons and publications—or the "party line," as Professor Arthur Leonard, of New York Law School, put it—it was not without exceptions. One came from Leonard himself. Writing in the *New York Native,* Leonard first laid the epidemiological groundwork for the non-epidemic among heterosexuals by using New York City Department of Health statistics. He did the job so well that it was difficult for any reader to refute his statement that, "however much we may be enchanted by the 'party line' about heterosexual transmission that has finally focused the attention of the media, the public, and the government on AIDS, heterosexual men are, next to lesbians, probably the least threatened by AIDS *as a sexually transmitted disease* [that is, apart from IV-drug use]."[90]

"In the long run" he went on,

> I don't think it does us much good to continue insisting that heterosexual men are at serious risk for sexually transmitted AIDS, or that there will be a major shift toward heterosexual transmission in both directions. . . . The "party line" about heterosexual transmission may do more harm than good by deflecting attention from groups who need the most help in protecting themselves from this epidemic: gay or bisexual men, IV-drug users, and women whose sexual partners come from the first two groups.

Concluded Leonard, "The facts are bad enough without perpetuating mythologies of our own."[91]

The nation's foremost homosexual AIDS writer, Randy Shilts, has also spoken out on the subject of the exaggerated threat to heterosexuals: "The people getting AIDS today are the people who largely were getting AIDS three and four years ago," he said in 1988.[92]

Indeed, some homosexuals have reacted bitterly to the media's exaggeration of the AIDS threat to heterosexuals while often ignoring the plight of homosexuals. Wrote one:

> TV treats us to nauseating processions of yuppie women announcing to the world that they will no longer put out for their yuppie boyfriends unless these boyfriends agree to use a condom. Thus hundreds of thousands of gay men and IV drug users, who have reason to think that they may be infected with HIV, or who know that they are . . . are asked to sympathize with all those yuppettes agonizing over whether they're going to risk losing [an opportunity for intercourse] by taking the "unfeminine" initiative of interrupting the invading male in order to insist that he practice safe sex.[93]

Backlash

There was another highly undesirable fallout from exaggerating the risks to heterosexuals that even Leonard did not pinpoint. A dark but predictable side of human nature is that any mysterious epidemic will give rise to scapegoating. During the Black Death, Jews were blamed for causing the pestilence by poisoning the wells. Although Jews sickened and died at the same rate as anyone else, in many places they were seized and burned.[94] It was not until half a millennium later that Europeans learned that it was not Jews but rats and fleas that wiped out up to a third of their population. By asserting that AIDS is not a localized epidemic but one that, while hitting them first, was destined to hit everyone, homosexuals perhaps even *increased* their stigma. For now not only were their sexual practices and life styles in general looked upon with suspicion or outright disgust; but, indeed, they were setting themselves up as the rats and fleas of the new plague. Those already disinclined to homosexuality had a field day—several years of field days.

While quarantining never got off the ground, frustration at homosexuals perceived as plague carriers was enough to prompt a large increase in homosexual beatings. According to the National Gay and Lesbian Task Force,

> Negative attitudes toward gay people as a result of the AIDS epidemic contributed to the problem of anti-gay violence in 1987: 15 percent (1,042) of all incidents reported for last year, and five percent (40) of the physical assaults, were known to have involved verbal references to AIDS by the

perpetrators or were directed against persons with AIDS. As in 1986, nearly two-thirds (63 percent) of the local groups reporting anti-gay episodes in 1987 believed that fear and hatred associated with AIDS has fostered anti-gay violence in their communities.[95]

In New York City alone, reported attacks on homosexuals jumped from 176 in 1984 to 517 in 1987, with much, if not most, of the increase attributed to AIDS.[96]

Among AIDS-related assaults:

- A Brooklyn homosexual was assailed by three youths who shouted, "You faggots give us AIDS!" then knocked him to the ground, and kicked him in the face and side. "Don't make him bleed!" cried one of the youths. "If he bleeds on you, you'll get AIDS!" They left him lying in the gutter.[97]
- A male nurse, walking on a lower Manhattan street, was attacked by a man with a hammer who thought he had AIDS. The nurse was hospitalized for a month.[98]
- In San Francisco, a youth who admitted beating up a homosexual man called a gay-crisis hot line hours later and asked whether there was any chance he had contracted AIDS in the attack.[99]
- Members of New York's Gay and Lesbian Big Apple band were pelted with eggs during a ninety-minute outdoor concert in Queens by 30 youths who, one said, feared the band was "bringing AIDS into the park."[100]
- Yelling "Diseased faggot!" a gang of teenagers assaulted a homosexual man on the streets of Seattle and raped him with a crowbar.[101]
- A man was walking through a supermarket parking lot with his groceries when someone shouted, "You faggots are killing us with AIDS!" He was pushed, bashed in the head with a chain, kicked, and beaten to the ground with a skateboard. The victim's jaw was broken and had to be wired for several months in order for it to heal.[102]

Of course, it is impossible to say whether all of these acts were really prompted by fear or loathing of AIDS. Some assaults on homosexuals no doubt would have occurred anyway; AIDS just provided a handy excuse.[103] But no doubt some of the beatings were over AIDS. As the journalist D. Keith Mano, who, incidentally, didn't buy into the "everybody's going to get it" theory, put it:

Gay men . . . stand to AIDS as the Broad Street pump stood to cholera. About this there is understandable ill-feeling. We have all been inconvenienced to a degree. One of those street hoods might have lost some sexual opportunity because Miranda or Chi-Chi wouldn't do it without rubber assurance.

Concluded Mano, "This isn't a good time to be gay."[104]

Certainly it seems that many homosexuals who spread the myth of the heterosexual epidemic did seem to miss an important point. If there were a heterosexual "breakout," it *could be* an inevitable occurrence; one that would occur regardless of whether there was a single homosexual in the United States. But the other way of looking at it is the way Mano's hoods did: that homosexuals are the vectors of plague; that but for them, there would be little or no AIDS here. On the whole, the homosexuals accomplished their task. In league with the democratizers, the media, the alarmist doctors, and their unwitting allies, the conservative moralists, they pumped up the nation's fear and pumped up the research funds. But just as the conservative moralists were shocked to find heterosexuals accepting their prescription for fear without accepting their proscription on premarital sex, so too would the homosexuals have to deal with unexpected fallout from their deceptions.

It would seem that if any group had an excuse for exaggerating the threat of AIDS to heterosexuals, it would be the homosexuals. While some homosexuals stridently demanded a cure for AIDS so they could march right back to the bathhouses without fear of infection, many just wanted to live. With some authorities citing infection rates as high as 70 percent to 90 percent in some homosexual communities,* not only did many homosexuals simply assume they were seropositive without bothering to get tested, but they assumed that even if they were not seropositive, probably most of their friends were. If heterosexual fear were needed to prime the research pump, then so it would be. However understandable this motivation, it does not alter the truth that, like their heterosexual alarmist counterparts, they were deceivers nonetheless.

---

*For example: "Current estimates indicate infection in sexually active homosexual men in San Francisco and New York to be 70–90 percent";[105] and, "In New York City, it is estimated that . . . 70 percent of homosexuals and bisexuals carry the virus."[106]

15

AIDS
Goes to Hollywood

While propaganda has a long history, celluloid and videotape and the realism they impart have added a new dimension to the trade. In fact, one of the first full-length dramatic motion pictures ever made was D. W. Griffith's *Birth of a Nation* (1915), which many people viewed as depicting the heroism of the Ku Klux Klan. Eisenstein's *Potemkin* (1925) revealed the horror under which many people lived and worked in czarist Russia. During the Great Depression, such films as *Our Daily Bread* (1934) and *The Grapes of Wrath* (1940) pushed the cause of socialist collectivism; and when the nation went to war, it did so with explanations provided by such as Frank Capra's *Why We Fight* (1942–45), John Huston's *Battle of San Pedro* (1948), and the John Wayne film *Sands of Iwo Jima* (1949). More recently, the 1980s saw a spate of antinuclear movies—*The China Syndrome* (1979), *The Day After* (1983), *Testament* (1983)—along with such counterreactions as *Red Dawn* (1984) and the *Rambo* series.

The involvement of the entertainment industry in the fight against sexually transmitted diseases actually predates public cinema. In 1913, the social hygiene campaign (promoting morality to prevent venereal disease) came to Broadway with *Damaged Goods*. The play followed the tragic story of George Dupont who, though warned by his physician that a recently incurred syphilitic infection forbids his forthcoming society marriage, ignores the advice after consulting a quack. The result of his folly is that he infects his newborn child, his wife, and the wet-nurse.[1]

It was thus inevitable that Hollywood would get into AIDS. And while the industry was slow to warm to the subject, when it did so it was with a vengeance, launching probably its greatest concentrated propaganda effort since the Second World War. This time, however, the enemy was not the jackbooted Nazi or the treacherous yellow Jap, but the prejudice and ignorance surrounding AIDS. The prejudice was the fear of casual contagion from homosexuals, and the "ignorance" was that this was somehow a homosexual disease that heterosexuals need have little fear of contracting.

Early in the government's anti-AIDS blitz, it began calling on well-known actors to make public service announcements. Ted Danson of "Cheers" told us: "Anyone. Any type can get it."[2] Jimmy Smits of "L.A. Law" declared: "AIDS has touched all of us."[3] But heterosexual AIDS did not really hit Hollywood until 1988, a year after it had already peaked in the news media. One film released that year, *Casual Sex?*, begins with Lea Thompson speaking to the audience: "I remember a time when sex was fun, when I said, 'That was great. What's your name?' Now sex is scary."[4] Indeed, the very title of the movie reflected the new concern. When the show originally appeared as a play, the title had no question mark. As it turns out, both Lea Thompson's character and that of her best friend end up having sex with two men apiece, some of whom they barely even know. Apparently throwing in the question mark, a few condom jokes, and a single allusion to AIDS (without saying the word) was enough to give this sexy romp an SC rating (Socially Conscious).

Some producers insisted that what the customer wanted was less sex. "I don't think many people are writing sex-oriented scripts, because they're not in demand," said the screenwriter Leslie Dixon of *Outrageous Fortune* fame. "*Risky Business* [in which Tom Cruise turns his parents' house into a temporary brothel] could not be made now. Everybody's got to be thinking, 'Are all these kids gonna get diseases from these women?' Besides, the hero is too unrepentant."[5]

One writer quoted the executive vice president of production at Columbia studios as saying, "Every script we look at where [AIDS] might be an issue, questions get asked: 'Would so-and-so have that kind of casual involvement.' Even James Bond only slept with two women in the last movie, instead of the usual six."[6]

Several movies in 1988 were reportedly "desexed" en route from script to screen. Originally the script for *Vibes* contained a scene described as "fairly raunchy" between the stars Jeff Goldblum and Cyndi Lauper. But neither the director nor those of Lauper's fans who were polled seemed too happy about it. The scene was dropped, but the

movie flopped anyway. In *Bull Durham,* considered one of the sexiest
movies of the year, a major scene was originally shot in a whorehouse,
with the star, Kevin Costner, surrounded by prostitutes. But, recalled
the writer-director of the film, "the reaction [by preview audiences]
was so overwhelming, we reshot it in a poolroom."[7]

Asked if he thought the movie industry was acting responsibly in the
face of AIDS, Screen Actors Guild Chairman Jack Valenti stated, "Oh,
absolutely. . . . I think casual sex is almost verboten in movies today."[8]
Nor was desexualization of the cinema simply the result of a *zeitgeist.*
In fact, in May 1988, the Director's Guild sent its membership a list of
guidelines (which it described as a "resource") "regarding the depiction
of AIDS and AIDS-related issues." Among the eleven points: "Indicate
consequences of unprotected sex," said one. "Recognize and respect
abstinence," said a second. "Depict casual sex only if it is important to
the story," said a third.[9]

The guidelines did not sit well with all directors; indeed, one referred
to the list as the "new Hays Code."* "I'm living my life ignoring it
[AIDS] and I'm making my films the same way," said another. "They
took smoking out of movies. Now are they going to get rid of kissing and
sex? Men and women have enough trouble getting together without
this. What will happen to instinct?"[10]

Some filmmakers opted for a "sex isn't everything" approach. Such
was the case with *Cocktail,* in which Tom Cruise plays a bartender.
Everybody assumes that bartenders go home with a different girl each
night, especially when they look like Tom Cruise. Not this one,
though. "*Cocktail* is the first post-crash movie," said the screenwriter
Heywood Gould. In Cruise's world, "there's sex all over the place.
He tries to hustle rich older women, but he finds that it's not for
him. He's rejecting promiscuous sex while endorsing family life and
working-class values."[11]

Still, if *Cocktail* was a positive portrayal of the importance of the
family and traditional values—the carrot, as it were—the hit movie of
1987 portrayed the stick. *Fatal Attraction* did for adultery and one-
night stands what *Reefer Madness* was supposed to do for marijuana. A
man with everything going for him—a beautiful, loving wife, a darling
little girl complete with pet rabbit, a new home in the 'burbs—never-

---

*From 1922 to 1966, the Hays Code, named after Will Harrison Hays (1879–1954), an
attorney, politician, and motion-picture executive, prevented the showing of not only
nudity and explicit sex but even of certain allusions to sex: for example, a film could not
show a husband and wife in a single bed, and couples "necking" on a couch had to have
at least one foot each on the floor.

theless risks it all for a couple of nights of passion with a svelte but not especially attractive co-worker. He tries to leave his one-weekend stand at just that, but she does not see things his way. Before the movie is out, she has boiled the bunny, kidnaped the kid, washed the man's car with acid, and tried to turn his wife into strip steak. A man who risks everything near and dear for a night of passion. It almost sounds like . . . AIDS?

But if the movies chose to speak more in terms of metaphors or the humorous allusions of *Casual Sex?*, the small screen was decidedly more direct with its message. In some cases, promiscuous characters had their sex lives seriously toned down. Sergeant Christine Cagney of CBS's landmark "Cagney & Lacy" police series was for several seasons a sexually freewheeling woman. But, said the executive producer, "It became clear to us that we were sending an improper or irresponsible message to the public."[12] The plan to reform the detective consisted of having her go celibate for the first half of the season. Then she would have her first "blue-collar relationship" which would reflect her gradual awareness of the dangers of unsafe sex.

Other TV programs gave unabashed lectures to their audiences. In one episode of the immensely popular yuppie NBC series "L.A. Law," the attorney Douglas Brackman is humiliated when a woman with whom he has cavorted barges into the law offices to berate him. Later, in the men's room, he encounters the law firm's premier womanizer, Arnold Becker:

BRACKMAN: Don't start.
BECKER: [*Shrugs*] Hell hath no fury. I just hope you used protection.
BRACKMAN: If you mean you think she might enmesh me into a paternity situation, I can assure you I made certain she was on the pill.
BECKER: Not her. You. A Condom? AIDS, Douglas? The second coming of the black plague?
BRACKMAN: AIDS?
BECKER: If you're going to practice surgery, take it from someone who knows: Never operate without your gloves on.
BRACKMAN: What are you talking about? Heterosexuals aren't at risk. I read an article about it in *Playboy*.

At this point Becker berates Brackman for believing everything he reads (television, perhaps, is an inherently better source of medical information?) and launches into his mathematical formula, presented in chapter 6, concluding "any time you hit the sheets with someone new, you link yourself up virally to about half the world population."[13]

One might think that an attorney at a high-priced Los Angeles firm would see the inanity of the likelihood of a single act of intercourse exposing one to the diseases of half the world's population. Yet, when confronted with such simplistic arguments supporting a heterosexual epidemic, TV fall guys invariably fell apart.

One "Designing Women" segment, called "Killing All the Right People," wrapped a tremendous number of heterosexual AIDS clichés into one half-hour show, notwithstanding that it concerned a *homosexual* friend of the attractive quartet who has been diagnosed with AIDS. The victim, a handsome, masculine twenty-four-year-old man, is lauded by the women individually just before he makes his entrance. Upon so doing, he quickly gets down to the point. He has AIDS and he wants the designing women to design his funeral.

After overcoming the shock, one woman exclaims to him, "I didn't even know you were gay!" He replies, "Well, I am, but you don't have to be. You should have seen the hospital where I was just in. On one side of me I had this sixty-five-year-old grandfather who got it from a blood transfusion, and on the other an eighteen-year-old girl who got it from her boyfriend who got it from a girl he used to date."[14]

(The section up to here was rebroadcast as the introduction to "Geraldo" 's "Women and AIDS" segment.)[15]

> "Is your family here?" asks another of the sympathetic young ladies.
> "No," he replies, "they're pretty upset."
> "I can imagine."
> "Actually, they're more upset about the gay part. They didn't know."[16]

Despite the heavy-handedness of the propaganda, or more probably because of it, homosexual groups were unabashed in their praise of the episode. As a result of the show, producer Linda Bloodworth-Thomason's series won the Award of Merit from the Alliance of Gay and Lesbian Artists, and was given the first Humanitarian Award from the Funders' Concern About AIDS. *USA Today* called it one of "Designing Women's" "most accomplished episodes" and said "it is a sure bet for Emmy consideration this year,"[17] while Surgeon General Koop called it "the best thing I've seen done on AIDS in movies or TV."[18]

If there was one reason to praise "Designing Women," it was that it actually featured a homosexual. More often than not, Hollywood AIDS victims were anything but. Stated one wire story:

> The subject of AIDS . . . is now becoming a hot topic in entertainment programming. In the next two weeks, TV characters will contract AIDS on

the medical show "St. Elsewhere," the youth-oriented sitcom "Mr. Belvedere," and the light drama series, "Hotel." Most AIDS cases have occurred in male homosexuals and intravenous drug users, but the three series chose to create stories around examples of AIDS transmissions that are statistically much smaller (e.g., Dr. Bobby Caldwell will get AIDS from a female carrier of the disease after they've had sexual relations).[19]

For some doctors, the last finally went too far. Dr. Caldwell was the plastic surgeon and resident hunk at "St. Elsewhere," played by *People* magazine's "Sexiest Man Alive," Mark Harmon;[20] and when Harmon decided to leave the show, "St. Elsewhere's" producers decided to sacrifice Dr. Caldwell on the altar of AIDS awareness. Caldwell had never shown a hint of homosexuality or of sleeping with drug abusers; and after the diagnosis, he gave a little monologue about loneliness and simply not taking care to find out his partners' histories.[21]

It turned out to be not quite as simple as all that. As soon as NBC announced Caldwell's upcoming demise, calls and letters began streaming into the studio protesting that the show was misleading because female-to-male transmission was extremely rare. Among the critics was Dr. B. Frank Polk of Johns Hopkins University, who was also among the original critics of the original study of Dr. Robert Redfield. In asking that the script be revised, Polk wrote to "St. Elsewhere's" executive producer: "The plot as it stands is very misleading in that it suggests that this kind of transmission is common. In fact, if it happens at all, it is very uncommon." He continued, "It is absolutely the wrong message. To present it would arouse undue concern and fear among a population already frightened by this disease." A Johns Hopkins spokesperson stated, "People really believe those characters. They're always saying, 'But I saw it on television, and they wouldn't say it if it weren't true.' It will just start again with a round of scare stories."[22] Of course, that was the whole idea.

"St. Elsewhere" having struck a blow against heterosexual promiscuity, the producers of a new series, "Midnight Caller" (about a cop turned radio-talk-show host), did likewise with bisexuals and one-night stands. In it, a white middle-class bisexual infects two beautiful white middle-class women whom he has picked up from a singles bar. He has slept with each one only once. The odds against such an occurrence are about 1,000,000 to 1—but, after all, this is Hollywood.

Having now informed every woman in America who has ever had a one-night stand that she is quite possibly, for one night's folly, going to die horribly, the show ends with the disc jockey preaching, "We can't let hysteria overrule common sense."[23]

Naturally, *USA Today* loved the show. "By suspensefully showing us the persons *most at risk Midnight Caller* might have courted charges of tastelessness," its reviewer wrote of this Tinseltown terror (emphasis added). "But it's a powerful hour with an integrity of its own."[24]

The Casual Transmission Threat
that Ate Hollywood

But if, in the case of AIDS and the question of who's at risk, art in Hollywood didn't exactly imitate life, perhaps the artists believed it did. After Rock Hudson's diagnosis, a kiss between himself and Linda Evans on "Dynasty" claimed national attention. Evans was reportedly terrified—as, indeed, was much of the film industry. Not that the rest of the film industry had kissed Rock Hudson, but if such a macho man could prove to be homosexual and infected, then how could anyone be certain that other seemingly masculine actors were not leading closeted lives? Indeed, it was a certainty that they were—in a profession acknowledged to have more than its share of homosexuals, none of Hollywood's leading men or even actors of moderate fame are openly homosexual. Thus, deep kissing was suddenly thrown into the category formerly reserved for actors who do their own stunts. The Screen Actors Guild demanded that actors be informed of kissing scenes in advance, although after a while the rule was no longer enforced. For a scene in *Glory Days*, a teen film made in Seattle, the director Martha Coolidge employed several hundred eager young extras. But she was exasperated by her search to find two for a simple boy-girl kissing scene. She finally found a couple going steady who were willing to touch lips for the camera.[25] In another film, *Dudes,* released in 1987, Penelope Spheeris filmed a love scene in which she "shot it so they did the dialogue, kissed, and I cut away so audiences could assume the rest." Speaking a short time later, she said if she were making the film today, "I'd shoot it so they didn't even kiss. I wouldn't ask an actor to kiss another actor, even though they say you can't get AIDS from kissing."[26] Perhaps she could just show titles as in the silent films saying, "Couple kisses."

The so-called "Hollywood kiss" also began "rapidly disappearing at dinners and cocktail parties," reported "Nightline."[27] The Hollywood columnist Marilyn Beck also reported that "[Hollywood] restaurant business is down, that the kissie-kissie Hollywood cocktail parties are no more, that [persons] are using straws when they go to cocktail parties instead of drinking out of glasses." As if she hadn't already made the point, she added, "There's hysteria out here, and this is an emotional community. I mean, we've discovered this before."[28]

As to actual intercourse, the weekly tabloids had regular updates on which stars this month were swearing off sex indefinitely—from Sylvester Stallone[29] to Julio Iglesias. The *Globe* stated that Iglesias had claimed to have had sex with three thousand women but has now gone stone celibate. Iglesias allegedly told the *Globe,* "I make love only in my dreams. And I get my goose bumps from singing on the stage to 6,000 women. . . . I'll not take risks with casual relationships anymore. I don't even have a girlfriend."[30]

It is tempting but probably unwise to laugh off the effect of scandal sheets such as the *Globe.* Regardless of the ridiculousness of much of their contents (and the *Globe* appears to be far less so than most, with few claims about flying saucer invasions and baboons with human heads), people who read them probably believe them or at least perceive themselves as capable of reading effectively between the lines to get the true story. And *Globe* readership is a massive 1.6 million.[31] It is doubtful whether anything I have ever written on AIDS has had as much direct effect as one article in the weekly tabloids.

Homosexuals and Hypocrisy

The sense of panic was clearly evident in Hollywood's treatment of homosexual actors. As *TV Guide* put it,

> In spite of all the charity events, all the benefits, all the right words, the campaign to create an awareness of AIDS has apparently also created exactly what it didn't want: an intensification of the already widespread prejudice against homosexuals in Hollywood. The community that is so publicly supportive is privately becoming more oppressive. "In the '70s, actors were on the verge of being openly gay," says Mark Locher, the public relations director of the Screen Actors' Guild. "Since the AIDS epidemic, people have been pushed farther into the closet than ever before."[32]

One homosexual actor diagnosed with HIV-related illness stated, "The one thing we need is to make a safe place in this world for people who have AIDS, and it's not safe for people to have AIDS in Hollywood."[33] Indeed, the Actors Guild received calls from gays concerned about a possible backlash that could cost them their jobs, and *Newsweek* reported there was "dark talk of possible mandatory blood tests for gays."[34]

Yet even as it discriminated against homosexuals, Hollywood persisted in its do-as-I-say-not-as-I-do attitude. In addition to its many efforts to portray homosexual AIDS victims sympathetically, in late 1986 one could go to three movies in a day that portrayed homosexuality in a positive light: *Kiss of the Spider Woman* (1985), *Desert Hearts* (1985), and *My Beautiful Laundrette* (1985). And while actors and actresses lived in terror of kissing, they also made public service announcements, such as the one where Meryl Streep declared: "The fact is, there isn't a single case of AIDS on record caused by casual contact." Who was Streep addressing? Us? Or the star in the next trailer?

Blue Movie Blues

If the film industry in general was worried about AIDS, one wonders what the reaction was in that part of the industry devoted to the depiction of sex, the X-rated filmmakers?

John Holmes was considered by many in the industry to be the "king" of pornography.[35] In 1981, at the age of thirty-seven, he claimed to have slept with over fourteen thousand women, and he had a filmmaking career spanning eighteen years and one thousand films and sixteen-millimeter loops.[36] Even by the standards of his profession, Holmes was sleazy. Also in 1981, he was arrested as an accomplice in a Hollywood massacre involving the fatal bludgeoning of two men and three women. He was acquitted due to lack of evidence, although he later admitted to having been present, albeit not of his own free will.[37] Thus it seemed only fitting to many observers when, in March 1988, Holmes made X-rated history again, this time by becoming the industry's first (publicized at least) death from AIDS. Like the coal miner with black lung or the soldier who dies of his wounds, Holmes suffered the perils of his job; but unlike mining or soldiering, it was a job that holds little honor outside its own circles. The tsk-tsking sounded like a chorus of cicadas.

But was it one or more of those women who did Holmes in? Somewhat lost in the final controversy of Holmes's life was that some of those alleged fourteen thousand women were men; indeed, evidence was readily obtained, insofar as he had made pornographic movies with men. His wife (yes, he was married; she, too, was a blue movie actress) later admitted to these films, but added that it was "her feeling" that Holmes was infected while making heterosexual movies.[38] It also came out that Holmes had been an intravenous-drug abuser, addicted to cocaine.[39] Far from indicating the entry of heterosexual AIDS into the pornographic movie industry, as some people implied,[40] Holmes engaged in activities that put him in all of the highest risk groups for AIDS.

As a last unsavory testament to Holmes, it was revealed that he had continued to make films even after he had been diagnosed—a revelation that apparently made his partners none too happy. Which makes one wonder how X-rated actresses in general have reacted to the presence of the disease, considering how many average citizens were terrified of contracting it from a fellow worker under conditions that bring them no closer to them than discussing weekend plans over a water fountain. One soft-core magazine has interviewed many of them on the subject, coming up with a broad array of responses. Some stars have heeded the call for monogamy, such as "Kascha," who says, "I'm very afraid of AIDS and that's one of the big reasons why I will only work with one partner. [My partner] and I have been tested and now we're both strictly monogamous."[41] Others have gone in for risk reduction. Barbara Dare says, "I don't do anal. . . . I've always said that I'm going to save that for the man I marry."[42] Old-fashioned values yet survive.

Angela Baron, a German import, says, "I'm really afraid . . . that's why I always use protection. Most performers use various types of protection."[43] We are not told what form of protection she uses, but porno filmmakers rarely allow use of condoms; close-up shots make them obvious, and inasmuch as the whole idea of porno is fantasy, the presence of a device to prevent disease and pregnancy hardly contributes to the atmosphere. Angel Kelly gives insight into what "protection" may mean: "Most of us . . . go to a doctor regularly and try to stay healthy through nutrition, vitamins, and exercise."[44]

Others, however, are more nonchalant or are fatalistic. "I don't think there's a real fear as far as performers go. However, the media has blown the whole thing so out of proportion that people, in general, are afraid to have sex," says Sheri St. Clair.[45] And Krista Lane concedes, "A lot of people are afraid but my theory in life is if it's your time to go, it's your time to go. I hope it doesn't become an epidemic in the business. I hope that we're safe enough that we don't get it. I think I have a better chance of staying away from it working in the industry than if I go around picking people up at bars."[46]

Despite the X-rated filmmakers' general disdain for condoms and safe sex, the industry was not without its consciousness raisers. In 1987, the Mitchell Brothers produced the first "safe sex" porno movie, *Behind the Green Door—The Sequel.* The idea was the brainchild of Margot St. James, founder of COYOTE (Call Off Your Old Tired Ethics), a prostitutes' rights group, who approached the Mitchells during the Meese

Commission hearings. Recalled St. James, "I said, 'You guys should take the offensive here before they shut you down. Show that you're responsible citizens—help men get over their prejudices against rubbers. Make it smart and sexy to wear them.' "[47]

They would do so with a vengeance. For the female lead they chose a fresh face in the business, Elisa Florez. Florez (who prefers the moniker "Missy"—which was "Missy Manners" until Judith Martin filed a cease-and-desist order) was in and of herself something of a sensation since she was previously a page for conservative Mormon Senator Orrin Hatch and a member of a prominent Utah Mormon family, which promptly disowned her upon her film debut.

Florez and other performers in the *Green Door* sequel followed strict guidelines during the making of the film. All men wore condoms, and all sexual organs were slathered with nonoxynol-9, a spermicide that has also been shown to be effective in killing HIV. The movie includes such scenes as a bearded hermaphrodite engaging in cunnilingus with a rollicking fat lady, carefully keeping a thin latex dental dam between himself and his corpulent partner.[48] In another scene, six comely vestal virgins surround Florez and fall upon her with their vibrators. Florez herself was a driving force behind making the film just as "safe" as possible. She says she was "terrified of possible exposure," and insisted that each of her partners wear two condoms in case one broke. Nonoxynol-9 was placed between the man's penis and the first condom and then between the two condoms as well. "In fact," says Florez, "a lot of men say they like the sensation of two condoms better than one. More friction."[49]

While Florez vowed that her first porno film would be her last ("I've made my statement"), she continued to serve as a safe-sex spokeswoman for heterosexuals. She said her next project would be to see that every buyer of her video also receives a complimentary Missy Safe-Sex Kit, which includes a pair of latex gloves, a packet of nonoxynol-9, several types of condoms, and dental dams—plain and chocolate flavored.[50]

The advent of affordable video cassette recorders and recorded videotapes will no doubt go down as one of the most important phenomena of the 1980s. A significant share of the market for tape sales and rentals are educational videos. Everything from aerobics to improving one's golf swing to *How to Beat Speeding Tickets* can be purchased on videotape. Sometimes the tapes are a surrogate for those too lazy to read; other times, as with aerobics or golfing, they provide illustration impossible to get from printed matter. It was not surprising, then, that AIDS instruction would make its way onto videotape as well. A broad array of such tapes were produced, some aimed at schools, others intended for private consumption. Of the latter, the quality varied greatly. On the one hand were such videos as Home Box Office's *Everything You and Your Family Need to Know About AIDS,* which—despite repeating a few clichés, such as the "There are no risk groups, only risk behaviors"—was fairly professional and responsible. Others, such as Morgan Fairchild's *Safer Sex for Men and Women: How to Avoid Catching AIDS,* were, well, about what one would expect.

On the extreme of perniciousness was *AIDS: Changing the Rules,* if mostly because of the notoriety it received from featuring the son of the President of the United States, Ronald Reagan, Jr., who, like his siblings, succeeded in cashing in on his famous father. (His older brother, Michael, took part in commercials for weight-loss plans which were disguised as talk shows with Reagan as host. His sister, Patty Davis, in what may have been a publishing first, published a *novel* "as told to" another author.) Ron, Jr., a ballet dancer at the beginning of his father's first term, parlayed his family ties into commercials and a job as political reporter for *Playboy.* His television debut was on "Saturday Night Live," in which he imitated Tom Cruise in *Risky Business* by doing a dance in his underwear.

Reagan admitted that the purpose of the AIDS video was to shock,[51] and it does. AIDS victims in advanced stages of decimation are shown, as are numerous crying individuals and many other disembodied voices declaring, "I have AIDS."[52] Reagan begins his narration saying, "The rules that run all of our sexual lives have changed. Now gay men and IV drug users are not the only ones in danger. The number of AIDS cases due to heterosexual contact is not that large yet, but it is growing fast." The most poignant scene comes when a white, apparently middle-class woman tells viewers, "I have AIDS." "Jack always said he was faithful to me," she says, imparting her sense of betrayal. Here it was: living, breathing proof of heterosexual transmission, the monster come out from shadows. Well, not exactly. Actually, the producers had so much trouble finding a heterosexual woman victim (presumably a white one) that they had to hire an actress.[53]

But no matter, for the video's heart was in the right place. Thus, the *Washington Post* editorialized that it "is not just another program. It's an exceptionally good presentation, artfully directed at heterosexual adults and addressing in explicit language the full range of questions and myths about AIDS."[54]

No License to Teach

In times of crisis, people will look anywhere for leadership and guidance. Unfortunately, many looked to Hollywood. There was, of course, nothing wrong with movies featuring less sex and more of an emphasis on traditional and family values. Any other time such a metamorphosis might have been welcome, but in the context of AIDS it helped contribute to the general hysteria. The need for traditional values will always be with us: AIDS will not. Worse, Hollywood's example was clearly exemplified by "Do as I say, not as I do." Hollywood sought to teach us how AIDS is transmitted, yet those same actor-teachers in their personal lives exaggerated the threat not only of heterosexual intercourse but also of casual contact. At a time (1985) when some Americans were nervous about kissing, Hollywood was thrown into a panic. Three years later, when most of those who had earlier feared kissing were laughing at such fears—either because they comprehended that it was virtually impossible to contract HIV that way, or because they simply realized they had more to worry about than living in fear of a kiss of death—Hollywood's panic had only slightly abated.

At the same time the medium that has endeavored to improve the image of homosexuals—by portraying them as masculine (or in the case of lesbians, feminine) "people like us," by always taking special care to present homosexual AIDS victims as sympathetic, and even submitting all homosexuality-related scripts beforehand to a homosexual group,[55] the Gay Media Task Force, for what even liberal actor Paul Newman described as "cleverly disguised censorship"[56]—nevertheless has discriminated against homosexuals to an extent rarely still found in other occupations.

During the AIDS crisis, the American people turned to the government for leadership and found demagoguery and special-interest catering. They turned to the media for information and found yellow journalism. They didn't turn to Hollywood, Hollywood came to them, bringing confusion, deception, and hypocrisy posing as social responsibility. Its crusade to convince the public to "get the facts" was based far less on science than on fiction. What we should have learned from this experience is, if you want to be entertained, go to a movie. If you want to learn, stay home and read a book.

16

The Death of the
Sexual Revolution (Again)

If heterosexuals with AIDS obstinately refused to begin showing up in the obituaries, one death showed up time and time again—that of the "sexual revolution."

• "[AIDS] will certainly end the sexual revolution," declared the deputy director of the Centers for Disease Control, Donald Francis.[1]

• "Farewell, Sexual Revolution, Hello, New Victorianism," declared the title of one of the editor's commentaries in *The Futurist*.[2]

• "Bid a sweet farewell to the sexual revolution. Casual sex and one-night stands are now for daredevils. For desperately seeking singles, the mating dance is now infected by fear of the fatal virus,"[3] stated Geraldo Rivera.

• "Barring the development of a vaccine, swingers of all persuasions may sooner or later be faced with the reality of a new era of sexual caution and restraint," warned *Time*'s "Big Chill" article.[4] Quoting the Health and Human Services Secretary Otis R. Bowen as saying, "I can't emphasize too strongly the necessity of changing life-styles," *Time* declared, "To America in the '80s that means rescinding the sexual revolution of the past quarter-century."[5]

Yes, if anything was clear about AIDS, it was that the disease had brought the sexual revolution to a close. While the height of the media heterosexual terror occurred as early as 1987 and had abated somewhat by 1988 with the attack on Masters, Johnson, and Kolodny, it had by no means disappeared. In 1989, television news shows still declared, "The fear of AIDS has put the big chill in the twenty and thirty-something crowd. . . . With the advent of dread diseases, we may have to return to the morality of the 40s and 50s."[6]

And who else could describe the situation better than sleaze TV?

"Scared Sexless"—Terrifying Titillation

Of all the television news presentations on AIDS, the most outrageous was NBC's "Scared Sexless," which aired in December of 1987 and was hosted by Connie Chung. The tone was set immediately with a clip from the 1967 film *The Graduate,* where Dustin Hoffman smiles coyly, and says, "Mrs. Robinson, you're trying to seduce me." Said Chung in an attempt at profundity, "We were free, then promiscuous. What we became we are. But free love came at a cost. So, we've begun the trip back."[7]

What followed was a fairly amazing conglomeration of clips and testimonials. A few doctors made appearances; but for the most part, expert testimony came from the actors Alan Alda, Goldie Hawn, and Hal Linden and the football star Marcus Allen. The statements of numerous terrified heterosexuals were thrown in for flavor and to drive home the theme of the show. What could have been a serious documentary was instead made into "Circus of the Stars."

After the usual perfunctory talk about heterosexual transmission, which included the usual "it goes from a man to a woman and a woman to a man" without any discussion of efficiency of transmission, the show bashed singles bars, made a pitch for living together without being married (Chung called it "auditioning for a spouse"), suggested that AIDS is responsible for the declining divorce rate (which started declining well before the AIDS scare), and titillated the audience by asking Gloria Steinem—completely out of the blue—"Can you . . . share with me: When was your first sexual encounter?" Replied Steinem, "Actually, I had several first sexual encounters, since I revirginized myself."[8] And so it went.

Call such a show whatever else you want, but call it successful. Reported *TV Guide:*

The audience's response to this late 1980s-style "documentary" was equally perverse [to that of the show itself]: the Nielsen numbers revealed that "Scared Sexless" achieved a 17.5 rating and a 30 share—almost one-third of all households watching television during that hour. . . . It was the highest-rated such NBC News program since "UFOs: Do You Believe?" in 1974.[9]

Print reporters eagerly joined in chronicling the demise of the sexual revolution, pumping out articles with such titles as "Spread of AIDS May Send Sex Mores Back to the '50s,"[10] "For Many Singles, the Party Is Over,"[11] "Looking for Love in the Era of AIDS,"[12] and "The New Dating Game."[13] They usually began something like this:

> As AIDS and the fear of it increasingly infect the nation, a new movement toward safer sexual practices is starting to gather momentum among heterosexuals. It promises to work a major change in male-female relationships and bedroom behavior if, as some health officials warn, the fatal disease reaches epidemic proportions in the general population.[14]

When *USA Today* wrote about singles, it treated the topic as practically synonymous with AIDS. In one issue, it offered "a potpourri of questions and the experts' answers." "Question" number one: "I like being single, I like my freedom and my independence. And I just wanted to let you know that I always use a condom—you have to in this day and age—and my female friends are asking their men to use condoms, too."[15] A few pages away, the newspaper informed us, quoting a psychologist, that "in the AIDS era, singles are not . . . 'interested in one-night stands. They want relationships.' "[16] How many singles? All? Most? Some? Few? Two? Does this mean that before the AIDS era, they were not interested in relationships? Any combination of these could be correct. The sentence doesn't mean a thing. It's not Newspeak; it's Junkspeak. It's light, airy, slides down the throat easily, and has no nutritional value whatsoever.

Defining the Sexual Revolution

Yet while everyone could agree that the sexual revolution was dead, it seemed that no one had ever given a definitive description of what this revolution was. To be sure, we all go to movies in which the leading man and woman bed each other within the first twenty minutes. And we have all read article after article, novel after novel, on how cheap and easy sex is—or, until recently, was—in these liberated times.

So it comes as something of a shock to find out that, according to Masters and Johnson (working in an area closer to their expertise), fewer than 5 percent of sexually active heterosexual adults below the age of forty had 6 or more sex partners in any given year;[17] while according to another study by the sex therapists, this one consisting of 425 heterosexual adults, most of whom were middle-class whites, the group reported a yearly mean of 3.8 partners for men and 2.6 for women.[18] And it may be shocking to find that a larger 1988 study by the National Opinion Research Center found that even lumping in homosexual males with heterosexual ones, 76 percent of males reported only 1 or no sex partners in the last twelve months; for women, this figure jumped to 85 percent.[19] A 1986 study of male and female heterosexuals in England and Wales found a mean of 0.91 partners over the previous year.[20] One of the largest (over two thousand questionnaires) and best-known studies, published in *Sexual Behavior in the 1970s,* found that the median number of coital partners for single males under twenty-five in the past year was 2, while single males of twenty-five to thirty-four had a median of 4 coital partners a year. For single females, the medians were, respectively, two partners in the past year for under-twenty-fives, and three partners for those in the twenty-five-to-thirty-four-year-old decade. Comments the author, Morton Hunt:

> This sounds a trifle more like the swinging single life that has lately been made so much of, but one must remember that only a small fraction of adult males and over nine-tenths of all females have married by the halfway point in the 25–34 decade, and thus premarital intercourse behavior for this age bracket is not typical of that of the great majority of Americans.[21]

While noting that virgins are considerably rarer than they were almost fifty years earlier, Hunt nevertheless cites figures that "suggest that the youngest group is, in a way, even less inclined to casual premarital coitus than its predecessor."[22] Hunt writes that

> recreational sex is a reality, but we think it does not clearly appear as a separate entity in our data or in most of our interviews because for most people it is not a viable alternative way of life. . . . [While casual sex] meets the needs of many somewhat older single people on occasion, . . . for the great majority of Americans at the present time, the recreational philosophy of sex is viable only for brief periods; to meet their deeper needs for enduring love, security and intimacy, they turn to the romantic philosophy of sex.[23]

For much of America, post-teen virginity never disappeared, nor did any of the institutions of courtship. Many "children of the sexual revolution" were thus no doubt mystified to read that AIDS was going to restore times "when young people went steady, got engaged and later maintained a monogamous marriage." Granted, monogamous marriages are not as common as they used to be, but "used to be" here refers to Victorian times, not the 1950s. And when they heard the experts declare, "The glow is off single life,"[24] these children wondered where the glow had been. For many of them, being single and playing the dating game was usually a discouraging business, especially as more and more singles became too wrapped up in their studies or work to even leave themselves time to date.

Yet reporters would print stories about pseudonymous young men who claimed to have formerly "bedded two or more women in the course of a weekend," but said, "now you have to work at it . . . movies, dinner, and then you have to convince them you're clean. It's hell!"[25] None of the children of the sexual revolution were given the chance to suggest to the reporter that the story about two or more women in a weekend was some young man's masturbatory fantasy. It was, to say the least, irritating to many people to read reporters cackling gleefully about the end of a party to which they hadn't even been invited.

The fiction of heterosexuals hopping from bed to bed to bed was more than just cheap erotica for the news media and Hollywood. It was also to a great extent necessary to maintain the larger fiction of a heterosexual epidemic. After all, the perception of the heterosexual epidemic was so heavily linked in the public's mind with casual sex and promiscuity in general that to take away this image would weaken, if not destroy, the whole heterosexual AIDS image. The obvious solution was to make reference to the very real homosexual sexual revolution and tie it to the alleged heterosexual one.

Solemnly declared the then-mayor of San Francisco, Diane Feinstein, "We can no longer be a promiscuous society."[26] Reigning over the city that had the largest number of bathhouses and other businesses catering to homosexual sexual abandon of any city in the world, the response should have been, "What do you mean, *we?*" But it wasn't. Instead, the remark was lapped up by a nationally syndicated columnist who not only sympathized with the Moral Majority but had formerly worked for the organization—Cal Thomas.[27]

One semantical problem, of which the democratizers took full advantage, is that *promiscuity* is a very subjective term. Some people think of promiscuity as bad; others, as good. Some think having two sexual partners a year is promiscuous; others think of it as severe sexual deprivation. But comparing heterosexual promiscuity with homosexual promiscuity, at least in the pre-AIDS era, is not just a gross simplification; it is simply wrong. In the pre-AIDS era, promiscuity among male homosexuals was a badge of honor. Before the publicity surrounding AIDS, much of this aspect of homosexual life was concealed from most of the public. As a result of the writings of homosexuals like the journalist Randy Shilts (and, before AIDS, writings of the playwright Larry

Kramer) as well as of homosexual critics, the public is considerably more informed. What we know now is that many, perhaps most, of the male homosexuals in large urban areas had so many sexual partners as would boggle the heterosexual mind; as noted earlier, approximately 1,100 on average for early sufferers of AIDS.[28] Obviously, normal heterosexual-style courtship procedures could not allow such vast numbers of partners. Special institutions were established. Homosexual bars had darkened backrooms, where sex was readily available. The author David Black described what happened when health inspectors went into the Mine Shaft, a Greenwich Village homosexual bar:

> The place smelled sour. It was crowded with men dressed like cowboys, bikers, construction workers; some wore only jockstraps, others wore nothing. *S/M demonstrations . . .* read a sign. *The Mineshaft's school for lower education.* There were gym horses, and a cross for mock crucifixions. Inspectors saw men giving and getting [oral sex], sodomizing and being sodomized. Just as some inspectors were about to enter a backroom, they reportedly heard what sounded like a whip and screams. They decided to investigate no further.[29]

In public restrooms, "glory holes" were cut in the dividers between cubicles to allow completely anonymous fellatio. Parts of parks or woods were designated for "cruising," culminating either in outdoor sex or a trip back to the house for a quickie. But the ultimate institution for quick, anonymous sex with many partners was the bathhouse. Here men could cruise darkened halls, checking out other men in cubicles and, if they found one who looked attractive, negotiate through looks and gestures the kind of sex they wanted. The number of one's partners was limited only by his physical endurance. Even before AIDS, notes Shilts,

> the bathhouses were a horrible breeding ground for disease. . . . A Seattle study of gay men suffering from shigellosis, for example [a parasitic disease most efficiently transmitted by ingestion of feces], discovered 69 percent culled their sexual partners from bathhouses. A Denver study found that an average bathhouse patron having his typical 2.7 sexual contacts [per visit] risked a 33 percent chance of walking out of the tubs with syphilis or gonorrhea.[30]

Shilts writes that homosexuals who had racked up as many as 20,000 [*sic*] sexual partners engaged in high-risk (anal receptive) acts long after it became apparent that a horrific, always-fatal illness was spreading from person to person through the homosexual populations of New

York, San Francisco, and Los Angeles.[31] Scorning advice to limit partners and avoid high-risk activity, most homosexuals continued going to
bathhouses, readily infecting themselves with the AIDS virus, then
subsequently passing the virus on.

It is not just that these outlets for sex existed; they became institutionalized. Plato's Retreat in New York and Plato's Retreat West in Los
Angeles, both of which consisted of various rooms for anonymous
heterosexual encounters, existed but were celebrated by the media
because they were so unusual. A tiny percentage of heterosexuals in two
cities used them. By contrast, the bathhouses were an important part
of life for many, if not most, homosexuals in cities where they existed.
The homosexual author Dennis Altman even rhapsodized about the
baths and promiscuity: "The willingness to have sex immediately, promiscuously, and with people about whom one knows nothing and from
whom one demands only physical contact can be seen as a sort of
Whitmanesque democracy, a desire to know and trust other men in a
type of brotherhood."[32]*

The sort of promiscuity that characterized the homosexual communities of the United States in the late 1970s and early 1980s, and which
still continues among many,[34] is a creation uniquely homosexual. It may
well be that many a heterosexual male would, if he could, go to a place
where he could have free sex with any number of beautiful women
already disrobed and lying in wait. The fact is that he cannot.

"It never made any sense that AIDS would become a heterosexual
disease," Shilts told one journalist.

> It's not the biology that argues against it. It's the sociology. Gay activists
> don't want to admit that no heterosexual man could hold a candle to a
> moderately active gay man. Heterosexuals have never had institutions like
> bathhouses to amplify the contagion. Singles bars are very different. There
> was a social milieu in which this disease spread, and to ignore those factors
> is foolish.[35]

---

*This statement, incidentally, was criticized by a fellow homosexual not on the grounds
that it promoted decadence or disease, but that such sex was not democratic: "Anyone
who has ever spent one night in a gay bathhouse knows that it is (or was) one of the most
ruthlessly ranked, hierarchized, and competitive environments imaginable. Your looks,
muscles, hair distribution, size of [penis], and shape of [buttocks] determined exactly how
happy you were going to be during those few hours, and rejection, generally accompanied by two or three words at most, could be swift and brutal."[33]

A Man Can Die Only Once, But the Sexual Revolution . . .

If all of the talk about the death of the sexual revolution sounded somewhat familiar to readers, it should have. Half a decade earlier, the newsmagazines had already declared an end to this alleged revolt. "Those remarkable numbers [of infections] are altering sexual rites in America, changing courtship patterns, sending thousands of sufferers spinning in months of depression and self-exile and delivering a numbing blow to the one night stand," declared *Time.* AIDS? No, herpes. "The herpes counterrevolution may be ushering a reluctant, grudging chastity back into fashion," suggested the magazine in an issue that featured a scarlet *H* splashed on the cover. Concluded the article, "Perhaps not so unhappily, it may be a prime mover in helping to bring to a close an era of mindless promiscuity. . . . For all the distress it has brought, the troublesome little bug may inadvertently be ushering in a period in which sex is linked more firmly to commitment and trust."[36]

In fact, herpes is a relatively innocuous infection (except in children born with it): it never leaves the body, but usually causes only one severe eruption, if that. Once people realized this, and that the "remarkable numbers" were simply gross estimates with little bearing in reality, it took the wind out of the sails of the mini-hysteria. But the newsmagazines knew pretty prose when they saw it, so five years later, in a tribute to recycling, they dusted it off and used it again, this time for AIDS.

Of course, the reason the media can keep proclaiming the sexual revolution dead is because in the sense that the media presented it, it was never alive. Bob does not go home with two girls a weekend any more because Bob never did. Sally is now in a monogamous relationship for no special reason other than that she always was. Like the heterosexual AIDS epidemic, the myth of the sexual revolution as musical beds had an element of truth. But for the greater part, it was a media fabrication which served to sell movies, books, and articles but could not hope to live up to its own reputation. And so it died. Again.

17

Lies, Damned Lies, and Statistics

"Our problem is that we are a nation that tends to look at statistics," said Admiral James D. Watkins, chairman of the President's Commission on the Human Immunodeficiency Virus. "We say that, on the basis of today's photograph, tomorrow will be okay. But the statistics could be very misleading. Over the next 10 years, we may find that the heterosexual aspect of this disease is very serious."[1] The admiral was half right. We are a nation that loves statistics. We hate generalities. We want to know exactly how many people are doing what, how often something happens, and precisely what will be the result if something does or does not happen. Note the popularity of *Harper's* "Index" section, a listing of pure statistics, now imitated by *Playboy* and other magazines. But the problem is not in relying on statistics; it's in whether the statistics are accurate or, more precisely, whether they are being accurately interpreted. It may be true that saying "We have X cases of AIDS today" doesn't tell us much about AIDS cases ten years down the road, but that is a function not of the statistics themselves, rather it is one of their interpretation. Often in the AIDS epidemic, statistics were lacking. Far more often the problem was that they were simply misinterpreted, either willfully or through sheer ignorance.

It was in late 1986 that the media's efforts to terrify the heterosexual population began the new upswing that would take the nation to the height of the heterosexual AIDS scare. The media had been straining at the reins for some time. In April 1983, *Newsweek* quoted a doctor declaring, "AIDS is creeping out of well-defined epidemiological confines."[2] In what was to become the most infamous headline of the AIDS hysteria, *Life*'s July 1985 cover declared, "Now No One Is Safe From AIDS."[3] A month later *Newsweek* warned, "Once dismissed as the 'gay plague,' the disease [AIDS] has become the No. 1 public-health menace"[4]—even while *Time* proclaimed that "the threat to heterosexuals [appears] to be growing."[5]

It was in 1986 and 1987, however, that the press proclaimed that all hell had broken loose.

• *Newsweek,* 24 November 1986: "The nation's heterosexual, drug-free majority cannot possibly take reassurance from [the fact that homosexuals and drug addicts still make up most cases] for AIDS . . . is not 'their' disease but ours."[6]

• *U.S. News & World Report,* 12 January 1987: "The disease of *them* suddenly is the disease of *us.* The slow death presumed just a few years ago to be confined to homosexuals, Haitians, and hemophiliacs is now a plague of the mainstream, finding fertile growth among heterosexuals" (emphasis in original).[7]

• *Time,* 16 February 1987: "The proportion of heterosexual cases . . . is increasing at a worrisome rate. . . . The numbers as yet are small, but AIDS is a growing threat to the heterosexual population."[8]

• *U.S. News & World Report,* 20 April 1987: "Now, however, the disease is spreading so rapidly beyond homosexuals and drug abusers that the old rules no longer apply."[9]

• *U.S. News & World Report,* 15 June 1987 (Michael Kramer, chief political correspondent): "With an approximate seven to ten year latency period before the symptoms become evident, compelling evidence of a breakout of AIDS may come too late. That's a 'breakout' into what the government calls 'the general population.' That's you, Mr. President. That's heterosexuals. Put most simply: AIDS is a fatal disease—always—and *everyone* is at risk."[10]

What had happened?

When AIDS was first detected in 1981, there was little media attention other than from homosexual publications such as the *New York Native, Christopher Street,* and the *Advocate.* The reason, it is generally agreed, is that there were few cases outside the homosexual and intravenous-drug-abuser populations, two groups not readily accepted into the average American home. By the end of 1982, however, the media began discovering an angle that they could get their teeth into—stressing the possible extension into sympathetic or "innocent" populations—babies, hemophiliacs, and blood-transfusion recipients. There were also hints at danger to the general population.[11]

Still, media coverage remained slight until Dr. Anthony Fauci, director of the National Institute of Allergies and Infectious Diseases, in a *faux pas* he is still trying to live down, wrote an editorial for the 5 May 1983 issue of the *Journal of the American Medical Association,* stating that, based on the findings of a New Jersey pediatrician, AIDS might be transmissible by "routine close contact."[12] At last AIDS had become a media event. A review of media coverage via the computerized bibliographic news service Nexis revealed that during the second and third quarters of 1983, AIDS news coverage quadrupled to about 700 articles each quarter. But reassurances were given to contradict Fauci's statement; and by the first quarter of 1984, coverage dropped to 321 articles, with no significant rise for seven more quarters, even though it was during this period that the disease-causing virus was discovered and a blood test was announced. The scientist and media-watching AIDS journalist William Check noted all of this and concluded, with a touch of understatement, "Apparently, what really appeals to editors is raising the specter that AIDS is about to break out of major risk groups."[13]

"If previously healthy straights were getting a fatal disease for which there was no cure and the number of cases was doubling every seven or eight months or so, the story would be in the papers every day," said a reporter to another AIDS journalist, David Black. "You know, like the Iran hostages: *Day four hundred and seventy-two.* So many sick, so many dead."[14] But for the most part, it seemed heterosexuals weren't getting sick, and so long as they weren't, the media had little interest.

Suddenly, however, it seemed that heterosexuals in droves *were* getting AIDS and becoming infected with the virus. Heterosexuals "just like you and me," with no risk factors other than good old-fashioned heterosexual intercourse. Beginning in late 1986, the media spread the word that the proportion of heterosexual transmission cases had doubled in one year from 2 percent to 4 percent and would shortly equal 9 percent or 10 percent of the AIDS cases. Nobody was *seeing* these additional cases, to be sure; but they existed nonetheless. They existed on paper, with the trail of paper leading right back to the doors of the Centers for Disease Control in Atlanta. What the media did not tell us about those three different percentages—2, 4, and 9 or 10—was that the CDC used three different definitions for this group, each more expansive than the one before.

Category 1 to Category 2: 2 Percent to 4 Percent

The 2-percent figure, group 1, included only native-born Americans, excluding Africans and Haitians who had recently moved to the United States. The CDC originally classified Africans and Haitians into separate risk groups because the patients in these groups always denied using IV drugs or engaging in homosexual activity, making it appear that in their native countries something was going on that did not match heterosexual infection patterns in the United States. As the classification turned to stereotype, the number of American tourists to Haiti dropped from 70,000 to 10,000 within a single year.[15] Before the epidemic, tourism was the country's second largest source of income in a precarious economy, directly and indirectly supporting 25,000 jobs.[16] According to a *New York Times* report, when one American returned from Haiti, the customs officer was so worried about the possibility of catching AIDS, she said, "'Open your passport. I'm not touching it.'"[17] Even healthy Haitians in the United States found themselves being shunned.[18] The Haitian government reacted with understandable bitterness, asserting that most of the Haitian cases were simply cases of homosexual transmission, and lobbied the Public Health Service and its subunit, the Centers for Disease Control, to "redesignate" this category.[19] All Haitian/African groups were then lumped into the "undetermined" category in April 1985.[20] In July 1986—perhaps embarrassed by its swelling number of "undetermined" cases, perhaps concerned that persons would look at this category's growth as evidence of casual transmission, or perhaps in a deliberate effort to increase the appearance of a threat to heterosexuals—the CDC threw all of these cases into the heterosexual category. This despite strong evidence that many of the Haitians probably acquired the illness homosexually, and that much of the transmission among Africans also was not attributable to heterosexual activity.

Thus, the sudden "doubling" of heterosexual cases from 2 percent to 4 percent of all AIDS cases that so excited the media represented, in fact, not even a single additional case by the old standard: it was exclusively attributable to the CDC's reclassification of existing cases. To compare the 2-percent with the 4-percent figure was the proverbial comparison of apples and oranges.

Category 2 to Category 3: 4 Percent to 9 or 10 Percent

But if the 2- and 4-percent pairing is apples and oranges, then the 9- or 10-percent one represents grapefruit. This figure came out of the

Public Health Service Coolfont conference held in Berkeley Springs, West Virginia, in June 1986. Within the next four months, two reports presented at that conference were released in medical journals. Although they were based on the same conference, the two reports read differently. One—written by CDC's chief statistician, Dr. Meade Morgan, and its AIDS program director, Dr. James Curran—stated that by the end of the year an estimated 2 percent of cases would be heterosexually transmitted. The report went on to say, "An estimated seven percent of cases diagnosed in 1986 will be among heterosexual contacts, *persons born outside of the United States, and persons with no identified risk factor...*" (emphasis added).[21] It concluded this section: "The proportion *in these groups* is projected to increase to nearly 10 percent in 1991" (emphasis added).[22] The conclusion of the article as a whole, however, made no mention of either category 1 or category 2. Instead, it simply stated that by 1991, "Cases in 'other heterosexual men and women' are projected to increase to more than 7,000 (nearly ten percent)."[23] Because medical journal articles are often technical, it is probably not unusual for a reporter simply to flip to the conclusion. Thus, many reporters no doubt saw the "increase to nearly 10 percent" language, without noticing the earlier statistical manipulations.

The other report, which had appeared one issue before in *Public Health Reports,* listed no authors but went under the official title of the "Coolfont Report." It made no mention whatever of categories 1 or 2. Instead, it simply stated, "Additional cases in heterosexual men and women are projected; the 1,100 (7 percent of the total) for 1986 will increase to nearly 7,000 (more than 9 percent) by 1991." It did immediately add, "This group includes patients who reported heterosexual contact with an infected person or someone in a risk group. It also includes patients in groups in which epidemiological studies suggest heterosexual transmission as the major risk factor."[24] This last sentence is code for all Haitians, Africans, and undetermineds.

As questionable as was lumping Haitians and Africans with heterosexuals, throwing in undetermineds was far more so. *Undetermined* simply means that the source of exposure is unexplained. The patient either had no idea what the source was, blamed prostitutes without identifying anyone specific, refused interview, died before being interviewed, or simply had not been interviewed yet. It hardly follows that someone who has died or has not been interviewed is therefore likely to be a non-IVDA heterosexual. But because some researchers thought a substantial portion of these unexplained contacts might be attributable to heterosexual contact, the statistician who created the 9/10-percent figure, according to the CDC's Chief Statistician Dr. W. Meade Morgan, lumped the categories together to form a "worst case" scenario.[25] That the public health authorities would throw *all* of these cases into the heterosexual transmission category demands explanation. That the language of one report was terribly confusing, and the other simply deficient, also demand explanation. Unfortunately, the only one Dr. Morgan could offer was that "the report was prepared in only a day and a half to two days.

"It was probably an omission [to fail to state that the undetermined were lumped in with the heterosexuals]," Dr. Morgan told me. "It should have been put in there, but if somebody called we'd set them straight."[26] Calling for verification, however, is something the media almost universally neglected to do.

The Media's Heterosexual AIDS Explosion

Armed with statistical "proof" of a dramatic increase in heterosexual cases, the alarmists and the media went wild. The sex therapist Helen Singer Kaplan used the jump from 4 percent to 9 percent to declare in her book, "IT IS NOT TOO LATE TO PROTECT WOMEN, BUT IT'S CLOSE."[27] The author Chris Norwood used just the 9-percent figure (for 1991); then stated that, in her opinion, "the real possibility is that heterosexual infection will account for 15 to 20 percent of all cases by 1991."[28] *USA Today* used the 10-percent figure for 1991 in one article sidebar, "Infection Will Spread Outside High-Risk Groups," without jumping from an earlier figure but without specifying the composition of the category.[29] *Consumer Reports* used the 7-percent figure to indicate heterosexual transmission, again without jumping from an earlier figure but without specifying what was included in the 7 percent;[30] as did *Glamour* in informing its readers that there will be 7,000 cases of heterosexual AIDS in the next four years.[31] *U.S. News & World Report* in 1986 used the same 7- and 9-percent figures in an article titled "AIDS Goes from Bad to Worse."[32] (A year later, the magazine stated, "To be sure, the percentage of Americans who have gotten AIDS through heterosexual transmission has remained at four percent since 1984.")[33]

USA Today also used the category 1 to category 2 jump to declare, "Cases Rising Fastest Among Heterosexuals."[34] *Savvy,* a woman's magazine, mashed all of the figures into a sort of goulash, telling the readers it sought to terrify that of those Americans who now carry the virus, "as many as seven to ten percent acquired it through heterosexual contact."[35]

Since, when the CDC first started keeping tabs on heterosexual transmission, that category was 1 percent of the total, some in the media chose to use the older figure to give the new one even more emphasis. Thus, the *Washington Post* used a jump from 1 to 4 percent as the basis for blaring across page 1, "Data Shows AIDS Risk Widening; Increase in Cases Among Heterosexuals Is Causing Concern."[36] *Money* magazine approvingly quoted Dr. Margaret Fischl as saying, "When heterosexual cases go from one percent of the total to four percent, that is enough to intervene with massive education."[37] The Associated Press, with the self-fulfilling title "Fear of AIDS Spreads among Heterosexuals," used the 4-to-10-percent jump.[38] UPI also cashed in with an article headed "Women Stampeding AIDS-testing Clinics," which informed readers "in 1986, heterosexual victims increased from 2.5 percent to 4 percent of the total."[39] *Newsweek*'s Tom Morganthau, in his 1986 "Future Shock" article, used the 4-to-9-percent jump.[40] Mickey Kaus of *Newsweek*, faced with the first rumblings of dissent in 1987 (what he called "the pooh-poohing of the epidemic"), hauled out the 4-to-9-percent jump to declare that AIDS was "hardly a 'small health problem.' "[41]

The award for the biggest jump goes to an AP story that leaped both categories at once, declaring that the heterosexually transmitted figure was 4 percent presently, but "has climbed from less than one percent in late 1985 and by 1991 is expected to reach 10 percent."[42] *Cosmopolitan* was a close runner-up, telling its readers in a 1987 article that "two percent of reported AIDS cases have been linked to heterosexual contact, and this number is expected to soar to nine percent within the next four years."[43]

Notwithstanding my exposé of this statistical horseplay in the November 1987 issue of *Commentary*[44] and the large amount of publicity it received, the media continued to use the inaccurate figures. *Newsweek* used the 4-to-9 jump in December 1987 even though the writer quoted from the *Commentary* article in discussing another subject.[45] (I wrote to the magazine to point this out, but the letter went unprinted and unanswered; *Newsweek* published no correction.) The *Village Voice* used the 4-to-9 jump in February 1988;[46] and *American Health* used it in June of that year, in an article that was nonetheless essentially *anti*-alarmist.[47] As with *Newsweek, McCall's* had obviously become aware of the statistical-jump fallacy, but thought the opportunity too good to pass up. So, in its March 1988 issue, it stated, "Heterosexual contact currently accounts for four percent of all AIDS cases; by 1991, it is estimated that five to ten percent of all cases will have been heterosexually acquired."[48] Slick, but just as wrong.

Katie Leishman asserted in the *Atlantic* that the heterosexual transmission percentage increased "by over 200 percent in one year." A
letter to the editor pointed out that this figure necessarily included
throwing in the Haitians. Leishman, to her discredit, replied, "The
CDC's report of a doubling . . . *excluded* the reclassified Haitian
cases."[49] But Leishman had not said in her piece that the heterosexually
transmitted portion was *doubling;* she said it had increased by over 200
percent—a *tripling*. Further, her article explicitly stated that the result
of the 200-percent increase was that the heterosexual caseload was
1,079 "or four percent of the 28,523 cases reported."[50] This calculation
must have included the Haitians and Africans, since the category for
native-born heterosexual transmissions included only about 500 cases at
that time.

So ingrained was the CDC's numerology that some homosexuals
could barely contain their glee in using it to batter heterosexuals over
the head. Sneered the "Media Watch" columnist for the *New York
Native*, "now that AIDS is everywhere, a certain percentage of
the prattle is worthwhile." Thus saying, he went on to praise both
Leishman's piece and *Time*'s "The Big Chill." Heretofore, said the
columnist,

> Our opinion-formers did everything in their power to promote the idea
> that AIDS only struck gay men and drug users. . . . Even now, news shows
> such as the *MacNeil/Lehrer NewsHour* continue to provide a forum for the
> debunked debate. Several weeks ago, a blond fundamentalist nitwit from
> Chicago was given much airtime as a qualified debater on [the show]; she
> asserted that most of the four percent heterosexuals in America are "Afri-
> cans or Haitians" and, therefore the correct figure is only one percent. No
> one bothered to correct this racist lie.[51]

(It might be well to ask why the writer thought it necessary to note the
color of the woman's hair.)

The director of the Sex Information and Education Council of the
United States, Anne Wellbourne Moglio, told the audience of "Geraldo"
that "a year ago it was one percent of the AIDS cases, now it's four
percent. That's a 69 percent increase in one year's time among heterosexual individuals."[52] Later in the show she mocked those who insisted
that the heterosexual problem was exaggerated: "We want to deny this
is a problem—it's not us, it's not happening to us, this is a—they're
playing games with numbers."[53]

Did the Government Intentionally Deceive the Media and the Nation?

Clearly, the Public Health Service misled the media, even if it was just as clear that the media had wanted to be misled. Surgeon General Koop was a prime offender. At about the same time he was telling the media that it appeared AIDS might be "exploding" into the heterosexual population, he told interviewers for magazines and television news shows that AIDS cases over all are "going to increase nine-fold . . . between now and 1990. But among heterosexuals there are going to be twenty times as many cases, so that perhaps 10 percent of the patients will be heterosexual."[54] He explained, "The curve for heterosexuals contracting AIDS is going up more than twice as fast because they are not taking the precautions homosexuals have learned are essential."[55] The real reason, of course, was the fallacious 4-percent-to-10-percent jump.

Health and Human Services Secretary Otis Bowen was also not beyond using the made-up numbers. In a mid-1987 article he stated that 7 percent of total adult AIDS cases were then heterosexual.[56]

Dr. Anthony Fauci is regarded by many persons as a hero in the fight against AIDS and as a straight shooter, despite his gaffe on casual transmission.* Nevertheless, when early in 1987 the columnist George Will asserted to Fauci on national television that heterosexually transmitted AIDS was not exploding, Fauci boldly replied, "That's not correct. The percentage of individuals who have gotten AIDS by heterosexual transmission is about four percent now. It is projected that that number will be up in 1991 to about 10 percent."[58]

Although all of the aforementioned doctors worked for the Health and Human Services Department and the Public Health Service, none was directly under the CDC, the source of the confusing numbers. However, one doctor who did work directly for the CDC, Mary Chamberland, addressing the Third International Conference on AIDS in Washington in 1987, told her audience of researchers and reporters that, yes, heterosexual cases now accounted for about 4 percent of the total and that one victim out of ten could be heterosexual by 1991.[59]

Finally, the numbers hysteria reached such a point that Dr. Harold

---

*Indeed, when then–vice-president George Bush was asked during the 13 October 1988 presidential debate to name a personal hero, he named Fauci.[57]

Jaffe, then-chief AIDS epidemiologist at the CDC, felt compelled to call a press conference at the same meeting. Supported by a few other non-PHS epidemiologists, including B. Frank Polk from Johns Hopkins University in Baltimore, Jaffe said that many scientific leaders in AIDS had overstated the risk to heterosexuals in the absence of data. Declared Jaffe, "Those who are suggesting that we are going to see an explosive spread of AIDS in the heterosexual population have to explain why this isn't happening."[60] It was a challenge that should have been put forth by Jaffe's boss, James Curran; but Curran, while doing little to foster alarm, would do nothing to squelch it. For a long time, among prominent officials of the PHS, Jaffe would stand virtually alone. William Check, writing in 1985 of the media's desperate efforts to stir up heterosexual fear, asked "Where are the public health officials who should be taking aggressive action to maintain a correct perception of this disease's spread?"[61] The answer he would receive, in short order, was that many of them, especially those working for the federal government, were busy providing the media with just the alarmist fare they were searching for.

Whatever the purpose of the CDC officials who came up with the contorted statistics that launched the heterosexual "explosion" scare, it is incontrovertible that with the exception of Jaffe they nonetheless stood back and watched as magazine after magazine, newspaper after newspaper, and government official after government official announced to the nation that official projections showed a tremendous increase in the proportion of heterosexual cases. If the deception was not planned, no decision was made to halt it. And if it was not planned, it could not possibly have been more successful had it been.

The Real Heterosexual Increase—Still No Cause for Alarm

But if the 2-percent to 4-percent to 9- or 10-percent jumps were apples to oranges to grapefruits, the Coolfont report did predict heterosexual increases *within* the categories as well; and although these increases were not nearly as dramatic as those created by jumping from one category to another, they deserve attention. Thus, it was predicted that the native-born heterosexuals category would increase from about 2 percent to 5 percent by 1991; the native-born heterosexuals plus Africans and Haitians category, from 4 percent to 5.3 percent; and the third category, consisting of these two groups plus the undetermineds, from 7 percent to 9 or 10 percent. *Time* and other periodicals expressed concern, using the correct Coolfont estimate that category 2, then at 3.8 percent, would increase to 5.3 percent.[62] Similarly, other magazines have avoided the projections and simply looked at actual caseloads to find heterosexuals making up an alarmingly larger proportion of cases. Warned *U.S. News & World Report:* "The numbers *are* climbing. During 1986, AIDS cases transmitted through heterosexual contact increased by 135 percent—a much bigger gain than was seen in any of the traditional risk groups."[63] It was a trend that would continue through 1989. But was it cause for alarm?

The primary consideration here is that our numbers are coming from a pie chart: that is, they are expressed not in absolute terms but in relative ones—relative to the other slices in the pie. Since all of the slices have to add up to 100 percent, if one slice grows the others will shrink accordingly; if one shrinks the others necessarily grow. This redistribution of the pie takes place regardless of whether the size of the pie itself is growing, shrinking, or remaining the same. To use another metaphor, if one measures the distance between the surface of a river and the bridge overhead, then comes back a day after heavy rains and finds that distance reduced, it probably would not be wise simply to assume that the bridge has somehow pulled itself closer to the water.

The writers of "The Surgeon General's Report on Acquired Immune Deficiency Syndrome" couldn't understand this. That report stated, "About 70 percent of AIDS victims throughout the country are male homosexuals and bisexuals. This percentage probably will decline as a heterosexual transmission increases."[64]

In fact, heterosexual transmission was not increasing at all; the rate of increase in the heterosexual transmission category had been decreasing for several years. It was simply decreasing at a slower rate than the homosexual category. As the homosexual slice of the pie narrowed, the heterosexual slice widened. To look at another example of this phenomenon, consider a 1988 CDC *Morbidity and Mortality Report* on the changing patterns of hepatitis-B transmission. The report noted that in 1982 homosexuals made up the second largest risk category (the largest being "no known source") at 20 percent. But by 1986 this percentage dropped to 9.[65] In the meantime, the "heterosexual activity" group jumped from 15 percent to 26 percent. Did this mean heterosexual hepatitis B was increasing dramatically? Again, according to the logic of the media and the surgeon general's report the answer was clearly yes. In fact, the answer was no. Heterosexual transmission did increase, but just slightly. What accounted for the change was that homosexuals, by reducing their risk for AIDS, coincidentally reduced their risks for hepatitis B.[66] Their slice of the pie shrank, while that of heterosexuals and IVDAs increased.

The salient point is that while pie-chart figures give us an idea of how one group is faring in comparison with others, it tells us absolutely nothing about cases or infections within that group itself. Thus, it is possible for a country to have 90 percent of its infections fall within the heterosexual transmission category, and yet there would be no cause for alarm. How? Let's say country A, with a population of 50,000,000 people, tests every one of its citizens and finds only 10 to be infected, of whom only 1 was homosexual. Consider country B, also with 50,000,000 inhabitants, where testing reveals that there are 1,000,000 infections, of which 90 percent are homosexuals. According to the logic of the surgeon general and the parroting press, country A has a terrible heterosexual AIDS problem, since heterosexuals make up 90 percent of the AIDS chart. Conversely, country B has a significantly smaller heterosexual problem, according to this logic, since there heterosexuals make up only 10 percent of the figures. Yet there are only 9 infected heterosexuals in the entire country A, and their prevalence is less than 1 in 5,000,000 for the general population. Country B, on the other hand, has 900,000 infected heterosexuals and their prevalence is almost 1 in 50.

As a real-life example, in Japan at present most cases of AIDS have been found in hemophiliacs; that is, hemophiliacs make up a majority of the pie chart. Does this mean that hemophiliacs in Japan are at greater risk than hemophiliacs in the United States, where hemophiliacs account for only 3 percent of all cases? Applying the logic of the surgeon general's report, it would. In fact, it just means that, aside from hemophiliacs who were infected from clotting factor imported from the United States, Japan does not yet have much of an AIDS problem—and possibly never will, since homosexual practices and needle-sharing drug addicts appear to be much more infrequent there than in the United States.[67]*

---

*For another example, one can look at the Asian/Pacific Islander (API) category in the CDC breakdown: 8 percent of their cases came from blood transfusions, whereas among Hispanics, only 1 percent of the cases came from blood transfusions. Does this mean that (1) APIs receive many more blood transfusions? or (2) API transfusions for some reason tend to be HIV-contaminated far more often? It means neither. The explanation is that

How the Pie Chart Is Changing

As the epidemic progresses and the number of homosexuals being diagnosed with AIDS drops, the other categories will assume ever larger shares of the pie. Such has been the dropoff in homosexual cases that IVDA diagnoses in New York since 1 January 1988 are virtually equal to homosexual/bisexual cases diagnosed during that same time.[68] In the country as a whole, cumulative homosexual/bisexual cases represented 63 percent of all diagnoses at the beginning of 1988, but for cases diagnosed during 1988 the percentage dropped to 56 percent. IVDAs, being the second largest slice of the national pie, made up the difference by going from 19 percent cumulative to 24 percent for 1988 alone, although the heterosexual transmission category—including Africans and Haitians—grew slightly from 4 percent to 5 percent and, excluding them, to 3 percent.[69]

While some pundits and persons in the media have noted the change in the demographics, characteristically they have portrayed this transformation as negative for IVDAs and their heterosexual partners ("They haven't changed their ways") and neutral for homosexuals. In fact, these developments are more or less neutral for IVDAs and their heterosexual partners, and good for homosexuals. That is, the IVDA and heterosexual transmission rates of increase continue to slow, but the increase for homosexuals has slowed the most. Thus, for example, the *New York Times* in December 1988 reported with alarm that the heterosexual transmission percentage of the cases in New Jersey had increased almost 50 percent in the last year, but did not bother to note that heterosexual transmission was nevertheless slowing, just not slowing as rapidly as homosexual transmission.[70]

Expect this phenomenon to continue. In the years ahead, homosexuals will make up ever smaller slices of the pie, especially when their epidemic curve peaks and they are actually having fewer cases diagnosed each year than in the previous years. IVDA cases will take up most of the slack, but some of the increase will come in the heterosexually transmitted category, and perhaps from the blood transfusions and hemophiliac categories, since their peak of infections probably occurred later than did the homosexuals. As even IVDA cases peak and

---

whereas about 40 percent of Hispanic cases fall into the IVDA category, only 3 percent of the API category are IVDA. It is not that there's a greater problem with API transfusion recipients; it is that there is a lesser one with IVDA.

begin to decline, the heterosexually transmitted category will suddenly bulge until such time as it begins to peak and decline as well. (The heterosexual curve, reflecting as it does primarily women who have sex with IVDA men, will necessarily lag somewhat behind the IVDA curve.) Will the media report this heterosexual transmission bulge as merely a growing slice in a rapidly shrinking pie? Or will there be another round of headlines: "The Heterosexual Breakout Here at Last!" Don't bet against it.

18

The Media and
the Doctors of Doom

On 20 July 1988, readers of "The Nation's newspaper" *USA Today* received one of the worst jolts of the AIDS crisis. "By 1991, 1 in 10 Babies May Be AIDS Victims" read the teaser on the first page. By this time, readers were beginning to tire of stories on heterosexual transmission, but discussions of infected babies had become quite the rage. As was usual with any aspect of heterosexual AIDS, *USA Today* led the nation's newspapers in sounding the alarm. And as usual, *USA Today* was wrong. The story quoted Dr. James Oleske, the same doctor who had foolishly assumed that the children he was seeing with AIDS in 1983 might be getting infected through casual transmission, and whose assumption led to Anthony Fauci's infamous editorial on the subject noted in the previous chapter. Now Oleske was back making foolish assumptions, this one being that not only would the pediatric AIDS situation in the New York City–Newark area (where Oleske works) keep getting worse, but that the problems of this area, with about one third of all the nation's pediatric cases,* could somehow be extrapolated to the nation as a whole. Even still, Oleske's statement as quoted in the paper was simply that 1 of 10 babies *admitted to hospitals* by 1991 might have AIDS.[2] *USA Today* should have asked a few good questions, found the statement lacking, and eschewed a story. At the very least, it should have quoted another doctor with a countervailing view. Instead, it slapped a teaser on the first page indicating that over 300,000 babies would be born with HIV in 1991. The next day, *USA Today* ran

---

*By the end of January 1989, New York City alone had 402 of the nation's 1,355 reported pediatric AIDS cases.[1]

a tiny little correction which no one could possibly have seen who wasn't looking for it. This affair shows in a nutshell what happens when an alarmist doctor links up with media craving ever more alarmism.

AIDS is called a syndrome because, rather than killing directly, it usually does so by devastating the immune system, which allows opportunistic infections to do the killing. *Pneumocystis carinii* pneumonia and fungi choke off the lungs, Kaposi's sarcoma rots the skin and other organs, cytomegalovirus eats away at the retina of the eyes. Almost nine years after the first news stories on AIDS started trickling in, most Americans are vaguely familiar with these symptoms, yet remain ignorant of another aspect of the epidemic as insidious a destroyer of vision and clear thinking as AIDS itself—the syndrome of those opportunists in the medical fields and their collaborators in the media who put their own interests in fame and spectacular articles ahead of the public's right to know. Let me turn a spotlight on some of those doctors and the media who made them famous.

William Haseltine

Haseltine is a virologist at the Dana-Farber Cancer Institute, Harvard School of Public Health, whose expertise in that specific field is unquestionable. Unfortunately his greatest claim to fame seems to be his constant willingness to make headline-gaining apocalyptic predictions about the epidemic. William Check, co-author of *The Truth About AIDS*, in an article in the *Review of Infectious Diseases* criticizing media coverage of AIDS, cited Haseltine as his prime example of the doctor who becomes an authority through sheer quotability and outrageousness.[3] Some of Haseltine's statements—arguably his most important ones because they are statements of fact rather than just predictions—have been demonstrably grossly inaccurate. "[HIV is] as easily transmitted from a man to a woman as it is from a man to a man," he told one reporter.[4] "Outstanding citizens" in New York City who visit prostitutes have a 1-in-5 chance of contracting the virus and taking it home to infect their wives, he said on another occasion.[5] But Haseltine's false etiology is merely the backdrop for the apocalyptic statements for which he has become famous, asserting that the AIDS epidemic will produce an "enormous" and "frightening" effect on world health which public health officials may be "relatively powerless to contain."[6]

Haseltine splashed onto the national scene when he took advantage of an invitation to testify before Congress in 1985 to spread his world view on AIDS. Two years before, Haseltine's colleague at Harvard, the microbiologist Myron Essex, had declared, "In short, AIDS is clearly a serious threat to the entire population."[7]* Now it was Haseltine's turn. In a statement that was tremendously long by the standards of congressional hearings, Haseltine began, "We are now engaged in another deadly episode in the historic battle of man versus microbe."[9] In his written testimony, he went on to make the following statements:

1. "We now know that a spread of the disease in the United States and Europe was preceded by a massive spread of disease in central Africa."[10]
2. "In central Africa—within the so-called AIDS belt—over ten million people are now infected, accounting for almost one tenth [*sic*] of the entire population."[11]
3. "We can expect that unless immediate and effective measures are taken, virtually all intravenous drug users in this country and around the world will be infected within the next few years."[12]
4. "There is accumulating evidence that infection is transmitted from prostitutes to their customers."[13]
5. "More than one million Americans are now infected with [HIV]. Official estimates are that one in ten Americans will be infected with the virus in the foreseeable future."[14]
6. The scope of HIV infection will include "all hemophiliacs."[15]
7. "At present, there are 150,000 heterosexual people infected, representing 0.03 percent of our population infected with the virus. Half of these heterosexuals have no known risk factors associated with the disease including homosexuality, use of intravenous drugs, or membership in any of the ethnic groups which are known to be infected with these viruses [Haitians]."[16]
8. "It is estimated that 1,000 to 2,000 new cases of infection with the AIDS virus occur every day in the United States."[17]

In fact, as noted elsewhere in this book, every one of these alarming statements has proven false. Furthermore, there was no reason to think they were true at the time Haseltine testified. Indeed, some of them appear bold prevarications. For example, while Haseltine cites an "official" estimate of 10 percent of Americans infected in the "foreseeable future," the first official estimate of U.S. seropositivity came out a year *after* Haseltine's testimony, at the June 1986 Coolfont conference—and then made no estimate of future levels of seropositivity. No official estimate of future seropositivity has *ever* been made by the Public Health Service or the Government Accounting Office, the only official U.S. bodies that would do so. The 1-in-10 figure is pure fiction.

---

*On another occasion, partially in reference to himself, Essex said, "The fact is that the dire predictions of those who have cried doom ever since AIDS appeared haven't been far off the mark."[8]

Not incidentally, Haseltine concluded his statement by making a pitch for tremendously increased funding for AIDS research. Later he would call for a "Manhattan Project," to develop therapies to treat the disease.[18]

Now, here was a man who spouted figures on everything from prostitute spread to African seropositivity to hemophiliacs to drug abusers, and rarely cited authority for his assertions, instead relying on his known expertise for looking at viruses in a laboratory. Yet, at that moment, Haseltine was anointed an expert on AIDS epidemiology and transmission by the media. His statement that "five percent of United States soldiers reporting to venereal disease clinics in Berlin are now infected with the AIDS virus" was treated by the press as if he himself had conducted the study. "Prostitutes Transmitting AIDS to U.S. Soldiers," blared the *Washington Post*, citing Haseltine's testimony and identifying him only as an "AIDS researcher at the Harvard Medical School."[19] In fact, he had merely heard about the study, and cited it to his advantage. The article left no doubt in the reader's mind that such transmission was occurring, and provided no space to those who, like Harold Jaffe, challenged the notion that the soldiers were being infected by prostitutes.[20]

Haseltine also appeared on a network television program later that year with such AIDS experts as Jaffe and Dr. Paul Volboerding, head of the AIDS clinical unit at San Francisco General Hospital. In that appearance, Haseltine contradicted the other panelists' assertion that anal intercourse is a special risk factor for AIDS.[21] How many women watched that show and took Haseltine's remarks to heart cannot be known.

Haseltine even ruffled the feathers of the CDC's AIDS director Dr. James Curran, who rarely seized the opportunity to criticize someone for overplaying the scope of the AIDS epidemic: "Haseltine will say something different from the *ex officio* people and he would accuse us of underestimating the problem. That's the whole issue of disinformation. The public hears all of these different things and they think that nobody knows anything."[22]

Robert Redfield

If there were a father of the heterosexual AIDS scare, it would have to be Dr. Robert Redfield, an infectious disease specialist at Walter Reed Army Hospital in Washington, D.C. Although references in the popular media to a possible "breakout" go back as far as 1983, and the

Centers for Disease Control published their first report on heterosexual transmission in 1981, Redfield was the principal researcher on the first heterosexual partner study presenting evidence of HIV transmission.[23]

When Redfield spoke, people listened. He made a hit with such statements as: "As AIDS enters the heterosexual population, I think it will repeat the rate of spread that occurred in the homosexual population during the last four years."[24] A survey of articles by the big three newsmagazines and major city newspapers reveals that articles on heterosexual AIDS rarely went without a quote from Redfield, sometimes countered with quotes from CDC officials or others but often standing alone. Although his popularity has clearly diminished with the passing of time and the obstinate refusal of the heterosexual explosion to show up, he still continues to pop up occasionally in the newspapers. Along with Haseltine, Masters and Johnson, and a large variety of other alarmists, Redfield testified before the President's AIDS commission, spouting warnings then, as he did in 1985, of impending heterosexual doom. Redfield was highly revered by conservative congressional staffers and may have been the doctor with the most influence on White House and Education Department AIDS policy during the Reagan administration, more so even than members of the Public Health Service. He also served as unofficial chief medical advisor to a moralist group, Americans for a Sound AIDS Policy, in conjunction with whom he maintained a busy schedule addressing evangelical Christian groups.

Like Haseltine, Redfield was not shy about making his own estimates about national seroprevalence, telling eager reporters that the AIDS virus was "likely to be present in the blood of five million to 10 million U.S. persons by 1991."[25] *Newsweek,* in fact, built a whole article around the prediction.[26] And while the CDC in 1987 was unsure enough about its data to refuse to project cases beyond the end of 1991, Redfield that year did not hesitate to declare in a written address that "MORE AMERICANS WILL DIE OVER THE NEXT 15 YEARS FROM THIS VIRUS THAN LOSS [SIC] THEIR LIVES IN THE LAST FOUR WARS."[27] (About 800,000 lives.)

Also like Haseltine, Redfield did not feel that Africa was beyond his ken, telling the *Washington Post* in its exclusive profile on him, "In some central and East African nations, the infection has already gone so far that it is not unreasonable to predict the death of a quarter of the entire population."[28]

Redfield discovered, as did the alarmists in general, that every silver cloud could be found to contain a dark lining. In May 1987, the results of the first fifteen months of military recruit testing were made available, revealing that infection rates among applicants to the armed forces had maintained a stable rate of 1.5 per 1,000 tested. This was surprising news to many who, like Redfield, had predicted a steady increase in seropositivity, if not an explosion. Dr. Timothy Dondero, chief of the HIV Seropositivity Branch of the CDC's AIDS program, declared, "Clearly there's no evidence for [an] explosive rise in level of infections."[29] Good news for most of the population, but not so for Dr. Redfield, who, according to the *Washington Post,* "was less optimistic about the new findings. He said that when test results among recruits were analyzed by age and race, they showed that infection rates had increased significantly among some groups, particularly black men born between 1962 and 1967."[30] Indeed, they had. But if the overall seropositivity level remained steady, and yet it rose in one group, doesn't that mean it must have fallen in another? Of course, but Redfield did not want to talk about that.

As with Haseltine, not only did this foolishness not dissuade the media from using Redfield as an expert source, it attracted them. Wrote Check of the media reaction to Redfield:

> At the [first international] AIDS conference in April [1985], one survey generated considerable alarming press coverage. This was the report that perhaps 30 percent of a group of military personnel with AIDS admitted to no risky behavior. Dr. Robert Redfield, the chief investigator, speculated that these men could have contracted AIDS from their frequent contacts with prostitutes. . . . One might have asked whether nationwide AIDS statistics showed that frequenting prostitutes is commonly reported (it is not). But even a reporter not familiar with the nuances of AIDS epidemiology could easily have obtained qualifying comments at the meeting, which was attended by practically every world expert on AIDS.

"Such caveats," wrote Check, "were only rarely included in stories reporting Redfield's work."[31]

Ironically, Redfield's single greatest supporter in the media, a person whose loyalty to his most outlandish notions was unwavering, was Check's own co-author for *The Truth About AIDS,* Ann Guidici Fettner. ("It's a long story," Check told me, recounting how he and Fettner had been put together by the publisher.)[32]

For example, Fettner, in attacking an anti-alarmist piece in *Playboy,* wrote in 1986,

> Redfield even questions whether IV drugs are a realistic vehicle for transmission of the so-called "AIDS virus." [This was while Fettner was still denying that HIV was the AIDS etiological agent.] His reasoning is intriguing: If

several thousand health care workers have been accidentally inoculated with infected blood and sera, and if the virus is so easily passed by IV-drug users in that fashion, why have so few . . . health care workers become infected?[33]

Two years later, in a self-interview in the *Village Voice,* she repeated Redfield's "intriguing" reasoning.[34] But a far better word than *intriguing* would be *shallow.* Any time a syringe is used in an injection, the downward motion of the plunger creates a vacuum, so that the plunger retreats slightly into the syringe, often drawing a little bit of blood back as well. This is true whether the syringe is being used by a health-care worker or a drug abuser. But when drug addicts share needles, the subsequent abuser fully depresses the plunger, injecting all of the first abuser's blood in the syringe into the vein of the second abuser. When a health-care worker suffers a needlestick injury, the plunger is not being pushed down. By far the most common way of receiving a needlestick is during attempts to recap the needle prior to disposal. The plunger is never touched. The result is that the health-care worker who gets accidentally stuck tends to get a much smaller dose of blood than a junkie sharing needles would get.[35] This is the case even if the abusers are not engaging in a practice called booting, in which blood is *intentionally* drawn back into the syringe and injected in a large volume into the second user's arm.

That needlesticks can efficiently transmit a virus is proven by data showing that 12 to 17 percent of all needlesticks in which the patient had hepatitis B resulted in a transmittal of hepatitis B to the hapless health-care worker.[36] As stated earlier, the reason HIV is so infrequently transmitted this way is that HIV infection requires a much greater viral load than does hepatitis-B infection. A drug user who intentionally empties the contents of a syringe into his arm gets a vastly greater load of virus than does a doctor or nurse accidentally sticking their fingertip. It is the need for a large viral load of HIV—and hence its comparative inefficiency—that has contributed so much to keeping AIDS away from the non-IVDA heterosexual population. Amazingly, through his ignorance of the mechanics of inoculation, Redfield has turned one of the best indicators of why heterosexual transmission is rare into an argument for heterosexual transmission.

Whatever can be said of Redfield, he cannot be accused of flip-flopping, as could many of the alarmists who worked for the Public Health Service. In 1985, Redfield said, "This is a general disease now. Get rid of the high risk groups, anyone can get it."[37] Two years later, with the statistics concerning AIDS in risk groups versus non-IVDA heterosexuals stating exactly what they did in 1985, he was still declaring, as if for the first time, "I think the risk groups should be abandoned." The reporter obligingly entitled his article, "AIDS researchers say 'High-Risk' Designation Becoming Obsolete," although the only researcher cited was Redfield.[38]

Of course, Redfield's continuing call for abandoning the risk categories was more than just consistent. After all, what better way to cover his being disproven than effectively to destroy the evidence? Further, remember that the fall-back position of the alarmists is that, failing to make their case for a rapidly growing heterosexual problem, they could simply declare that nobody really knows what's going on. This would allow them to pull out their "we must therefore err on the side of caution" argument.

Another favorite Redfield line for wiping out evidence was, "I'm concerned not by how people get infection, but how they can transmit this virus to other individuals."[39] It is a line that impressed reporters, but pray, what better way of telling how a virus is transmitted than by determining how carriers were infected in the first place? Indeed, is there any other way of telling?

It could be said of Haseltine and Redfield that if they hadn't existed, the media would have created them. But in a real sense, the media *did* create them. They took an obscure virologist and a heretofore-unknown army infectious disease specialist, neither of whom appeared to have the least experience in epidemiology, and turned them into national authorities because they could not find anyone else to say such irresponsible things. The doctors gave the media what they wanted—scary quotes and bizarre interpretations of data; and the media gave the doctors what they wanted—attention.

But whatever else can be said of them, they were consistent in holding fast to their original position. While Fettner earned money writing articles allaying the fears she had earlier spread, while Krim turned against her fellow alarmists Masters and Johnson, while the public health officials from the surgeon general to Anthony Fauci acted as if they had been saying all along that there would be no dramatic increase in heterosexual cases, William Haseltine and Robert Redfield talked the same line in 1988 as they had years before. Just as wrong, with less evidence than ever, but consistent to the end.

The Good Guys—Forgotten, But Not Gone

The number of doctors working on some aspect of AIDS is virtually countless, and growing all the time. But only a limited number have been trained in, and have devoted their lives to, studying transmission patterns of disease. Of these, a limited number have chosen to specialize in AIDS. So why did the media keep going to sex therapists, to virologists, to doctors who treated AIDS symptoms, in fact to virtually anyone willing to say something alarming, for expertise on the AIDS epidemic as an epidemic? This when there is a select group of doctors who have specifically trained for and devoted their lives to the study of epidemics—the epidemiologists?

At the top of anyone's short list of top sources for AIDS transmission information would be, it would seem, Rand Stoneburner, Harold Jaffe, and Alexander Langmuir. Stoneburner, originally an epidemiologist for the CDC in New York, moved over to the New York Department of Health in 1984 to head up the AIDS research program in the city with the largest number of AIDS cases of any in the world, along with the largest number of heterosexually transmitted cases. Jaffe was the chief AIDS epidemiologist for the CDC, essentially the top-ranking AIDS epidemiologist in the nation. He worked on the earliest studies of AIDS transmission, having conducted "risk factor" interviews at one time of 75 percent of all the living AIDS patients in the nation—four years before Redfield came onto the scene. Alexander Langmuir (who is a veteran of the Spanish flu pandemic) personally institutionalized infectious disease epidemiology in the practice of public health after he came to the CDC in 1949. The techniques he established are now used as standards, not only in the United States but throughout the world.[40]

All three of these men were ready, willing, and highly able to counter the onslaught of AIDS alarmism. Yet while Jaffe was often quoted on the epidemic, it seems he was just as often misquoted. Stoneburner was rarely quoted outside of the *New York Times,* and even then rarely on the specific question of the scope of the epidemic. Langmuir, for his part, was virtually ignored. Instead, the media took a specialist in treating infectious diseases and a virologist and crowned them as experts in epidemiology. It would be much like a sportscaster going to a football coach to get a prediction on the World Series that baseball coaches refused to make.

The media never asked Jaffe about the mechanics of viral replication, or if they had, he would have referred them to a virologist, perhaps Haseltine. The media never asked him about the stages of AIDS illness, or if they had, he would have referred them to an infectious disease specialist familiar with the area, perhaps even Redfield. When I asked Stoneburner to testify before the U.S. Commission on Civil Rights, he would do so only under the condition that he only be asked to discuss the epidemic in New York City. Thus, while Haseltine the virologist was gladly throwing his opinion around about prostitute infections in Berlin and seropositivity levels in Africa, Stoneburner the epidemiologist would only discuss the epidemiology of the disease in his own city.

There is little question that Haseltine and Redfield were competent in their own areas; it was simply that they were grossly ignorant in at least this one area outside of their own—and entirely unwilling to admit it. Far from having the humility to admit their ignorance, they willingly grasped at the brass ring of fame by venturing into an area that just happened to be the one that the media considered most exciting and that consequently grabbed most of the headlines. Unfortunately, it seems, humility was a trait far more associated with the epidemiologists. Time and again, they let the Redfields and Haseltines of the country rule the headlines, saving their ripostes for the back pages (letter section) of the medical journals, and for the occasional intrepid reporter who thought to call an epidemiologist for a comment on epidemiology.

In a two-page *Washington Post* interview on the subject of AIDS and heterosexuals, Myron Essex agreed that the virus is more easily transmitted from man to woman: "Per sexual act, a female is three times as likely to become infected as a man. That is my estimate. That is not based on statistics with known sexual contacts." What else it could possibly be based on, one cannot imagine, except that the words "wild guess" come to mind. Still, Essex said, ultimately this means nothing because males "generally have three times as many partners as females. That automatically negates the efficiency-of-transmission issue because the male is three times as likely to become exposed to an infected female."[41] In fact, a moment's pause for reflection would reveal that every time a man is having heterosexual intercourse, a woman is, too; thus, on the whole women have just as many male partners as men have female partners. In fact, since surveys repeatedly show fewer women having coitus than men, it means that each *sexually active* heterosexual woman has on average *more* partners than does each sexually active heterosexual man. It is simply unthinkable that an epidemiologist who specializes in AIDS or any other sexually transmitted disease would make such a foolish statement. Yet the *Washington Post* granted Essex a large section of its health section to make such statements about transmissibility. Indeed, no AIDS epidemiologist was ever given a formal interview in the *Washington Post*. No AIDS epidemiologist would have delivered up such juicy misinformation as would a Myron Essex.

The point is not that only an epidemiologist could acquire expertise in epidemiology, nor that an epidemiologist would necessarily be responsible—a few, albeit *very few,* might actually qualify as alarmists. The point is that the media simply assumed that anyone with an M.D. who worked in any field remotely related to AIDS was qualified to speak as an expert on epidemiology. It would never have occurred to them to go to an ear, nose, and throat doctor for information on artificial insemination, or to a dermatologist for information on spinal taps. Yet they did not think twice about going to a doctor who looks at viruses under a microscope for information on whether prostitutes were spreading that virus, or asking a doctor who treats symptoms how many millions of Americans, now healthy, will have those symptoms in five or ten years. Thus, just as the media played fast and loose with its statistics, whether out of ignorance or intent, it did so, too, with its choice of experts. And the average reader, watcher, or listener lay paralyzed in confusion.

Masters and Johnson's Last Stand

By the middle of 1988, most of the media had finally grown tired of the endless forecasting of a heterosexual AIDS explosion. *Time,* in fact, had declared, "While heterosexual transmission is possible, it does not happen easily. . . . If AIDS were creeping into the heterosexual population, it would most likely be doing so in New York City, . . . yet . . . the spread of the disease [there] has been surprisingly circumscribed."[42]

But just when many thought it was safe to go back in the bedroom, along came the sex therapists Masters, Johnson, and Kolodny with the Klaxon sounding: "AIDS is breaking out. The AIDS virus is now running rampant in the heterosexual community. Unless something is done to contain this global epidemic, we face a mounting death toll in the years ahead that will be the most formidable the world has ever seen."[43]

Now, this was alarming stuff, even by the standards of AIDS alarmists. Mathilde Krim and New York Commissioner of Health Dr. Stephen Joseph both blasted the book, with Krim calling a press conference to denounce it and Joseph saying the book could only cause hysteria.[44] Alexander Langmuir declared, "This is the most venal, damaging thing that has happened in AIDS in five years."[45] An unidentified "senior scientist" at the National Institutes of Health said, "Only a fool would publish something like that. There is no data to support it at all."[46] Dr.

Elizabeth M. Whelan, executive director of the American Council on Science and Health, said, "Tens of millions of heterosexual Americans who in past years have had multiple partners may have been needlessly terrified, agonizing over the possibility that they have already been exposed to the disease."[47]

Yet the venerable sex researchers had their supporters as well. One was their fellow sex therapist Helen Singer Kaplan, who portrayed the trio as martyrs: "This will probably kill them. They know they'll be attacked, but they care more about the public than they care about themselves."[48] But, with few exceptions, it seems that the defense of Masters and Johnson was from the right side of the political spectrum. The *Washington Times* columnist John Lofton wrote a column that, while making no effort whatsoever to substantiate anything in *Crisis*, merely attacked the single criticism that the work had not been submitted to peer review, and repeating instance after instance in which expert "peers" had been wrong before.[49]* The idea was that Pasteur's critics had been wrong, thus Masters and Johnson's could be as well. The conservative Thomas Sowell, who, like Lofton, had written his share of alarmist columns, also kicked in with a defense, which said little more than that Masters and Johnson were being picked on.[51] The Birchite *New American* came to the sex therapists' defense with its AIDS regular Kirk Kidwell, and Hopkins and Johnston at the conservative Hudson Institute relied on the *Crisis* study some months later in coming up with their own dire predictions.[52]

The foundation of cards upon which Masters, Johnson, and Kolodny based their thesis was a study of 400 men and 400 women, age twenty-one to forty, who claimed to have had no homosexual relations and no history of IV-drug use, and of whom 200 of each sex claimed only to have had sex with 1 partner while the others averaged slightly more than 10 partners each. Their blood tests resulted in a seropositivity rate of .25 percent for the monogamous subjects; but among those with multiple partners, a whopping 7 percent of women and 5 percent of men were positive.[53]

Fortunately, the only thing running rampant here was Masters, Johnson, and Kolodny's ignorance of survey-research methodology. The mistakes lay at two ends. First, the sampling was grossly unscientific, on the order of high-schoolers doing a class project. Subjects were recruited through childbirth classes, bulletin board announcements on university

---

*That there was by no means a consensus on the right, or even at the *Washington Times,* that the sex therapists were prophets is evidenced by the *Time*'s editorial, which blasted not only the sex therapists but the "heterosexual AIDS myth" as a whole.[50]

campuses, and fliers at singles bars and singles dances.[54] Since the subjects all had to volunteer, the group was self-selected, which in and of itself destroys the purpose of measuring a sample of the general population. Finally, the selection of only four cities—New York, St. Louis, Atlanta, and Los Angeles—while perhaps convenient, served no scientific purpose.

Yet, with the arrogance that permeated the book, Masters and Johnson nonetheless criticized as being skewed blood-bank testing and military testing,[55] both of which show substantially lower infection rates.

That the sex researchers neglected to re-interview their subjects already destroyed their study's validity. But if uselessness could be multiplied, the sampling problems would have done that. Indeed, Kolodny admitted to ABC News's "Nightline" that, "Ours is not, in any manner, what could be termed a representative sample of the broad heterosexual population."[56] Which raises the question: What good was it? The blood-bank and the military testing, while they are skewed toward those individuals inclined to give blood or who joined the service, nonetheless consist of millions of individuals. Further, while they cannot be used as exact correlates of the general population, at least they can be compared with the previous year's figures for that same group, indicating whether the prevalence rate is growing in these subpopulations and perhaps in the population as a whole. Thus by Kolodny's first statement, the Masters, Johnson, and Kolodny study served no purpose at all—save, of course, to terrify.

Not content, however, to warn of the dangers of heterosexual intercourse, Masters, Johnson, and Kolodny, in a chapter entitled "Can You Catch AIDS from a Toilet Seat?," warn about sharing toilet seats, drinking glasses, eating utensils, and restaurant chefs who cut their fingers. It was this, along with the sex therapists' call for mandatory premarital testing, that drew the wrath of Mathilde Krim, who was not entirely upset with their position on heterosexual infection: "I don't disagree with their sense of alarm. Heterosexual transmission does occur and as long as it can happen, people need to be concerned."[57]

"It is *theoretically* possible to be exposed in a restaurant under certain circumstances," Masters, Johnson, and Kolodny warned.[58] In fact, they were careful to use the word *theoretically* in all of these instances. Nevertheless, when the otherwise-ignorant reader comes away from reading *Crisis*'s exhortation that, "if you use a drinking glass or eating utensils that were previously used by an infected person and weren't cleaned properly, there is a small, as yet undetermined risk,"[59] because of the general inability to understand the concept of risk, he or she is less likely to think, "One in 20 million," than, "That's the last time I eat out."

Crisis was the high-water mark in AIDS cynicism not because it was the most outrageous book on the subject (Gene Antonio beat them hands down on that), but because Masters, Johnson, and Kolodny had the best reputation of any of the alarmist authors. As it happens, that reputation may have been undeserved. Two psychologists, Bernie Zilbergeld and Michael Evans, writing in the August 1980 *Psychology Today,* reviewed the work of the sex therapists and came to the conclusion that

> Masters and Johnson's [sex-therapy] research is so flawed by methodological errors and slipshod reporting that it fails to meet customary standards— and their own—for evaluation research. Although every study is open to criticism, Masters and Johnson have gone far beyond the allowable limits of nonperfection. From reading what they write it is impossible to tell what the results were. Because of this, the effectiveness of sex therapy . . . is thrown into question.[60]

As with pop sociologist Shere Hite, what Masters and Johnson had been writing was so interesting and so convenient for so many that few people ever sat down to look at the methodology behind the results. With Hite it took three books before the public caught on; with Masters and Johnson it seems it took a bit longer.

A large royalty advance and a chance to be under the spotlight one last time was probably incentive enough for the sex therapists, but there turned out to be another. A week after *Crisis* came out, the *Wall Street Journal* reported that Masters had been given $25,000 seed money the previous year by a pharmaceuticals company to develop a spermicidal vaginal jelly to protect women from HIV.[61] Nevertheless, this may well have been nothing more than a happy coincidence.

Newsweek magazine, by excerpting the Masters and Johnson book,[62] established itself as the flagship of irresponsible AIDS journalism. (William F. Buckley, Jr., noted wryly that this was the same magazine that some years earlier had published the forged "Hitler Diaries.")[63] That in an accompanying article[64] the magazine pointed out that the *Crisis* thesis was controversial, and quoted several critics, no more excuses the magazine than if it excerpted a book by the Ku Klux Klan "proving" Negro intellectual inferiority, then labeled the underlying study controversial, and printed opposition quotes. (In lesser-known developments, *Good Housekeeping,* obviously stuck with a contract to excerpt *Crisis,* felt so uneasy about stamping a seal of approval on it after all the negative publicity that it commissioned a doctor to write a short rebuttal which it ran after the excerpt.[65] *Redbook,* too, had purchased part of the book and published it, doing no more than simply asking, "Are Masters and Johnson spreading needless panic? Or are they sounding a necessary alarm?"[66])

One of the most intriguing aspects of the Masters and Johnson controversy was, however, the way the other two major newsmagazines turned viciously on their brother for promoting a point of view (the heterosexual transmission aspect, at least) that they themselves had thrust onto terrified readers only months earlier. *Time* ripped holes in the sex therapists' methodology and cited "the danger that they would divert attention and resources from the real heterosexual epidemic— the one raging in the inner city among IV drug abusers." The magazine also pointed out the sex researchers' early suspicious work.[67] *U.S. News & World Report* likewise blasted Masters, Johnson, and Kolodny but could not resist taking a swipe at *Time* as well for having devoted a cover to Shere Hite's most recent book before her cover was blown.[68] Incidentally, one of the co-authors of the *U.S. News & World Report* piece was the same reporter who seven months earlier began a *USA Today* heterosexual doom article with "Dozens of studies indicate that spouses spread the virus to each other more than half of the time by vaginal intercourse"[69]—a statement as scary and as false as anything that Masters, Johnson, and Kolodny wrote in *Newsweek.*

Like so many piranha, the newsmagazines went after heterosexual readers first; then having gotten all the meat possible from those bones, they turned on each other. And like the bad guy who, upon being shot on a boat on the Amazon river, falls into the water and is devoured amid blood-curdling screams, Masters and Johnson got exactly what they deserved. They were forced to cancel their national tour, the book sold poorly, and they will probably never publish another book again. But, as Willard Gaylin, president of the Hastings Institute, a center for biomedical ethics, said of the sex therapists, "They are riding the crest of a wave they didn't create. Hyping the anxiety of the general population was a calculated policy of the AIDS establishment—a political move necessary to garner support and get people to take the disease seriously." He added, "The problem with that position is that you pay a price when you compromise the facts, even for a good end."[70] The problem is that, while the bad guys who fell in the water got their due, the piranha have gotten off scot-free.

19

An Epidemic of Media Hype

While the statistical jumps and doomsaying doctors were the linchpins of the media AIDS hysteria, they were by no means the only things the media had at their disposal to create massive numbers of AIDS cases out of thin air. Herewith a few of those techniques:

1. Mix and Match:

Take an outrageous statement and put a quote by an authority next to it, making it look as if the authority made the statement. Thus, the Canadian magazine *MacLean's* stated in 1983, "According to health officials, at the present rate of infection, in three years AIDS could claim 100,000 victims; in five years, 1.6 million. Says Dr. Harold Jaffe, a member of the AIDS task force in Atlanta: "Looking for a quick fix is not very realistic."[1] The first statement was ridiculous (five years later there were about 75,000 cases in the United States and Canada, not 1,600,-000); the second statement was right on the money. In fact, Dr. Jaffe was virtually always on the money. Which is why he would never have made a statement such as the one linked to his name. But the reader of this article would naturally assume that one of the noted "health officials" was Dr. Jaffe of the Centers for Disease Control.

2. The Glass Is Always Half Empty:

Where there is necessarily an upside and a downside, talk about one while ignoring the other. For example, the evidence is that HIV is transmitted more efficiently from men to women. Instead of doing articles emphasizing that men are at reduced risk if their partner turns out to be seropositive, the media presented articles saying women were at greater risk. This is the same technique the media uses each national election year when it talks about the Republican "gender gap." All this means is that Republican presidential candidates tend to get a smaller proportion of female votes than male votes. The flip side, of course, is that the Democratic candidates get a smaller proportion of male votes than female votes, but this flip side is virtually ignored.

3. Present Old Information as New (and Alarming):

One *USA Today* story in late 1988 well illustrated this technique as well as technique two. In the story, titled "Women's Risk of AIDS on the Upswing," the president-elect of the American Women's Medical Association was quoted as saying, "Our efforts to educate about sex and the effects of sex have to be redoubled."[2] The reader trembles. There is new danger for women, and experts are calling for drastic action to head it off. The reader might be surprised to hear that, in fact, women's cases were "on the upswing"; that is, they constituted a slightly growing percentage of AIDS cases, pretty much since the CDC began keeping track in 1981. But through use of an alarming title and a carefully placed quote, the newspaper was able to breathe fresh life into a story over six years old. In fact, *USA Today* could have run a similarly titled piece every six months or so since the inception of the epidemic.

Concerning technique two, since, as the story noted, the so-called upswing simply meant more of the new AIDS cases consisted of women than previously, it was equally true that for men AIDS was on the "downswing."* Did the story mention that? No. Did the paper run a separate piece on men making up a smaller portion of cases? No. Did it, on that occasion or any other, come to the conclusion that, since men were making up fewer of the new cases than previously, their "risk" was going down? No. That would have been more accurate. It would have been honest. It would not have been news.

Even though the first official report of heterosexual transmission dates back to 1983 and heterosexual infections either from needle sharing or intercourse have been traced back to 1977, from 1983 on the media and the doctors it quoted kept saying *now* heterosexual transmission is occurring, as if this were a new and alarming aspect of the disease.

---

*In fact, this was just another facet of the pie chart phenomenon discussed in chapter 17. The rate of increase for both men and women has been steadily declining, but it has been declining faster for men than women, the result being that women are gradually making up a larger slice of the pie.

Thus in early 1985, the ABC News correspondent Mike von Fremd told "Nightline" 's audience, "There is *now* evidence that AIDS may be transmitted by heterosexual contact" (emphasis added).[3] In mid-1986, the ABC correspondent Jeff Greenfield announced, "AIDS has moved outside the gay and drug categories. Experts say it can *now* be transmitted, although infrequently, through heterosexual intercourse" (emphasis added).[4] Not to be outdone, Surgeon General Koop announced in July 1987, "However, we *now* also have reports of the AIDS virus occurring among heterosexual men and women who are not IV drug abusers" (emphasis added).[5]*

4. Declare Any Statistic to Be Alarming:

The media proved that any statistic can be made to seem alarming. For example, America's college campuses were often portrayed as prime breeding grounds for AIDS. Many argued that when AIDS hit the white heterosexual middle class, it would hit there first. Thus, at the urging of the surgeon general, the CDC undertook a special blind study at twenty university health centers. When the survey was about one-fourth completed, the CDC released the preliminary figures, and *USA Today* blared, "High AIDS Level Found on Campus."[7] The article had Gary Noble, a CDC AIDS official, expressing severe disappointment and quoted Sherry Bell, a health educator at the University of Texas's student health center in Austin, saying, "It tells me college students are not really thinking that they are at risk and that they are not cleaning up their behavior."[8] *Newsweek* chimed in, with the president of the American College Health Association declaring, "If that figure is true, it's alarming."[9] The magazine subtitled the piece, "College Campuses Offer Students No Sanctuary," as if someone had suggested that being on a campus were tantamount to vaccination. *Barron's*, in 1989, in a weak but earnest effort at convincing pharmaceutical investors that the epidemic was not soon about to take a downturn, cited as evidence little more than that heterosexual cases had doubled in the past year (not pointing out that two years previously they had been doubling every six months), along with the campus blood sampling.[10] *U.S. News & World Report* probably went the furthest, trying desperately to revive

---

*Also in August, Koop stated that AIDS "is everyone's problem, and it will become increasingly everyone's problem because the AIDS virus and the complications of AIDS in the form of opportunistic infections have now crossed into the heterosexual community."[6]

the worries of a heterosexual explosion in its article "A Scary Little Survey of AIDS on Campus":

> Many Americans went through a period of high anxiety two years ago when the rapid spread of AIDS among heterosexuals in Africa stirred fears that the same thing might happen here. Health officials gave some credence to the "heterosexual breakout" threat for a time, and then dismissed it as unsupportable by U.S. data. But last week, a new report about AIDS infections on college campuses revived such worries with a jolt.[11]

Thus, just eight months after running Masters, Johnson, and Kolodny through the ringer for needlessly terrifying the American public, while ignoring its own role in promoting hysteria, *U.S. News & World Report* was at it again.

But what was this terribly high percentage that had *USA Today*, *Newsweek*, and *U.S. News & World Report* reporters waxing trepid? It was 3.1 per 1,000, or about 0.33 percent. By contrast, the CDC had estimated that anywhere from 0.63 percent to 0.94 percent of the total U.S. population from fifteen to sixty-four was infected. While we would certainly expect fewer infections among college students related to needle sharing, there is no reason to expect campuses to have fewer than their share of the other risk groups. Indeed, assuming that about 4 percent of the men on a given campus are exclusively homosexual as sex researcher Alfred Kinsey would have asserted[12] and thus that 2 percent of the entire student body is exclusively homosexual males, this would mean 20 practicing homosexuals per 1,000 students. A seropositivity rate of only about 15 percent among these men (at a time when official figures put San Francisco male homosexual and bisexual seropositivity at 50 percent) would account for every infection in the survey, without there being a single infected bisexual, hemophiliac, blood transfusion recipient, or needle sharer, much less a non-drug using heterosexual. But the media could not conceive of those infections as being anything but heterosexually transmitted. Indeed, ABC's "20/20," in its 1989 heterosexual terror offering, declared that the figures indicated "What's happening to her [Alison Gertz, an AIDS-diagnosed heterosexual woman featured on the show] is happening to more and more young women and men—heterosexuals."[13] The innocent viewer, who was subsequently treated to views of carefree white heterosexuals on campus grounds, hardly could have known that the CDC college survey statistics provided no risk factor data since the sampling was blind, or that neither "20/20" nor any other news organization at that time had been given information even as to the gender of those testing positive.

In late May of 1989, three days after the "20/20" show, the final figures came in. Out of a total of 16,861 students tested, 30, or slightly less than 2 per 1,000, were infected, a third lower than the preliminary results. Of these, 28 were men. If the number of men and women tested were equal, this would leave a male-to-female ratio of 14:1, *greater* than the current male-to-female ratio of AIDS cases of 12:1. (In fact, more women than men were tested, hence the ratio is even greater than 14:1.) The female infection rate was 2 per 10,000[14] which, assuming even both of the positive women were infected through intercourse—not a good assumption since most AIDS cases in women are from other causes—would not be alarming. (Recall that Masters, Johnson, and Kolodny claimed to have found an infection rate of 7 percent or 700 per 10,000 in its study group.) These figures imply that heterosexually acquired infection in campus men is probably 1 per 10,000 or less, a rate less than one-tenth that of military recruits (see chapter 2). In short, it was wonderful news. But almost no one would know this because once again the media had insisted on lumping heterosexuals in with homosexuals. Thus the *New York Times* and *USA Today* gave the gender breakdown but gave no explanation as to what it meant. No distinction between homosexuals and heterosexuals was offered, nor was the infection rate for females only given.[15] The *Washington Times* went even further by not informing its readers of even the gender breakdown.[16]

In a similar fashion, *Newsweek* wrote in a sidebar entitled "Generally, the News Is Not Good," that random blood screening from four hospitals found that 3 out of 1,000 samples were infected.[17] But why is this figure "not good news," implying that it is bad news? We simply are not given enough information to justify a conclusion either way. If they were inner-city hospitals, the news would probably be good; if they were rural hospitals, it might be bad. In fact, the CDC was not releasing information about the location of the hospitals. The only reference point the piece gave the reader was that the figure was almost twice as high as the military recruit figure. The reader was not told that military recruits do not comprise a random sample but are instead a cohort that knows it will be tested and rejected if found to be seropositive. Thus, we would expect their figures to be comparatively lower.

5. False Perspective:

Present figures in a vacuum that need to be looked at in perspective, or put them in a false perspective. For example, there is the constant comparison of numbers of AIDS victims to deaths in the Vietnam War. As wars go, casualties in Vietnam were comparatively light. (A much smaller United States lost about 500,000 in the Civil War.)[18] At any rate, why compare epidemic deaths to war deaths? A more apt comparison would seem to be to pit the number of AIDS victims against victims of other diseases, such as cancer (1,000,000 victims a year, almost half ending in death), or heart disease (over 750,000 deaths a year) or victims of other epidemics—the Spanish influenza epidemic of 1918–19) killed over 500,000 Americans in a much smaller nation. The only times AIDS was compared to other diseases was when AIDS *projections* were being used. When it came to actual cases, nobody wanted to hear about cancer deaths or heart disease deaths, much less about deaths from past epidemics.

6. *Oversimplification* ad Absurdum

Another statistical trick was to present national seropositivity figures as if they were representative of the population as a whole. Thus one reporter began his story, "One in 30 of all young and middle-aged men in the United States is already infected with the AIDS virus,"[19] citing a CDC estimate put forth by James Curran. (Mathilde Krim also used the "one in 30" figure, although she bothered to point out that "some" were homosexuals.)[20] The idea is that one could grab any 100 men off Main Street in Anywhere, U.S.A., and find 3 to 4 seropositives. The idea was enforced by the rest of the article, which talked about nothing but heterosexual transmission. What the reporter did not want us to know was that those infections, as with actual AIDS cases, were almost entirely made up of members of risk groups. Among heterosexuals "without specific identified risks," the CDC estimated an infection rate of about 2 per 10,000;[21] and the methodology for this was such as to make even that rate suspiciously high.[22]

The media also gave the CDC estimates far more importance than they deserved, again because of sheer oversimplification. When the CDC announced its figure on seroprevalence for the entire U.S. population, it qualified that estimate in two ways. First, it said it was just an estimate. Second, it gave a range on that estimate, saying it could be anywhere from 1,000,000 to 1,500,000. Both of these qualifiers are extremely important.

Yet, time and again one would read or hear that 1,500,000 Americans are infected. No use of the word *estimate;* no reference to the range. The reverence given to the CDC estimate was amazing. In this cynical age of ours, when it has become routine to question God's will and call top government officials—including the president—liars, the CDC figures were often treated with more respect and less skepticism than were the Ten Commandments when Moses brought them down from Mount Sinai.

Thus, while a few reporters would conscientiously use the words *CDC estimate* and provide the range of 1,000,000 to 1,500,000—in itself a tipoff that CDC did not have an extremely accurate handle on the figures—others would state flatly, "Currently, some oné million-and-a-half people in the United States have been infected with the AIDS virus,"[23] or, "Of the almost 1.5 million Americans who now carry the AIDS virus . . ."[24] Not incidentally, when one figure was given instead of a range, one could always count on the 1,500,000 figure being presented instead of the 1,000,000 figure. The use of *some* in the first sentence and *almost* in the second was a way of dropping the bottom figure and yet maintaining "journalistic integrity."

Fear from Thin Air

In late 1986, probably as a result of a widely-shown film clip of a pit bull attacking an animal control officer in California, the media began running stories about attacks by pit bulls (the actual name is American pit bull terrier), medium-sized dogs of extremely tenacious character who were capable of killing a human being and would sometimes die trying. There were in fact more fatal pit-bull attacks around this time than there had been previously, but dog-bite fatalities are themselves extremely rare (about a dozen a year for all breeds), as in fact are pit-bull bites.[25] But suddenly pit bulls practically owned the news. The *Reader's Guide to Periodical Literature* for 1985 lists no articles on the dogs, nor did the 1986 guide for the first six months. But from July of 1986 to July of 1987, ten listings appear. Television cameras were on the scene quickly after each pit-bull attack anywhere in the country. Dog attacks committed by any breed were now called pit-bull attacks.[26] Pit bulls became the featured attraction of television magazine shows like "Nightline."[27] I was working at a newspaper at the time, and rarely did a day go by that there wasn't a blurb on the wire describing the latest clash of man and dog. City councils rushed to ban the ostensibly vicious canines and neighbors who owned the animals were threatened—albeit from a careful distance. Pit-bull owners then took to the airwaves to defend their pets as even-tempered and poorly represented by the other news-making dogs. But in the backs of their minds they probably knew that it was just a matter of time before the storm blew over. Sure enough, as quickly as it came, the pit-bull scare was gone. In a matter of months, pit bulls went from page 1 to right out of the newspaper. Today there are still pit bulls. They still attack people, albeit still rarely. But they no longer make news and hence inspire little more fear than any other strange dog would.

Perhaps a closer analogue to AIDS than the pit-bull terror was the missing children scare from 1983 to 1985. Here, as with AIDS, statistics played a major role in whipping up the hysteria. An attractive-looking fledgling newspaper named *USA Today*, in one of a series of emotion-wrenching editorials, informed its readers that "some estimates of lost children [per year] run as high as 2 million," and asked "how could it happen?"[28] On the same page it ran a piece by a Gannett columnist (Gannett owns *USA Today*) declaring "More than 100,000 children are abducted each year."[29] The editorials were accompanied by nightmarish cartoons, such as one depicting a little girl being carried away, Fay Wray-like, by a huge hand[30] or another depicting the United States with a gaping, widening hole in the middle with countless tiny childlike shapes being sucked down.[31] The hysteria reached feverish levels after showings in 1983 and 1984 of a television movie, "Adam," about a little boy who was kidnapped and decapitated. Reporters set to digging up every story of a possible kidnapping they could find. Milk cartons, grocery bags, and post office walls were plastered with pictures of missing children. Cynical leaflets with sales pitches on one side and pictures of missing children were stuffed into mailboxes. A national "Missing Children Day" was proclaimed by Congress, and demands for mass-fingerprinting of kids abounded. Children were taught that strangers were to be viewed as objects of terror, taught by parents who themselves now lived in terror. There were some critics of the hysteria, certainly, but they were vilified, accused of being callous and of "cavalierly dismissing the pain and suffering of families who had lost children."[32] *USA Today* reacted harshly to one such skeptic, declaring "It's no myth" and, setting up a straw man, added, "how can it be hysteria to search for the children we cherish? Trying to find a lost child is an act of love."[33]

If only *USA Today* had asked, "How could it happen?" in earnest, instead of rhetorically, it would have realized *it couldn't have*. If chil-

dren were disappearing at a rate 40 times that of automobile fatalities
in this country, each of us who could name two acquaintances killed in
a car should have been able to name about 80 missing children. But such
commonsense thinking was rare. It turned out that rather than 100,000
children kidnapped by strangers each year, the FBI reported that for
1984 the figure was 57. And the total of 2 million a year declared by
USA Today's unnamed experts to be missing? Thirty thousand, according to the FBI, most of whom were runaways or snatched by the losing
parent in a custody dispute.[34]

But as with AIDS, the myth lived past the revelation of the false
figures. *USA Today* admitted in an editorial that it had been duped
(which neither it nor any other periodical has done with AIDS) but, in
a fit of face-saving rhetoric, proclaimed that the campaign to rescue the
children was still valid.[35] The milk cartons, the billboards, the placards
would continue as before. Eventually, of course, the public got tired of
being bombarded with stories about missing children no one had ever
heard of. Today, milk cartons depict cows, and post office walls display
the photos of criminals.

During either of these manufactured crises, the average man on the
street would have worried greatly for the safety of his children from
both pit bulls and kidnapers, and most especially perhaps from kidnapers with pit bulls. No one was given any reason for there being more
to be afraid of this year than the previous year, when they had little fear;
people simply allowed themselves to be swept up with the tide in the
latest fear fad. The persons quoted in the *Washington Post* article in
chapter 6 about AIDS had also allowed themselves to be swept up.
Their fear was printed in a newspaper and circulated to hundreds of
thousands of readers among whom it stimulated yet more fear, like a
giant chain reaction. This year AIDS, a few years ago pit bulls, a few
years before that herpes, and a few years hence? Who knows?[36]

Virtually anything can be perceived as a threat; the fear is a matter
of emphasis. People who are terrified of flying because they might crash
will nonetheless drink and drive and do so without a seat belt. In part
this may be because we are more comfortable with death on the ground
than death in mid-air, but in part it's because while even fatal car
crashes often go unmentioned in the news, so much as an aircraft's
near-miss may make the front pages.

Ironically, people's fears may be inversely proportional to the actual
threats *because* those threats are so infrequent as to be more spectacular. A spokeswoman for the National Safety Council told me, with some
bitterness, of how parents were terrified of their children bringing

home poison-laced candy and apples with razor blades on Halloween night, even though they don't think twice about sending those children out with inflammable clothes and masks that obscure vision.[37] This even though razor apples are virtually nonexistent, and accidents caused by costumes are numerous. But because razor apples are so infrequent and hence spectacular, they draw all the attention.

The Dehomosexualization of AIDS

What the media, and everyone else allied with the democratizers, desperately wanted was a "heterosexual Rock Hudson." Said the Washington, D.C., sex therapist Martha Gross, "Because there is no Rock Hudson of the heterosexual world who has died of AIDS, straight men are able to hold on to their denial. They are not going to get scared until they see someone with the disease who is *just like them.* Only then will they say, 'Oh my God, if it happened to him it could happen to me.' "[38] Elizabeth Taylor, a friend of the late actor, reportedly said that heterosexuals would not take the disease seriously until a well-known white, middle-class heterosexual died of it. Nobody asked whether she had any volunteers in mind.

Nevertheless, there were heterosexual victims; and if the media lacked a Rock Hudson, they could at least keep the spotlight fixed firmly on those cases they did have.

The Center for Media and Public Affairs monitored media coverage of AIDS from 1 June 1987, the week of the Third International AIDS Conference, through 12 October, following the National Lesbian and Gay March on Washington. During this period, according to the center, TV news aired 100 stories, almost one a day. Coverage ran even heavier in the *New York Times,* which ran 150 stories.[39] Yet, if the news was voluminous, said the center in its newsletter, it nevertheless also had a clear slant: "Whether from discretion, aversion, or sympathy, the media minimized discussion of homosexual transmission. Only four sources mentioned sexual contact between males as a source of infection."[40]

Working under the assumption that "Television's unique impact stems from its visual element," the center coded the backgrounds of all patients who appeared on TV news, and used only information provided in the broadcast. It then compared the traits of TV's visual victims with real world data from the CDC. The result:

TV's visual portrait of AIDS victims has little in common with real life. Real world AIDS victims are eight times as likely to be homosexual as those shown on TV news (73 percent versus nine percent) and more than four times as likely to be black or Hispanic (39 percent versus nine percent). One in five actual AIDS victims uses intravenous drugs, a group never shown on TV. By contrast, female AIDS sufferers appear on TV news twice as often as they have in the real world (fourteen percent to seven percent). Thus, the risk groups the news audience see are very different from their real world counterparts.[41]

Clearly, the media had established an affirmative action program for those at low risk.

Steve Findlay was speaking for the entire industry when he said of his editors at *USA Today:* "They are big on covering AIDS, but clearly in the last year the editors are much more interested in heterosexuals and they don't want to hear about gays and drug users. It's a desire to shift the story in ways that may not be warranted."[42]

Enter now the Burks, the poster family of the AIDS epidemic. Patrick Burk was infected through hemophilia clotting factor. Unaware of his condition, he infected his wife, and she gave birth to a son, also infected. At the time the media discovered them, Patrick had AIDS, as did the child, and the mother had ARC. Only a four-year-old daughter remained uninfected. In the Burks the media found everything they wanted. The Burks were white and middle class. The original infection came not from such tawdry activity as drug usage, homosexual intercourse, or infidelity but from an "innocent" source—blood products. There was heterosexual transmission, and the one thing worse than heterosexual transmission—heterosexual transmission with an infected offspring. Patrick Burk was soon to die, but he would die famous. Within a short period of time, he and his family appeared in *Time,*[43] *People,*[44] the *New American,*[45] various women's magazines, and on "60 Minutes."[46] Although no article or show about the Burks ever made such a statement as, "The Burks are but one of many families so struck by AIDS," the implication was nonetheless there.

In fact, as noted earlier, infection of hemophiliacs' and transfusion recipients' wives is comparatively rare. When I was on a television talk show, one member of the audience attested that her husband had received a tainted transfusion, and that she had had intercourse with him for several years before he became ill and was tested—positive— for HIV. Nevertheless, she said, she tested negative. My opponents on the show, the sex therapist Helen Singer Kaplan and Dr. Thomas Quinn of Johns Hopkins University, told the woman that she was very, very lucky.[47] In fact, her odds of being infected were about 1 in 5; she was hardly an odds beater. The Burks, unfortunately, were. They beat them once by infecting the wife, and twice again: once by conceiving before realizing they were infected, and once by giving birth to an infected child (most children born to seropositive mothers are not infected). It may be belaboring the point to note that the reason the Burks kept appearing all over the place is that they were exceptional; indeed, when Patrick died, followed by his son, the media found no poster family to replace them. But for a brief, shining moment, the media had what they wanted: an audio-visual aid for white, middle-class heterosexual AIDS.

By mid-1989, there was a new poster person, Alison Gertz, a 23-year-old white girl who claimed to have been infected during one act of intercourse with a bisexual. Notwithstanding the usually fictitious claim of "only one time" there was reason to think she did contract it through intercourse, since her middle-class background hardly fit the profile of someone who shares needles in a shooting gallery. Gertz went public with her disease, and her story was quickly snatched up by the *New York Times*[48] and ABC's "20/20" (mentioned in this chapter). Here, at last, was something to throw back at those who were insisting that the threat of AIDS to most heterosexuals had been vastly overstated. Declared Gertz's father on "20/20": "I used to say . . . it's just a myth—but, boy, when it hit me . . . it's not a myth, it's not a hype, it's there and it's real."[49]

Clearly the man deserves our sympathy, more so his daughter. But no, the fact that his daughter was one of the very few white middle-class heterosexual AIDS victims in no wise makes myth the assertion that there are indeed very few white middle-class heterosexual AIDS victims. It should go without saying that they have to be *somebody*'s son or daughter. What we didn't see on "20/20" were the 20,000 fathers each year who lose white heterosexual daughters in automobile accidents, 10,000 of which could have been prevented if those daughters had perceived their actions to be risky enough to necessitate wearing safety belts. That, however, was not "20/20"'s concern.

Commercials

Of course, commercials did not need to employ any tricks of twisting facts and figures. They simply delivered a conclusion, right or wrong. The giant advertising firm of Ogilvy & Mather has been given $6 million by the U.S. government to produce a series of radio, television, and print advertisements about AIDS.[50] While I cannot claim to have seen every ad they produced, it can be said that their first press packet consisted of only one mention of homosexuals, and that was fairly vague.

Daniel Lara, an AIDS educator, is quoted saying, "We don't talk about AIDS because, one, we don't know about AIDS and secondly, to acknowledge the existence of AIDS we must acknowledge that other things are going on, such as men having sex with men. We don't talk about that." That appears to be as close to warning of the dangers of homosexual sex as Ogilvy & Mather would ever get.

When I asked a spokeswoman for Ogilvy & Mather why there were virtually no references to homosexuality, she replied, "You've got to understand this is a government-sponsored campaign. There is a fight going on in Congress right now about funds for explicit sexual references." The legislation she was talking about was a bill introduced by Senator Jesse Helms (Republican, of North Carolina), which would have forbidden federal spending on material that serves to promote immoral activity. The spokeswoman said, "This very well may preclude use of the word 'anal sex.' "[51] But it's difficult to see why unpassed legislation would affect an advertising campaign; or, indeed, why saying that anal sex is the top risk factor for HIV transmission is somehow promoting immoral activity. At any rate, long after the Helms bill had died unpassed, Ogilvy & Mather was still ignoring homosexuals.

Overseas, the propaganda effort was far more vicious. The British advertisement showing the Grim Reaper bowling over heterosexuals might well be the nastiest advertisement since Lyndon B. Johnson's "mushroom cloud" spot implying that a vote for his opponent was a vote for Armageddon. Another British ad:

> ANNOUNCER: Who are you sleeping with tonight?
> MAN IN BED: I don't know.
> ANNOUNCER: Who did you sleep with last night?
> MAN IN BED: I don't know.
> ANNOUNCER: Who slept with her last night?
> MAN IN BED: I don't know.
> ANNOUNCER: How did you get AIDS?
> MAN IN BED: I don't know.
> ANNOUNCER: It's not just gays who get AIDS you know. Sleep around and you're at risk. If you must sleep with more than one partner, you must wear a condom, because if you do get AIDS, what can the doctors do to save you?
> DOCTOR: I don't know.[52]

In the rest of Western Europe, heterosexual-targeted advertising was slightly less hard-sell but more risqué. Swedish television actually depicted couples in bed. The sides of Danish buses had drawings of naked men and women, with large pink condoms floating between them. As in the United States and Great Britain, public service messages acted as if heterosexual sex and needle usage were the only possible risk factors for HIV.

Misinformation in Microcosm

The single worst article of the heterosexual AIDS scare was by Katie Leishman, a freelance writer who specializes in women's magazine profiles of such public personalities as Princess Diana (*Vogue,* October 1988), Pee-Wee Herman (*The Atlantic,* May 1987), and wheel-spinner Vanna White (*McCall's,* October 1986). But Leishman jumped from fluff to fear with her *Atlantic* February 1987 cover piece, "Heterosexuals and AIDS," subtitled "The Second Stage of the Epidemic." The media critic Jude Wanniski wrote of it, and the other AIDS piece Leishman wrote that year in the same magazine, that they were "just weird" and "gave no evidence to support a heterosexual epidemic and interviewed lawyers and porno stars to get their views."[53]

Indeed, "Heterosexuals and AIDS" was a microcosm for an amazing number of fallacies, tricks, and just plain false information. First, Leishman used the 2-to-4–percent jump. In the same paragraph, she made the extraordinary statement: "No one has any idea how many people are infected but asymptomatic, or how much transmission is going on. It has been estimated that in California there are sixty cases of AIDS for every reported one, and reporting is more complete in that state than anywhere else."[54] Since at the time the article appeared, almost 9,000 cases had been reported, if Leishman or the fact checker had punched a few keys on a calculator, they would have found that this meant there were over 540,000 AIDS cases in California at the time. In fact, the CDC estimates national underreporting at about 10 percent, not 6,000 percent,[55] which would have meant that California had about 10,000 cases. No doubt what happened was that Leishman had heard that there were an estimated 60 *infections* for every case.*

Another fairly extraordinary error came in what is the most terrifying line in a terrifying essay: "Given the alarming accounts of hepatitis B and HIV contracted after a single encounter, it may well be that hepatitis and HIV are more readily transmissible than either gonorrhea or syphilis." Leishman added, parenthetically, "For gonorrhea the probability of transmission is about fifty-fifty in a single encounter with an

---

*In fact, when she was challenged on this by a representative of Gay Men's Health Crisis in New York, she said that was what she meant *and what she stated* but generously offered that she could "see how my wording allowed the interpretation that [the letter-writer] drew."[56]

infectious partner; for syphilis, even when a person still has a lesion, it is less than 20 percent."[57] Application of just a thread of common sense would show how wrong such a statement is. If transmission were better than 50 percent with HIV, AIDS would have been surging through the heterosexual population. Nobody would be writing "what if" articles; they'd be doing damage assessments.

In fact, there are three major problems contained in that one sentence. First, hepatitis B and HIV simply cannot be lumped together in one equation. As discussed earlier, hepatitis B is far more contagious than HIV. Just because there have been reports of each being transmitted in a single encounter, it does not mean they can be equated any more than hepatitis B and influenza can be equated, even though there are accounts of both of these being transmitted in a single exposure. Second, using "accounts" of transmission is both mathematically and scientifically flawed. Although there are "accounts" of persons winning at roulette after one spin of the wheel, what do they tell us about the odds of winning at roulette? Nothing more than "accounts" of persons failing to win even once, even after spinning the roulette wheel a thousand times. Of course, the way one determines odds is by spinning the wheel over and over; the more one spins, the more accurate the estimate. The Padian study (discussed earlier in chapters 2 and 4) found that on average it took about 1,000 spins of the wheel to transmit HIV from men to women. While this study was completed after Leishman's piece came out, Leishman actually *began* her article by talking about Dr. Peterman's study indicating transmission of less than 1 percent. Although she did not give us that figure, she did state that over a *period of time* actually only 8 of the 50 initially infected men gave the virus to their spouses and 1 of 20 women did likewise.[58] Thus, Leishman's own article contained a ready refutation of her dire statement.

Mixed in with all of this were the usual statements of "scared sexless" heterosexuals, none of whom, incidentally, had actually become infected, along with interviews of prostitutes talking about "blow jobs" and various other topics designed both to titillate and to terrify the reader.

As poor as media coverage of AIDS epidemiology was, it would be hard to imagine a worse article than Leishman's. Indeed, there wasn't one. And the media's reaction? "Heterosexuals and AIDS" was nominated for that year's National Magazine Award.[59]

Media Motivations

Clearly the media had accomplished the task of terrifying heterosexuals. In its May–June 1988 issue, *Public Opinion* magazine reported that while 8 in 10 Americans believed that AIDS will become widespread in the heterosexual population, only 22 percent believe that the media have exaggerated the health risk involved with AIDS.[60]

One of the most disturbing aspects of the heterosexual AIDS myth, because of its long-term implications, is the way the entire paradigm shifted so that that which demonstrably was not came to be perceived as that which incontestably was. Thus, the *Washington Post* magazine reviewer Charles Truehart, while praising Leishman's "Heterosexuals and AIDS" piece, stated the article "is not so much a revelation—it is common knowledge that the disease is spreading rapidly, and irrespective of sexual orientation—as it is a distillation of human behavior in the face of peril."[61] The cover of the French popular magazine *Ca M'Interesse* in March of 1989 featured a concerned-looking man and woman on the cover and a lengthy section inside urging quick preventative action and scolding the French for their "allergic reaction" to condoms. Nowhere in the article did the word "heterosexual" even appear; it was simply assumed that this was a heterosexual disease that perhaps affected some homosexuals as well.[62] The *Saturday Evening Post,* in an interview with the AIDS democratizer Elizabeth Taylor, asked, "How has the public's response to AIDS changed since the disease has spread quickly among the heterosexual community?" To which Taylor responded, "The spread of this disease into the heterosexual community has simply affirmed what has been true from the beginning—AIDS is a disease of high-risk behavior, not of high-risk groups."[63] How did an untruth become "common knowledge"?

This is hardly the first time such a shift has happened. It is now widely accepted that the Tet offensive in Vietnam in 1968 broke the back of the Viet Cong. The North had to take over the war effort, replenishing the ranks of the Viet Cong with northerners, and never again would the Viet Cong play the role it once did. Yet at the time it was universally accepted that Tet was a tremendous military defeat for the United States and its South Vietnamese allies, and the reason is that is the way the media, from Walter Cronkite on down, presented it.[64] Both Tet and the propagation of the heterosexual AIDS myth reveal in a microcosm the tremendous power the media has to inform, and to misinform. It did not start with AIDS, and it will not end with it.

There were always dissenters from the media line on AIDS, just as there were dissenters in the other groups that pushed the idea of the heterosexual epidemic. One bright spot was provided by ABC News's medical editor, Dr. Timothy Johnson. On one segment of the "Health Show," Johnson recognized that AIDS is a terrible disease and has a potential high-cost impact in some areas but then stated:

> However . . . the vast majority of Americans are not at risk for AIDS and probably never will be. Even if we accept the estimate that 1.5 million Americans are infected with the virus, that constitutes less than one percent of all Americans, and those 1.5 million are not evenly spread throughout American society but still very much concentrated in large cities, and even in those cities are concentrated among high-risk groups, especially homosexuals and IV drug abusers.[65]

Johnson did go on to emphasize the importance of prevention in eliminating the risk of non-IVDA heterosexual spread, as opposed to the virus's inherent transmission inefficiency, but concluded forcefully, "I personally believe it is time to stem irrational fear that suggests AIDS is literally already everywhere and that there is no chance to stop it from spreading."[66]

Among the national newspapers, the *Washington Times* was fairly consistent in its efforts to cover the epidemic without injecting alarmism. This included a two-part series in early 1987, at the very height of the media AIDS blitz, criticizing the notion of heterosexual spread. The other major newspapers would also run an occasional non-alarmist story, but these were few and far between and readily fell between the cracks of readers' memories when surrounded by stories of horror.

The role of sheer ignorance is not to be understated. In their rush to churn out AIDS articles and shows, the media had little time or inclination to ensure quality control. Periodicals that would never have considered having a writer with no science background do a detailed piece on controlled nuclear fusion would nevertheless unhesitatingly assign AIDS epidemiology articles to persons who, like Katie Leishman, had previously specialized in fluffy women's magazine articles. The problem was compounded when the editors themselves were also woefully ignorant of the subject. Indeed, this would often prove to be the case since magazines that had no business talking about AIDS epidemiology felt justified in doing so because of the selling value of the subject. Nobody doubts that the editors of *Money* know as much about mutual funds as those at the *New England Journal of Medicine* know about AIDS. But the latter did not publish articles on mutual funds, while

Money insisted on doing one on the heterosexual AIDS spread—an article that, not incidentally, turned out to be one of the worst such to appear. Like *Money,* magazine after magazine with no natural relationship to AIDS epidemiology or AIDS at all nevertheless scraped desperately for an angle and a reporter who could titillate their readers with this fascinating subject. *Gung-Ho,* a mercenary magazine, ran a story on AIDS as a military weapon, splashing "AIDS" on the cover of the magazine so large that it covered two thirds of the page. Other obscure magazines from *Dance* to *Skin Diver* tapped into the AIDS gravy train.

The role of sheer reportorial sloppiness in the mishandling of AIDS stories should not be underestimated, either. The Illinois *Rockford Register Star,* for example, informed its readers, "Nationally 1.5 million *cases* of AIDS have been reported to the Centers for Disease Control" (emphasis added). Reinforcing its error, it immediately followed up: "(It is not required that physicians report a person who has contracted the virus, only those suffering the effects of this disease.)"[67]

It is amazing the extent to which members of the media would simply repeat figures they had heard without checking them. Oprah Winfrey obviously had a hard time believing that 20 percent of all heterosexuals would be dead of AIDS within three years; yet she did not hesitate to give the figure to millions of listeners, exhorting them to "believe me."[68]* This tendency to repeat without bothering to verify the original source can explain much media disinformation.

While much sloppiness could easily have been eliminated, major pressures inherent in the nature of contemporary journalism push writers and their publications in the direction of hysteria-feeding inaccuracies. *Newsweek* or *U.S. News & World Report* editors would shudder at being compared to a weekly tabloid, yet they are not far apart. Both types of periodical operate under continual pressure to offer something the competition does not. In the case of tabloids, this often means having the most outrageous headlines. All the people who read these tabloids will, upon interrogation, tell you they don't believe the stories, yet they buy the tabloids nonetheless.

---

*Only later in the same show did she finally ask a health authority about the figure: "The statistics I read earlier in the show seem just out of whack—one out of five heterosexuals by 1990?" Incredibly, Dr. Martha Sonnenberg of the Infectious Diseases & AIDS Service, Cook County Hospital, seemed to confirm those statistics, telling Winfrey's audience, "The statistics are late '86, early '87, is less than five percent, between four percent and five percent [of the total number of people who have AIDS]. So that projection is not unreasonable."[69] How it is "reasonable" to get from saying that 4 percent of all cases in 1987 are heterosexual to saying that, by 1990, 20 percent of all heterosexual Americans will be dead of AIDS is, to say the least, not entirely clear.

There is assuredly a greater proportion of fact in "serious" news journalism than in a tabloid, but that does not mean the former is pure of any taint of fiction. Ask anyone who has ever been privy to an event later written up in the newspapers whether what was reported actually occurred. Chances are at least one element was incorrectly presented. The quotes, for one, are often doctored slightly. Most oral statements, when translated into print, resemble sausage before it has been wrapped: reporters take the liberty of cleaning it up. Compare, too, the writer who recollects dialogue he heard years or even decades earlier: its eventual transcription on paper may range from being 90 percent accurate to complete inaccuracy.

The question, then, is not whether fiction appears as fact in periodicals, but in what proportion it appears thus? It is undoubtedly true that weekly tabloids have high fiction contents; and that daily newspapers, weekly newsmagazines, and monthly popular magazines have lower fiction ones. Unfortunately, unless one has particular expertise in an area, it is difficult to tell how much is which in most articles in most magazines. Part of our presumption of a high fact content is certainly based on our opinion that daily newspapers, newsmagazines, and monthly magazines are kept in check by each other. But what if they all make the same mistakes, as so often was the case with AIDS?

Further, to what extent is veracity even valued by the reader? We know that the weekly tabloids, with their low fact contents, often have tremendously large readerships. Obviously there is something in these tabloids that the readers value above factuality. Is it safe to assume, therefore, that readers necessarily value factuality in newspapers and newsmagazines? Of all the reasons one might give for favoring *Newsweek* over *Time* or *U.S. News & World Report* over either, how many readers would declare that one is more accurate than the other? It would *seem* to be a good criterion on which to base magazine purchases, but the average newsmagazine buyer would probably list a half-dozen factors they look for in a magazine before it would occur to them to list veracity. Many, indeed, would not think to list it at all.

If *U.S. News & World Report* were to begin running stories like "Human Mother Gives Birth to Ape Baby" or "Rudolph the Red-Nosed Reindeer Found in Meat Freezer," it would lose its market (while quite possibly gaining a more lucrative one). Still, between the 100-percent fact content the newsmagazines and newspapers would like us to think they possess, and the 95-percent fiction content of many stories in the weekly tabloids, there is plenty of room in which to maneuver.

Even reporters for the most prestigious publications recognize that an exaggerated story often makes for a more exciting one. Janet Cooke learned this lesson early on. Finally she went so far as to create a fictional character, little Jimmy, an eight-year-old heroin addict.[70] Her story won the Pulitzer Prize in 1981; but when Jimmy's fictional character was exposed, she was disgraced and dismissed. She had gone too far. It wasn't that her story contained some fiction: virtually all do. It wasn't that her story was all fiction: narcotics exist, they are injected, and it would be foolish to claim that, in a nation of hundreds of thousands of intravenous-drug users, none of them is as young as eight years old. The problem was, first, that Cooke's Jimmy *did not* exist; and, second, she won a Pulitzer for the piece, thus attracting the attention that would eventually reveal her hoax.

The effect of the pressures is ably summarized in the words of science reporters quoted by Jay Winsten:

> I'm in competition with literally hundreds of stories every day, political and economic stories of compelling interest. In science, especially, we sometimes have to argue [with editors], pound the table, and say, "This is an important story. It turns a key of understanding, it affects a lot of people," or "it's just interesting, it's part of the unfolding romance of science." But we have to make that clear in our copy. We have to almost overstate, we have to come as close as we can within the boundaries of truth to a dramatic, compelling statement. A weak statement will go no place.
>
> In journalism the trick is to get as strong as possible a lead and story theme, without going overboard and being absurd so that you destroy yourself. There is always this tension of what is the strongest thing I can say about this story and still have it be accurate. It is not how wishy-washy, how cautious, how moderate I can make it, and get buried way back in the paper. The fact is, you are going for the strong. And, while not patently absurd, it may not be the lead you would go for a year later.[71]

William Check writes that stories on unusual modes of HIV transmission—such as a sanitation worker being allegedly stuck with a needle in the course of his work, or a nun who got AIDS through a transfusion—became stories chiefly because of their "man-bites-dog" flavor. "There was little of medical significance in any of these incidents," he writes, even if they were all true. In this respect, AIDS conforms to a rule stated by a long-time science editor: "[To the mass media] science news is basically entertainment."[72]

In retrospect, then, despite Jude Wanniski's criticism and my own, perhaps far from being the worst article of the heterosexual AIDS scare, Leishman's piece was the best. True, the core of the piece was completely fallacious. Everything in the article stemmed from the "fact" that AIDS was now running rampant in the white, heterosexual middle class. But *besides* that, the quotes she used were often entertaining (I've used some myself in this book to spice things up), and she interviewed some very interesting people. In a society that seems to place a low premium on fact and a high one on entertainment value, Leishman's articles are the kind we can expect.

In a thoughtful *Newsweek* article, Jonathan Alter notes that "serious news is often treated with gullibility and lack of follow-through":

> "It's as if there is an inflatable map of the world," says author David Halberstam. "One month the Falklands is the biggest thing on the map, then it's a flyspeck again." Whatever happened to Poland? Or the artificial heart? Much of this spasmodic quality is due to television. With some exceptions, TV lacks any equivalent to the inside pages of a paper. That means that when a story fades, it fades almost entirely, and the media's saturation coverage skips on to the next event, often passing over whatever new details arise that may fundamentally change the "old stories."[73]

So it was with the heterosexual AIDS explosion. When the major newsmagazines seemed convinced that such an explosion was occurring, they slapped it onto their covers, repeatedly. When they saw this was not the case, they either said as much somewhere fairly deep in the magazine or they said nothing at all. (An exception to the rule finally came in 1989 when *Time* gave a few pages over to John Langone.[74])

By the end of 1988, the heterosexual AIDS alarmists had all but worn out the public's attention. At that time, Dr. Harry W. Haverkos, something of an ally of Robert Redfield from early on, published a mildly alarmist survey article in the *Journal of the American Medical Association.* For example, he relied on Masters, Johnson, and Kolodny for determining prevalence of heterosexual infections as a source (perhaps the only medical journal article to do so), his only caveat being that the sex researchers did not submit their study to peer review.[75] Yet when the article came out, notwithstanding its appearance in one of the most prestigious of the medical journals, it was for the most part ignored.*

The explosion did not come, fortunately. Yet, like a balloon that has been blown up and then had the air released, or like a size-8 hat worn regularly by a size-7 head, things never went completely back to the way they were. While there may have been a general feeling among the public that some of the scare material was just that, the common "wisdom"—if that term be used—was still that AIDS poses a major threat

---

*For example, the *Washington Times* reporter Joyce Price ignored the alarmist message and concentrated on the very real problem of black heterosexuals and AIDS.[76]

An Epidemic of Media Hype

to the heterosexual middle class. And while at least during the time the alarmists were especially active the anti-alarmists could also claim some share of the media's attention, when the furor died down the anti-alarmists to a great extent disappeared off the airwaves and magazine pages as well. Anti-alarmism, after all, had simply been a reaction. While the alarmists were acting, it was much easier to oppose them. When Masters, Johnson, and Kolodny published their book, the media wanted an anti-alarmist reply.

In general, however, publishers were tired of the heterosexual AIDS question. They quit while the alarmists were ahead. Thus, just as Rome left its language and customs behind as it fell before the barbarian hordes, the media and the alarmists had left an impression that would last for years.

The problem, of course, is that the disinformation is still out there. For all the reasonably intelligent reader knows, the sudden dearth of stories on the heterosexual epidemic means not that there is a dearth of heterosexual cases, but that the media has simply grown tired of disseminating facts everyone must already know by now anyway. Six years after the intense media blitz on the Falklands, most of us still have a good idea of its location, climate, and population. We do not need constant reminders from the media. Why should it be any different with readers' assumptions about the heterosexual AIDS explosion? Especially when those media continue to find some sort of bad news for heterosexuals in virtually any AIDS study?

Apart from the pressures inherent in journalism, other motivations inclined many reporters to prepare stories fostering the impression of a heterosexual AIDS explosion, and still others influenced those the reporters were likely to quote.

The desire to democratize the disease undoubtedly had an effect. The group that the pollsters Robert Lichter and Stanley Rothman describe as the "media élite"—that is, reporters for such journals as the *New York Times*, the *Washington Post*, the *Wall Street Journal*, and the major networks—is decidedly liberal and very sympathetic toward homosexuality. While most Americans feel homosexuality is wrong,[77] of the media élite, according to the well-known Lichter/Rothman study, only 25 percent felt that homosexuality is wrong; while 76 percent disagreed with that position, and most of those "strongly disagreed." (The numbers do not add up to 100 percent due to rounding.)[78]

"Reporters have wanted to believe in heterosexual AIDS," says Randy Shilts. "There's been a gullibility. Reporters are always looking

for the local angle. The heterosexual angle did that for AIDS. Even if
AIDS isn't going to be a heterosexual disease, it could be in the mind
of some liberal reporters."[79]

Meanwhile, the sex therapist Helen Singer Kaplan titled the preface
of her extremely alarmist AIDS book "Why I Hate to Talk About AIDS,"
and in it began:

> For the last twenty-five years I have loved helping people with sexual
> problems and conducting research to improve theories and methods of sex-
> ual therapy. It is a joyful experience for me to help free a patient from a
> sexual disability that has cast a cloud over his or her life, or to see a couple's
> marriage improve as they begin to overcome their long-standing sexual dif-
> ficulties. I love telling people: "Enjoy, it's okay to have sexual feelings. . . .
> Sex is a natural function. . . . Sex is not dirty or harmful. . . . Don't give your
> kids sexual hangups!"
>
> But now I find myself warning people, especially our young women: "Look
> out! Sex with an infected partner is dangerous!"[80]

While Kaplan made no outright confession of her own guilt, she did go
so far as to imply a sort of national—or even international—guilt. Noting
that she is a "refugee of the Holocaust," she wrote:

> [I]f someone had warned us in the early 1930s at the first sign of the Nazi
> plague, *before* the Nazi Party became firmly entrenched, perhaps the trag-
> edy of the mass exterminations could have been prevented. We can't go back
> to that time, but it is still early enough to prevent a general AIDS
> *epidemic.* [81]*

That's a metaphor even Susan Sontag would not touch. But Kaplan's
efforts to spread the guilt for the Holocaust appears to signal her personal reservations about helping to give rise to conditions she now
believes are allowing the rapid spread of the AIDS virus.

Of course, when it comes to divining motivation, both sides can play
the game; and when someone declared that the risk to heterosexuals
was being overstated, the alarmists were often quick to assert that the
debunker was acting out of personal interest. On "People are Talking,"
a New Jersey television talk show on which both Kaplan and I appeared,
she declared that men downplaying the risk of AIDS to heterosexuals
did so because they did not want women to stop sleeping with them.[83]

*Kaplan again uses the AIDS-Nazi metaphor a page later: "You hear: 'Don't get hysteri-
cal, nothing is going to happen to you' and 'Relax, just use a condom. . . . Forget it, you'll
be okay.' That is exactly how I heard my parents and their friends talk, when the Nuremberg Laws were first passed: 'Relax, Hitler is crazy, he'll be gone by next year, just sit it
out.' "[82]

Similarly, when Geraldo Rivera discussed the issue on two shows in the same day, the "experts" he called upon to provide the view that the heterosexual risk was exaggerated were the *Playboy* publisher Hugh Hefner and the *Penthouse* publisher Bob Guccione,[84] as if to say, "Boys just want to have fun."

Clearly, some of the AIDS alarmists felt that telling the truth about AIDS was not in the best interest of the public. "You just can't tell these people that most heterosexuals are not at risk," one told me, "because then heterosexuals who *are* at risk will think you're talking about them." I disagreed, saying that it is possible to tell some heterosexuals they are at very low risk while warning others that they are at extremely high risk; that, indeed, misinforming the public now could be the worst thing to do. But the doctor had made a political decision, which was to disregard his epidemiological findings, and I did not doubt that this doctor's intentions were well meant.

The motivations of other doctors who manipulated the media, however, were often less salutary. Langone has written that with the high expenditures on AIDS

> comes visibility, the quality that can lead to fame for scientists. Although some researchers will tell you that they have more important things than AIDS to worry about, working on a disease that has a chance of spreading to the general public and therefore gets constant media attention is in itself an enticement: one gets the impression sometimes that a few of the scientists are the laboratory counterparts of military commanders who need a conflict to keep them in the limelight while they make their reputations.[85]

For persons such as this, presenting AIDS as a disease associated primarily with a small proportion of the population was wholly unsatisfactory. Langone says that when he mentioned to a virologist that anal intercourse is implicated in the majority of AIDS cases in the United States, the virologist pounded his desk and shouted in rage, "You're not helping your country at all by focusing on that!"[86]

It is hard to understand why, except in the limited instance of revealing military secrets, telling the truth to one's readers is not helping one's country. Fortunately, Langone refused to accept the virologist's idea of patriotism. Unfortunately, Langone was a rare bird indeed. With far too few exceptions, the sole ambition of reporters covering the heterosexual aspect of the AIDS crisis seems to have been sheer entertainment and sales. It is hardly a coincidence that the newspaper that has by far the worst AIDS coverage in the nation, *USA Today,* also has the highest circulation of any national edition. "You provide the prose poems; I'll provide the war," said Citizen Kane to a foreign correspondent, in a thinly veiled depiction of newspaper magnate William Randolph Hearst and his efforts to draw America into a war with Spain.[87] "You supply a grain of truth," the modern American media says, "and we'll supply the panic." In this case, it supplied an epidemic. Mr. Kane would have been proud indeed.

20

The Terror, Revisited

In previous chapters, we have seen the profit in making the myth. But where was the profit in buying into it? Why did people with seemingly nothing to gain so readily believe nonetheless that for which the evidence was always sketchy? Why, during the AIDS crisis, did America put its brain on hold?

Time and again, AIDS has been treated by a standard that, were it applied to anything else, would have been instantly recognized as patently absurd. We were told to multiply our sex partners by their sex partners by their sex partners *ad infinitum* to see our risks for exposure to HIV, but no one would think to tell us to multiply persons we've touched by the persons they've touched by the persons they've touched to see our risks for exposure to bubonic plague. We were told that 1 chance in 10,000,000 of getting AIDS is too high to risk having sex, even though none of us would consider shunning cars because our odds of dying in an automobile are about 1 in 5,000 a year. Why did we see the first as "playing Russian roulette," but not the second? Why, upon finding that condoms are not foolproof, did we make a huge fuss over eliminating "safe sex" in favor of "safer sex"? The first time someone died in a car while wearing a safety belt, did we insist on calling them "safetier belts"? Finally, who in his right mind would, upon being informed that there were twice as many flu deaths this month as last, whip out a pocket calculator and predict that the figures would keep doubling until everyone was dead of flu in the year 1998? (More on this next chapter.) Why would anyone in their right minds believe them?

The Cult of Fear

To a great extent, to be sure, the public's willingness to accept any and all alarmist propaganda was based on sheer gullibility with a pinch of stupidity. "I thought AIDS was a gay disease," said a man interviewed by *USA Today* in October 1985, "but if Rock Hudson's dead it can kill anyone."[1] Yet as time went on and the cases predicted continued to fail to appear, more and more of us should have asked, as did one skeptical writer, "But has anyone actually seen the [heterosexual] AIDS Demon?"[2] Yet we continued to believe in the demon—and, indeed, many will read this book cover to cover and still refuse to let go of their fear. Instead, they will scan the pages, looking for references to this study or that one that somehow can be construed to provide evidence that they might indeed have been infected during that one-night stand four years earlier, or that striking up a conversation with a gorgeous person making eyes at them might be the first step toward a horrible death. These heterosexuals hold their fear close to their chests as if it were a precious gem in a den of thieves. They constitute the single greatest allies the alarmists have. Anna Lekatsas, the New York City investigator responsible for that city's having such a low number of cases classified as heterosexually transmitted, comments, "What's really interesting is that this virus is not spreading rampantly, but people don't want to be reassured. I keep reading about doctors and other people getting hysterical over this. I guess it's something for people to obsess about or act out old fantasies."[3] Indeed, this obsession or fantasy of fear would prove to be crucial to the spread of the heterosexual AIDS myth.

Part of the explanation would appear to be that people react most apprehensively—and irrationally—to risks that are new or unfamiliar. The writer John Tierney gives an excellent example of this reaction:

Recently in New Jersey, outraged citizens prevented the disposal of some low-level radioactive waste (from a factory that made luminescent paint for watch dials) in an abandoned quarry. This threat was infinitesimal compared with something that researchers happened to be studying at the same time: the radioactive radon gas emanating from natural rock formations into many New Jersey homes. Researchers found that breathing the air in some New Jersey homes was equivalent to smoking three or four packs of cigarettes a day—yet even after the residents were told, most of them didn't plan to do anything about it. The rocks under their homes were a risk they could live with: something natural, something that had been around forever. But don't put any "unnatural" new poisons into the quarry down the road.[4]

If one were to conduct a survey of nondrug-using heterosexuals who had changed their lives substantially to avoid getting AIDS, one would probably find a seat-belt usage rate approximating that of heterosexuals who were not worried about AIDS. In other words, many heterosexuals terrified of AIDS do not bother to buckle up. Probably every person interviewed in that survey could name a friend or relative who had died in an automobile crash, while none could name a heterosexual who had died of AIDS. No matter. AIDS is new and marvelous; fatal automobile accidents are something we have grown accustomed to precisely because they are so very common. Nevertheless, while this may make such behavior more understandable, it doesn't make it any more rational. Says Tierney, "If I had to choose between never wearing a condom and never wearing a seat belt, I would keep the seat belt on."[5]

Another reason for willing acceptance of "the Demon" was offered by the author and medical doctor Michael Crichton, writer of *The Andromeda Strain.* In an article for *Playboy,* he recounted how many of his non–drug-using female friends were terrified of AIDS, even while his homosexual friend said he refused to stop engaging in unprotected anal intercourse. Crichton hypothesized that many of us have welcomed AIDS as an excuse to avoid intimacy: "Many heterosexuals accept the bad news almost eagerly, exaggerating the threat for their own purposes. Because in the end, it's easier to blame AIDS for the way you live than to face the uncomfortable truth that you're terrified of the very intimacy you say you desire."[6]

Disasterphilia

Yet there are plenty of reasons for those of us not seeking to avoid intimacy to welcome a terrifying AIDS scenario. As one friend of mine put it, "I know it sounds perverse, but when I hear of a disaster, I want it to be a really bad disaster." But if "perverse" implies a deviation from the norm, his thoughts are probably not. Many of us think of "based on a true story" horror movies as at least slightly scarier and hence more enjoyable than completely fictional movies. Disasters represent for us the ultimate horror movies. This cast of mind persists, notably, so long as we do not actually become the victims. We must be able to get no closer than the television or newspaper. One can be sure that those who predict a loss of a third of the world's population due to AIDS are fairly certain that they will not be among the tally.

David Black, in *The Plague Years,* writes of an AIDS conference he attended:

People were giddy with an anxiety near to joy, the same heightened emotion that comes when you wait for the firecracker to explode or for the midnight countdown to the New Year. I'd seen it when I was a kid during the Cuban missile crisis and when the United States had mined the harbors at Haiphong: the thrill of living on the edge of the apocalypse.[7]

It is the same thrill that Walker Percy had in mind when he noted that, in the week following the bombing of Pearl Harbor, the U.S. suicide rate "declined dramatically across the nation";[8] and that Sir Winston Churchill spoke of when he said, "Nothing in life is so exhilarating as being shot at without result."[9] One girl testified before Congress, "If there is such a thing as a high-risk group, it is teen America. And we at the Teen AIDS Hotline are working to save our generation."[10] Surely it's not every day that one is given the opportunity to save a generation. Susan Sontag has written,

> There is . . . a need for an apocalyptic scenario that is specific to "Western" society. And perhaps even more so to the United States. (America, someone has said, is a nation with the soul of a church—an evangelical church prone to announcing radical endings and brand-new beginnings.) The taste for worst-case scenarios reflects the need to master fear of what is felt to be uncontrollable. It also expresses an imaginative complicity with disaster. The sense of cultural distress or failure gives rise to the desire for a clean sweep, a tabula rasa. No one wants a plague, of course. But [having earlier quoted Harvard professor Stephen Jay Gould saying that AIDS may kill a quarter of us but "there will still be plenty of us left and we can start again"], yes, it would be a chance to begin again. And beginning again—that is very modern, very American, too.[11]

Compare the way the media handles economic news. If the economy is booming, it scrapes up experts willing to wring their hands and warn of the economy "overheating," with a consequent burst of inflation. If, on the other hand, economic growth starts to slow, there is no end of talk about an impending recession. But is an economy like a kerosene heater; can it overheat? That the value of a dollar is linked to the employment level is but an economic theory, nothing more, and one that fared none too well during the boom economy of the 1980s. Nevertheless, it contains a certain appeal. Apocalypses fill a need. They fill the newspapers and they fill us with a sense of meaning. In a free society, one can be sure that such demands will always be met.

The Sex and Death Allure

It is hardly a new discovery that sex sells. Overtly or subliminally, sex is used to sell everything from cars to vacation packages to pen-and-pencil sets to submarine sandwiches. But what the media discovered during the AIDS epidemic, as best represented by Connie Chung's "Scared Sexless," was that *antisex* could sell as well. Antisex has to be distinguished from lack of sex. "Ozzie and Harriet" was lack of sex: it wasn't that they explained in explicit terms what little Ricky shouldn't do, or that they tore down gorgeous centerfolds from his bedroom wall; the subject was just never broached. But when Alexis on "Dynasty" denies a salivating would-be suitor, that's antisex, and it can be downright sexy. An antimissile missile is still a missile and antisex is still sex; the antimissile implies the presence of a missile, and antisex implies the presence of sex. And just as a bikini on a shapely young woman can be far more tantalizing than seeing that same woman standing stark naked, so, too, can antisex be indeed sexier than the real thing.

But if Hollywood had only recently discovered that antisex could be sexy, it had long known that death could be. It has to be handled in the right way, to be sure, but as the phenomenal success of Anne Rice's vampire novels shows, the combination can be entertainment dynamite. The way to keep death sexy with AIDS was to allude to it, but not show it. Thus, while some of the more serious shows would depict AIDS patients in their last stages, those like "Scared Sexless" would get no closer to the death and debilitation of the disease than saying that it occurred.

Sex and death are often linked in popular culture. The stereotypical 1950s horror movie has a couple necking inside a car on a lonely hilltop as the monster silently approaches. The single most popular movie monster is the vampire, which traditionally was quite ugly and favored little children as victims, but in modern times has been converted to a tall, strikingly handsome male who favors beautiful women with lovely necks as victims. Even werewolves have been turned into sex objects, as demonstrates an entire series of *The Howling* films depicting voluptuous women who become wolves. Indeed, a whole genre of "exploitation films" has sprung up that consist of little else than softcore sex and hardcore killings. There would seem to be a "black widow" factor in many of us that somehow makes sex more exciting if there is a hint of death around. AIDS provides for some heterosexuals that hint of death. Proclaimed one woman's magazine, "For women who are single and dating, the AIDS epidemic can . . . present a cruel choice: love or life."[12]

If people find gambling exciting—and many do—what could possibly be more exciting than a game where love is the stakes and life is the risk?

The AIDS God

An acquaintance of mine provided, quite inadvertently, interesting insight into the state of probably many a heterosexual mind in the age of AIDS. Reacting to my assertion that the AIDS threat to heterosexuals was overplayed, he responded, "I don't care what you say, from now on I don't sleep with a girl till the second date." Well!

In an article in *Seven Days* magazine, Joseph Hooper wrote:

> There is something about the entire heterosexual AIDS debate that smacks of religion. Like God, heterosexual AIDS is basically invisible and heterosexuals are asked to believe in it with the understanding that if they don't, they will pay dearly. Atheists can take refuge in the hardheaded skepticism of a Michael Fumento, but I suspect most clean-living heterosexuals fall into the agnostic camp. They don't exactly believe they're at risk, but they will consider using a condom. Like going to church on Sunday, it's a minimum insurance policy. And the believers don't need a Bible, just last year's issue of *Time* "for those who are forever young, or venturesome, or lonely or simply careless." AIDS as Old Testament virus.[13]

I suspect that Hooper's suspicion is correct. Like my friend, heterosexuals wanted to do *something* to show that they were informed and properly fearful. Actions of little practical use, like waiting till the second date to have intercourse, served as talismans. If I wear this otherwise fairly worthless rock around my neck, the Evil Forces will spare me. If I wait until the second date to have sex, AIDS will spare me.

But these actions were probably more along the lines of a sacrifice. Treating a disease as if it has an intelligence is hardly a new concept. Such beliefs go back further than AIDS. One speaks, for instance, of "tempting fate," as if fate would get angry at you for trying its patience. Throughout history, people have made "contracts" with various forces of nature, including disease.

Still, no contract is valid without legal consideration. If you want Mother Nature to give you good crops, you have to give her something, too; and obeisance to AIDS took a variety of forms. One homosexual author stated that, at some level, he felt that if he continued to write about AIDS, he wouldn't get it. (He did.) When I asked a male nurse at the outpatient clinic at San Francisco General Hospital if, when he first started working there in 1981 (when the mechanics of transmission were still unknown), he wasn't afraid of catching AIDS from patients, his answer surprised me: "Actually, it was the other way around. I'm gay, and I knew I was at risk for AIDS. I and many of us working here convinced ourselves that if we worked with the disease it wouldn't strike us." That, too, was not to be; the day before I got there one of the staff succumbed to AIDS. But the fact that nature and disease have never been good about honoring contracts with human beings doesn't mean that the latter will stop trying to strike a deal. Hence, the sacrifice.

As a general rule, however, modern men and women do not care much for sacrifices. As recently as 1965, the Catholic Church required its faithful to abstain from eating meat on Fridays and to have only one meal on Good Friday and Ash Wednesday. To most of the world's population, having six days of meat a week would have been wonderful practically beyond belief. But for Europeans and Americans, it proved so onerous that the restrictions were cut back to apply only during Lent. Even this can be waived at the discretion of the bishop. What made heterosexuals' sacrifice to AIDS even worse was that, as Hooper pointed out, they weren't even sure a sacrifice was needed. It's one thing to scrimp and save for a new car or stereo system or some other tangible gain. It's another to give up something you love when you really have no idea whether there will be a payoff. You intrinsically realize that some people will have sex like bunnies and never get AIDS, any more than they've already gotten herpes. Why should you sacrifice what little sex life you already have?

The answer was to offer AIDS *something*, but nothing that would be really inconveniencing. With the logic of the little boy who, passionately hating spinach, decides that this is what he will give up for Lent, the nation is no doubt replete with heterosexuals who tell pollsters they have taken steps to avoid getting AIDS—but whose steps consist of not going out with women or men who wouldn't go out with them anyway, or using condoms about 10 percent of the time. At a glance, such apparently useless precautions seem patently absurd. But think again. For a low-risk heterosexual with high anxieties, what could be better than a virtually worthless palliative for a virtually groundless fear?

For many heterosexuals—like many Christians and Jews—the only thing they were willing to offer the virus was belief itself. This was the realm of pure superstition. Don't count your chickens before they're hatched, knock on wood when you talk about disaster, and don't act smug about AIDS not getting you. Remember that in the war movies it's always the soldier who says he knows he's going home in one piece who gets killed. The Harvard microbiologist Myron Essex hinted at the smugness effect when he said that many heterosexuals did not consider themselves at risk and thus would not take precautions, and "It is that alone which makes it certain that the infection will establish itself in the heterosexual population."[14] And, in a self-administered test in Chris Norwood's alarmist book in which the higher the score the greater one's risk for getting AIDS, the test taker finds that she gains four fat points if she answers one question by checking "I really don't think I could ever get it."[15] (Even though the test taker might be a cloistered nun.) Thus readers are informed that whatever their actions, the very act of not believing puts them at risk.

A failure to take action in accordance with one's own proclaimed fears extended beyond terrified heterosexuals. Over 300,000 people bought Gene Antonio's book extolling the dangers of airborne transmission of HIV. Assuming that Antonio believed his own writing or that anyone else did, they should have been wearing spacesuits in public— and at home for that matter, since one would never know whether his child or wife had been breathed upon by an HIV carrier. Yet there is no record of increases in sales of spacesuits at this time, or even of gas masks. (Early in the epidemic, some Hong Kong health care workers did wear such type suits when transporting AIDS patients.)[16]

In short, many people were willing to believe Antonio's assertions, but not to a point where they would greatly inconvenience themselves in acting upon its ultimate message. Avoiding public toilet seats and water fountains and writing angry letters to one's congressperson urging him or her to corral homosexual activities were one thing; cutting oneself off from society was quite another. Even in plague times, self-isolation for short periods of time was infrequently practiced. But with no *tangible* evidence that AIDS was the new Black Death, those who professed belief in the god Antonio created simply could not make their actions fit their fears.

Just as a combination of disparate motivations influenced those who exaggerated the scope of the AIDS epidemic, it stands to reason that a combination of disparate reasons influenced most of the American public to credit those exaggerations. While there are probably many reasons besides those I have touched on, it is beyond doubt that while the alarmists took us for a ride, many of us all too willingly got in the car and then refused to leave when the ride appeared to be over. As Walt Kelly's Pogo might have said: We have met the deceivers, and they is us.

How Has Sexual Behavior Changed?

To listen to the tantalizing media tales, single heterosexuals had either: (1) just about called it quits on sex and the sexual revolution; or (2), despite "the new realities," refused to call it quits on sex. Which was it? A 1988 Yankelovich Clancy Shulman survey for *Time* found that nationwide, of singles eighteen to thirty-four, 15 percent were personally "very worried" about getting AIDS, while another 15 percent were "fairly worried." Thirty-three percent were somewhat worried; and a slight plurality, 37 percent, were not worried at all.[17] But before one jumps to the conclusion that a lot of sexually active heterosexuals are carefree about AIDS, it must be noted that the 37-percent figure is not all that much higher than the number of singles who are celibate, and is far lower than the percentage who are either celibate or have been monogamous for the last twelve months.[18] For New York City, the fear level was even higher. A full 38 percent of eighteen-to-thirty-four-year-old singles were either "very worried" or at least "fairly worried" about contracting AIDS.[19] Still, one didn't need public opinion polls, nor did one have to believe the media's tales of terror, to realize that fear was in the air.

But fear does not always translate into action. Were heterosexuals actually acting upon their fears? The problem with ascertaining the answer to this question is that for the most part it depends on what heterosexuals wanted to say they were doing, as opposed to what they *were* doing. The media seemed to think that one of the best indicators was asking bartenders how many strangers meet and go home together—to which the answer was always, "Far fewer than before." Such a system provides titillating reading, but so many variables render it worthless. Similarly, the media provided anecdotes *ad nauseum* about how terrified heterosexuals were swearing off sex; but, again, the sampling is unknown to the reader. Did the reporter have to interview thirty people to get one juicy quote? Only two people? Did the frustrated reporter say to hell with it and make up the quotes, knowing no one would ever know? One surer way of determining heterosexual activity might have been to look at rates for non-AIDS sexually transmitted diseases. With that simple measure, it would appear that heterosexuals are having more sex, except that no doubt some of that increase—perhaps all of it—is attributable to declining resources spent on treating and tracing cases.

Thus, it appears we are left with simply asking heterosexuals. But even this is filled with pitfalls. Masters and Johnson reported that, in a

1986 survey they conducted consisting of 425 heterosexual adults, most of whom were middle-class whites, 72 percent of the women and 63 percent of the men said they had become more cautious about sex as a result of worries about AIDS. It was their interpretation, however, that many of the respondents did not seem to have translated this concern into consistent behavioral change; the authors noted that 47 percent of the women did not insist upon condom use; and 64 percent indicated that they had had unprotected intercourse at least a "few times" in the preceding year; 76 percent of the men indicated that they did not use condoms on a regular basis. On the other hand, 79 percent of the women and 74 percent of the men said that they were more selective in deciding with whom and when they would have sex. But what does this mean? A college woman might say, "Well, nowadays I would never sleep with a man who looks like he injects drugs"; yet it is quite possible she never would have before, even if only due to lack of opportunity on a middle-class Midwestern campus.

In the search for a more quantifiable measurement, interviewers ask how many partners one has had in the last year. Even though a sheer reduction in partners for most heterosexuals has little or no bearing on actual risk reduction, many people have been convinced that it is, thus it would seem to be at least a good indicator of action to reduce risk. And, sure enough, in the above Masters and Johnson survey, the mean number of partners for men decreased from the previous year from 3.8 to 2.5 and for women from 2.6 to 1.9.[20] In the Winkelstein study (see chapter 2), the San Francisco heterosexual men reported a decrease in partners from 2.8 to 1.8 over a six-month period.[21] The aforementioned New York City survey found that 22 percent of those surveyed had given up sex entirely.[22] This would seem to be good proof of definite action to reduce risk; but as Masters and Johnson concede, one really doesn't know for sure why the number of partners was reduced.[23] AIDS is a good guess, but nothing more. We also do not know whether the surveys were a representative sample, an important consideration since this *is* Masters and Johnson. Most important perhaps, we do not know whether there really was a partner reduction even among the study participants, because of a curious phenomenon pollsters refer to by the scientific term "lying." It means that when people being polled perceive there is no right or wrong answer ("Which detergent do you use?") they will tell the truth; but when they perceive there is a right or wrong answer, they have some inclination to prevaricate. Thus, at the height of the so-called energy crisis in the 1970s, one polling organization, asking what actions people were taking to do their fair share in alleviating the crunch, found an active and concerned citizenry who were inclined to make an extra effort to do their part. Nevertheless, it occurred to the polling organization to throw in a control question: Have you installed a thermidor in your car to get better mileage? Many of those polled said, indeed, they had. *Thermidor,* in fact, refers either to the eleventh month of the short-lived French Revolutionary calender or to a way of cooking lobster. It's an excellent question for a trivia game, but won't do much for mileage.*

Finally, there were polls that showed no risk-reduction activity even claimed. For example, despite the British government's terror campaign aimed at heterosexuals, surveys found little behavioral change in the number of sexual partners or in condom use.[25] In America, a survey conducted for the Alan Guttmacher Institute found that the proportion of girls fifteen to seventeen years old engaging in intercourse climbed from 32 percent to 45 percent between 1982 and 1987. It also found that the proportion of sexually active single women age eighteen to forty-four rose from 68 percent to 76 percent. Only 9 percent of unmarried adult women in 1987 reported their intercourse to be only infrequent—up 1 percent from 1982. Dr. Jacqueline Darroch Forest, vice president for research at the Guttmacher Institute, said the findings "run counter to the assumption many have made that emphasis on urging teen-agers to say no to premarital intercourse and AIDS have caused large proportions of heterosexuals to abstain from non-marital sex."[26] Condom use did nearly double among the women surveyed, but this sounds significant only until the actual percentages are looked at: 9 percent in 1982, 16 percent in 1987.

Thus, it really is unknown how significantly heterosexuals have changed their sexual habits. Certainly, some heterosexuals are having less sex because of fear over AIDS, and it's doubtful that any are having more sex because of it, but it remains unknown whether there has been any significant decline. It could well be that heterosexuals on the whole are having just as much sex as ever; they're simply a lot more scared about it.

If heterosexuals *are* having less sex, will AIDS have killed the "sexual

---

*More recently, the CDC reported on surveys in fifteen states to measure compliance with seat-belt laws. Everyone realizes that seat belts save lives, but many of us do not wear them anyway. When police officers in those states compared the percentage of persons in those states who told pollsters they always or nearly always wore seat belts with those who actually did (using scientific random sampling methods), they found that observed rates were considerably lower than reported rates.[24]

revolution"? There are those who say that the 1960s and 1970s were an aberration, and that AIDS, regardless of true risk, has brought a lost generation back to its senses. But it pays to remember that basically people who had a lot of sex before AIDS did it for one reason: they wanted to. That was something neither the moralists nor the self-appointed preachers in the media could comprehend. AIDS may have temporarily overshadowed that desire, and may continue to do so for years, so ingrained is the idea that heterosexuals are at high risk. But the desire to have sex will outlast the panic, leaving the moralists and the media preachers in search of a new disease or, preferably, a new approach.

21

The Incredible
Shrinking Epidemic

Eight years into the AIDS epidemic the death toll continues to mount. According to statements of some of our trusted doctors and commentators, what we have seen is little compared with what is to come.

Dr. Halfdan Mahler, former director general of the World Health Organization: We stand nakedly in front of a very serious pandemic as mortal as any pandemic there has ever been. I don't know of any greater killer than AIDS . . .[1]

Dr. Willard Cates, Centers for Disease Control: Anyone who has the least ability to look into the future can already see the potential for this disease being much worse than anything mankind has seen before.[2]

Dr. Stephen Jay Gould, professor at Harvard University and popular science writer: Yes, AIDS may run through the entire population, and may carry off a quarter or more of us.[3]

Theresa Crenshaw, member of the President's AIDS commission: If the spread of AIDS continues at the same rate, in 1996 there could be one billion people infected; five years later, hypothetically ten billion; however, the population of the world is only five billion. Could we be facing the threat of extinction during our lifetime? Even before our children are grown?[4]

Even though such views may not be accepted with the credulity that they once commanded, they still significantly influence public policy. Yet virtually all the early estimates of the size of the AIDS epidemic are proving to be grossly exaggerated.

The Unofficial Estimates

During the height of the media scare, no story on the AIDS epidemic was complete without a recital both of the shocking estimates of those now infected with HIV, and the still more ominous estimates of the soon-to-be-infected. Some of those estimates were arrived at by doing little more than pulling numbers out of a hat. Robert Redfield, for example, kept making reference to a figure of 10,000,000 infections in the near future,[5] as did William Haseltine;[6] but apparently nowhere in print have either of these doctors given any substantiation for the figure nor, for that matter, have the media challenged them to provide it. Similarly, in the same 1987 press meeting in which Surgeon General Koop told reporters, "If the heterosexual explosion follows the homosexual explosion, then we are in for unbelievable trouble," he also asserted his belief that the seropositivity level in the United States is probably "much higher" than the Public Health Service's top-end figure of 1,500,000.[7] What the fount of the surgeon general's special knowledge was we cannot know, although it seems clearly irresponsible for him to undercut the authority of his own PHS doctors by simply tossing off his own personal opinions at press meetings.

The media, eager for exciting news, repeated these numbers unquestioningly, often without even giving a source. For example, Michael Kramer, then the chief political correspondent for *U.S. News & World Report*, wrote that there would be as many as 10,000,000 U.S. infections by 1991 to support his declaration that "*everyone* is at risk" (emphasis in original). Redfield was mentioned later in the piece on a different subject, but no source for the 10,000,000 figure was even hinted at.[8] *USA Today* gave a 10,000,000 figure (by 1997) without citing a source. An accompanying graphic showed 10,000,000 to 15,000,000 infections by 2010, citing the Centers for Disease Control and "*USA Today* research," whatever that is.[9] Another figure of 4,000,000 current infections (as opposed to the 1,000,000 to 1,500,000 CDC figure) kept floating around, never with attribution.[10]

Many estimates of the extent of the AIDS epidemic used statistical formulae or models that, though superficially plausible, were utterly worthless. Among them were the "iceberg extrapolation," the "fixed doubling time," and the statistical "black box."

The iceberg extrapolation built upon CDC figures to give itself an air of legitimacy. Several CDC doctors said in 1985 that the actual numbers of seropositives may have been 50 to 100 times the number of AIDS cases reported in those areas;[11] or that for every AIDS case, there are 10 AIDS-related complex cases (ARC, a level of sickness between being asymptomatic and having full-blown immune deficiency); and that for every ARC case, there are 10 asymptomatic HIV carriers.[12] Graphically represented, these ratios look like a huge iceberg, with only the full-blown (or end-stage) AIDS cases showing above the water line. Such estimates of the ratio of asymptomatic cases to AIDS cases to ARC cases, and of ARC cases to full-blown AIDS cases, may once have been plausible, but they were made at a much earlier stage in the epidemic. In a group of 100 persons testing positive for the virus but without symptoms, or "asymptomatic seropositives," when the first person is diagnosed it means that the ratio of asymptomatics to AIDS cases is 99 to 1. A second diagnosis cuts that ratio in half, to 48 to 1, unless in the meantime a full 99 additional people have become infected. Unless the pool of those affected *doubles* before each new diagnosis, the ratio will inevitably go down. Hence, as the epidemic matures and susceptible populations become saturated, the ratio continually changes, until eventually the number of asymptomatics becomes less than the number of those with diagnosed cases. First prize for iceberg-theory terrorism belongs to Stanley K. Monteith, a California orthopedic surgeon who writes for the "AIDS Protection" chastity newsletter (mentioned in chapter 13) and is often called upon to do talk shows in his area. Monteith wrote in the newsletter,

> The CDC has estimated we will have 271,000 Americans dead and dying of AIDS by the end of 1991. They fail to add that for every person who has this disease, between 50 and 100 people will carry the virus. That means in four short years [his piece appeared in January, 1988], we will have somewhere between 13 and 27 million people carrying the virus.

Obviously Monteith's failure to account for a reduced ratio as time goes on, plus his insistence that even *past* diagnoses be added into the denominator, could easily be used to find half of America soon dying of AIDS. Indeed he asks, "what will happen with 50–100 million American carriers?"[13]

CDC AIDS Director James Curran, who may have introduced the whole seropositive/AIDS ratio concept, noted the declining ratio phenomenon,[14] yet it was often ignored by other supposed experts. Thus Masters, Johnson, and Kolodny estimated over 3,300,000 Americans were infected by late 1987, in part by using a 75-to-1 ratio (splitting the difference between 50 to 1 and 100 to 1).[15]* Another author uncritically used the early ratio to estimate that 5,000,000 Americans were infected with AIDS.[17] And in a review of the Masters, Johnson, and Kolodny book, Wayne Lutton, an AIDS-book author himself, exaggerated the number of asymptomatic seropositives by using the 100-to-1 ratio for AIDS cases diagnosed in mid-1988, and thus led readers to conclude that there might be 6,000,000 existing infections.[18]†

Another technique that exaggerates the scope of the epidemic also uses CDC figures. It plays off the case doubling time. Doubling time is a simple way of referring to the rate of increase in AIDS cases. If we observe that the number of cases is doubling every year, we say the doubling time is one year. If the doubling time goes from every year to every thirteen months, then the epidemic's rate of increase is slowing. The nature of an epidemic such as AIDS, based on behavior, is that the virus will initially pick off the "easy" targets. (In the case of AIDS, the easiest targets have been men who engage in receptive anal intercourse with numerous other men who also engage in receptive anal intercourse with numerous other men, since this activity has been shown to be by far the most conducive to transmitting the virus.) An epidemic will progress ever more slowly as fewer and fewer easy targets remain: that is, the caseload may increase from month to month, but the rate at which it increases is ever slower. For somewhat different reasons than with AIDS, this occurs every year with flu cases. Even though flu is casually contagious, only a fraction of the population gets it each year. The virus claims its victims and moves on, pulling them in at an ever slow rate.

This process has been observed with AIDS since the epidemic began. At first, cases were doubling every five months, but this rate quickly slowed to six months, seven months, and so on. By early 1989 doubling time was over sixteen months.[20] It is now certainly well over sixteen months, though it is hard to say since by definition we only know that it was sixteen months sixteen months ago, not that it still is. Obviously, freezing the doubling time—instead of allowing for its progressive slowing—and then extrapolating over a lengthy period of time will produce outrageous results. Despite this, or more probably because of it, some AIDS "experts" have done just that.

---

*"Since the cumulative total of cases of AIDS in the United States as of late 1987 was approximately 45,000, we can calculate (using the midpoint figure of 75 as multiplier) that the pool of infected people was approximately 3,375,000 as of that time."[16]

†Helen Singer Kaplan in her 1987 book also erroneously used the 100-to-1 ratio, but drew no conclusion nor called for the reader to do so.[19]

In *The AIDS Cover-up?*, for example, Gene Antonio used a twelve-month doubling time for AIDS cases and predicted that as many as 8,000,000 Americans would be infected by the end of 1987 and 64,000,000 by the end of 1990. Antonio erred not only in freezing the doubling time but in extrapolating from AIDS doubling time to HIV-infection doubling time. Because the incidence of AIDS follows, on average, several years behind the incidence of infection, it provides a picture of infection doubling time that is far out of date. And because, as we have seen, doubling time is increasing as the epidemic ages, the doubling time at any given moment for the infection rate would be far longer than that for end-stage AIDS.

Fallacious as such a concept seems, it is amazing how many people uncritically repeated the Antonio figures or methodology. A. D. J. Robertson, president of Research, Testing & Development Corp., used the same figures in a letter to the *Wall Street Journal* in 1985.[21] Notwithstanding his alarmism—or probably because of it—he went on to write several articles for various magazines, to testify before Congress, and to serve as an advisor to Gary Bauer at the White House. One Lyndon Larouche publication carried out the doubling time to the point at which all Americans were expected to be dead by 1993;[22] and a political group, Americans Against AIDS, claimed that AIDS could kill *"more than every single American alive today!"* (emphasis added).[23]*

Others have ignored the CDC estimates in devising their own computer models. One such model was devised by Anthony Pascal at the Rand Corporation, which found that from 400,000 to 750,000 Americans would be diagnosed with AIDS by 1991.[25] Another, by Kevin Hopkins and William Johnston of the Hudson Institute, estimated that by 1987 there were up to 2,900,000 HIV infections.[26] But these models were no better than the numbers fed into them, many of which were shaky estimates. Garbage in, garbage out. Economists call this "black boxing": you put figures into a black box and pull out whatever ones you wish. The Hudson Institute report relied on such discredited authorities as Masters, Johnson, and Kolodny and thus simply multiplied the errors of the sex therapists.[27] Models like the Rand Corporation's contained vast numbers of variables, in the apparent belief that the more factors

*David Black notes in *The Plague Years* the talk that the doubling increase was such that, if it continued at that rate and spread into the general population without check, it would in a decade kill everyone in the United States and in another decade kill everyone in the world ten times over. "The good news about that calculation is it makes the threat of a nuclear holocaust trivial," Black quotes an unidentified epidemiologist as saying: "The bad news is that it's only playing with numbers. No disease wipes out everyone."[24]

one has, the more fine-tuned will be the result. In fact, the opposite is
usually true. Each time different assumptions are used, new opportunities are created for miscalculations. Every mathematical operation
magnifies the effect of any inaccurately valued variable. If these estimates are then multiplied, the margin of error will be multiplied as
well. The result can be a model valid on paper but divorced from
reality.

One political scientist, who predicted that up to 10,000 men would
become infected by prostitutes in the next year, became upset when I
pointed out that there simply were not enough men being infected by
heterosexual intercourse—let alone from prostitutes—to justify such
numbers. While admitting that his original 10,000 figure was too high,
he nevertheless insisted that it was not just a wild guess because it was
based on a mathematical model. He failed to see that there might be
serious flaws in a model whose estimate he now recognized was too
high.

Sometimes those who came up with such models even saw ahead of
time that their conclusions would appear outlandishly high. A trick they
then employed was to present their absurd statistics, then say, "Even
if we cut this figure by X, we still have a major problem." For example,
one author used doubling time to assert that by the year 2010, 180,000,-
000 Americans could be infected, and added, "An absurd possibility?
The reports of concern discussed previously in this book suggest not.
Even if the above projection is off by 75 percent, 45 million Americans
may still be victims of the disease."[28] Gene Antonio did likewise with
his fanciful doubling-time figure. First, he predicted 64,000,000 infections by 1990, then said, "Even if the present estimated [estimated by
him] rate of AIDS virus transmission was cut in half . . . that means
15,187,500 [U.S. infections] by the end of 1990."[29] Hopkins and Johnston in the Hudson Institute report stated, "If studies such as that by
Masters and Johnson are anywhere near correct . . ."[30]

It's all quite appealing. These people aren't extremists, we are supposed to tell ourselves. Why, they're even cutting the figures to show
how conservative they are; yet they still make their point. Think again.
John Wayne Gacy was convicted of murder in the sex slaying of over
30 small boys. If he said that all of the boys consented to sex acts would
we say that "Even if Gacy were telling the truth only half the time, that
still means over 15 boys consented"? Of course not. Why, then, when
the methodology of a figure is obviously suspect, is it fair simply to adjust
the final number a bit? It is not. Just as there are no degrees of "destroyed," once the methodology of a model or study has been shown to

be lacking, the result is worthless. No amount of reducing or adding, dividing or multiplying, will be anything more than arbitrary.

The CDC Estimates: AIDS and HIV in the United States

But what of the "conservative" figures generated by official government bodies such as the CDC? In fact, even these have been overstated.

At its June 1986 meeting at the Coolfont resort in West Virginia, the CDC estimated that 1,000,000 to 1,500,000 Americans were infected with HIV. To get that figure, the CDC had first to estimate the size of the population at risk. That figure was based on the estimates of the prevalence of homosexuals in the population given in the 1948 Kinsey study of male sexual behavior,[31] an estimate of the prevalence of intravenous drug abusers provided by the National Institute of Drug Abuse (NIDA), and estimates of the numbers of hemophiliacs, blood recipients, and sexual partners of all of these. Other than the estimate of the number of severe hemophiliacs, whose reliance on clotting factor made them vulnerable to the AIDS virus but also fairly easy to count, all of the estimates were fairly soft.

Then the CDC had to estimate the extent to which each of these groups was infected. To do so, it could rely on little more than spot surveys conducted at such places as sexually transmitted disease clinics. This was already a recipe for trouble, in that attendees of STD clinics, far from representing the general population, represent those most likely to have any type STD. Most heterosexuals never get a sexually transmitted disease; and, indeed, many heterosexuals and homosexuals are celibate for much of their lives. Thus, a 50-percent infection rate at an STD clinic hardly means that 50 percent of the persons in that area should be considered to be infected. The doctors at the CDC knew this; yet knowing it, and being able to do something about it in terms of adjusting the final figures, were two entirely different things. Thus, the CDC tossed off the 1,000,000 to 1,500,000 figure probably more to satisfy the media's and the public's lust for hard numbers than for anything else. The epidemiologists I spoke to at the CDC said, off the record, that they had very little confidence about the accuracy of the figure one way or another.

Because of unsureness over the original estimate, and because of a dearth of information about how fast, if at all, the epidemic was spreading, the CDC was not quick to update its estimate. So the media and the self-appointed AIDS experts took it upon themselves to tack on their own estimates of new infections occurring since the CDC's. Masters and Johnson were among these, and used the resulting figure to corroborate their iceberg deduction of over 3,000,000 existing infections.[32]* Finally, in November 1987, the CDC tacitly admitted that the old figure was too high, but did so as surreptitiously as possible, not by reducing the old figure but by trotting out new data to show that the old figure was still good—a year and a half's worth of infections later.† (Actually, the CDC dropped the top end by 100,000 to 1,400,000.) It might be said that the CDC waited for infections to catch up to the earlier estimate. Even so, the entire conception of a growing pool of seropositivity may be false.

Current case demographics show that less than 3 percent of AIDS cases are attributable to native-born heterosexual transmission. Those who warn against taking this percentage as reassuring often invoke the long incubation period for AIDS. They suggest that there may be a much larger proportion of heterosexuals infected who have not yet shown up in the AIDS statistics. They ignore the flip side of this argument—that because of AIDS's long incubation, cases of actual illness will be diagnosed at increasing rates long after infections may have peaked. For most of the risk categories, this is clearly what has happened. Studies based on eight cohorts of homosexual and bisexual men in major cities indicate that the rate of new infections among homosexuals in major cities—the largest part of the CDC AIDS estimate—slowed to nearly zero (ranging from zero to 4 percent depending on the city) between June 1986 and the present.[35] New infections among IVDAs are also slowing dramatically. On the East Coast, where the "shooting gallery" phenomenon prevails, the IVDA population is so saturated with HIV that there is little room for new growth, except to the extent that there may be new "recruits" to the ranks of IVDAs. On the West Coast, where shooting galleries are much rarer, the overall infection rate is comparatively low (meaning there is room for many more infections)—but, then, so is the new infection rate. A study of Los Angeles IVDA reported in the January 1989 *American Journal of Public Health* found that of 800 tested, only 1.7 percent were seropositive, meaning few old infections and few new ones.[36] Thus, if the national

---

*Another sex therapist, Dr. Kaplan, also extended the CDC figure but, rather dishonestly, attributed it to the CDC itself: "The Centers for Disease Control estimates that two million Americans are now infected with the AIDS virus," she wrote in *The Real Truth About Women and AIDS*.[33]

†In fact the new number was actually somewhat lower—945,000 to 1,400,000—but, at least in informal writing, the director of the CDC AIDS program, James Curran, continues to use the old figure, as do the media.[34]

seropositivity figure was "almost certainly too high" in June 1986, as Curran puts it,[37] then it is quite possibly too high now.

Too high by how much, though? One method of trying to bypass the system of estimating seroprevalence for various groups and then stringing them together—the CDC method—consists of trying to extrapolate from a single group from which seroprevalence can be accurately gauged. Thus, the prevalence rate for first-time tested donors, 0.04 percent, multiplied by the size of the population fifteen to fifty-nine years of age (about 148,000,000), gives a national figure of about 60,000 infected.[38]* But this is clearly an underestimate since persons at recognized high risk are largely excluded from the blood donor pool. Military applicant figures are similarly skewed. Even the blood tests of hospital applicants so far performed tend to be skewed since the four hospitals originally participating were in metropolitan areas that have high minority populations and minorities have much higher seropositivity rates. Plans to conduct massive seroprevalence sampling across the nation continue to bog down.

The CDC has also tried to estimate infections based on the estimated incubation rate and the reported caseload, then adding 20 percent to account for unreported or unrecognized cases. But depending on which incubation or "progression" rate was used, this resulted in estimates ranging from 66,000 to 2,936,000 or, using only the "most likely" progression rate, 186,000 to 2,732,000.[39] Joel Hay, a health economist at the Hoover Institution, using what he believes to be the mostly likely progression rate, estimates only 500,000 to 800,000.[40] This number, he says, is similar to that confided to him by a top CDC official at the Fourth International Conference on AIDS in Stockholm. Hay says that when he announced his figure at a recent AIDS conference (at Johns Hopkins University), which included representatives from the CDC, nobody attempted to refute it.[41]

But while the number of infections will determine the number of AIDS cases in the long run, in the short run what counts are the cases themselves. Even here Public Health Service figures are not as solid as they might seem. At Coolfont, the CDC projected that 270,000 cases would be diagnosed through the end of 1991, or 251,000 cases from the beginning of 1986.[42] Unfortunately, this analysis is complicated by the CDC's adoption of a new case definition for AIDS. Under the new definition, which went into effect in September 1987, several new

---

*The CDC had used a slightly higher first-time donor seroprevalence in its calculations; since then, the seroprevalence has dropped, as noted in chapter 2.

symptoms of HIV infection are added to what defines AIDS, including such things as dementia and wasting syndrome. The result is that AIDS cases have increased about 30 percent above what they would have been under the old definition,[43] although in some areas, such as San Francisco, it's closer to 20 percent. If 130 cases are reported during one period now, one should assume that this would have been about 100 under the old definition. So, as Hay has pointed out, the redefinition of AIDS not only inflates the apparent rate of increase but also masks previous CDC overestimates.[44] Needless to say, the media ignore the new definition when talking about the rising number of AIDS cases; yet much of the increase in cases over the past two years is due to this.

In 1988, the PHS convened its scientists again and announced that it was extending the projected caseload figure to the end of 1993, predicting 450,000 cases by then. Curran told the media the new projections were unofficial but "pretty well set."[45] The figure of nearly half a million played the media well, grabbing its share of headlines. But in Stockholm a week later, Curran declined to make a prediction past 1992 and a figure of 365,000. "I'm not comfortable going that far [to 1993]," Curran later told me. "We're not publishing [the 450,000 figure]."[46] Indeed, it was not published when the figures were released in the CDC's *Weekly Morbidity and Mortality Report* in September.[47] But as far as most people were concerned, the figure had already been published. The CDC has published no retraction, has held no press conference to retract the figure. It is the 450,000 figure that was used first, and it is that figure that will be remembered and reused. Indeed, several weeks after the Stockholm conference, the editor of the *Washington Post*'s health section declared confidently, "No one is questioning the projection that about 450,000 Americans will be diagnosed with AIDS by 1993."[48]

Although the figure came out of a meeting (closed to the media, incidentally) involving some of the PHS's top scientists, epidemiology had nothing to do with the new estimate. In fact, the PHS analysis could have been performed with a pocket calculator. All that was needed was to determine the rate at which new cases were increasing.

As Dr. John Pickering of the University of Georgia has pointed out,

> If a model is to forecast reliably the incidence of an infectious disease over any extended period of time, then it must be based on the disease's underlying epidemiology, rather than on the mathematical functions that fit the existing incidence data.[49]*

*The full quote is: "[M]odels that are based on statistical fits to data are likely to have severe limitations in their ability to extrapolate and forecast future events, because their

The CDC figures are far shakier than one might think from the reverence with which they have been received. In fact, though the media treats the projections as if sacrosanct, CDC officials will tell you, as Harold Jaffe put it to me, "That's just stupid."[51] The figures are nothing more than a "best guess" path based on a range that estimates anywhere from 13,000 to 190,000 cases during 1992.[52] And the breadth of that range itself has only a 68-percent "confidence interval," meaning that there is 1 chance in 3 it will be incorrect.

Is the Epidemic Peaking?

But why is the CDC reticent about relying on its mathematical projections through 1993? Could it be that the epidemic would peak in that year or before? "Yes," Curran told me.[53]

Until recently the great unspoken words of the AIDS epidemic have been *peak, plateau,* and *crest.* While we have become accustomed to hearing only worse and worse news about AIDS and ever higher caseloads and estimates of caseloads and costs to society ("AIDS Without End" read the title of one otherwise staid article in the *New York Review of Books*[54]), the concept of the epidemic peaking is completely alien to most of the public. Indeed, Masters and Johnson, speaking on "Nightline" in defense of their controversial AIDS book, showed once again that when it comes to diseases they're not playing with a full deck: Masters stated, "We have never known of an epidemic, and historically there is no such positive history, of an epidemic that simply stopped without some manner of cure or vaccine constriction."[55] Yet from biblical times right up to the present, epidemics have been recorded as coming and going—all without the help of either cures or vaccines. Sometimes the disease will become endemic, only to flare up again as an epidemic. Some diseases seem to have disappeared off the face of the earth.[56] But *all* epidemics do peak, more or less along the lines of a bell curve. If the susceptible population is large, as it was when the plague struck a virgin population in the 1300s (the Black Death pandemic), the

---

functions do not necessarily encapsulate the forces driving the epidemic. While the AIDS outbreak may have increased exponentially up to now, clearly it cannot indefinitely continue to do so, if for no other reason than because host populations are finite in number. Models based on exponential functions might predict disease incidence successfully during the onsets of epidemics; however, without the ability to predict when incidence will level off, and possibly decline, such models will eventually fail. If a model is to forecast reliably the incidence of an infectious disease over any extended period of time, then it must be based on the disease's underlying epidemiology, rather than on the mathematical functions that fit the existing incidence data."[50]

peak will be very high. If the susceptible population is much smaller, as with childhood diseases such as polio or whooping cough, the peak will be comparatively lower. For extended epidemics, such as that of AIDS, the entire bell might be so stretched that the peak will actually be something of a plateau for some time, but eventually the cases must fall off.

The epidemiologist who has led the way in attempting to forecast such a peak (or "crest," as he prefers) is Dr. Alexander Langmuir. Langmuir notes that if one plots reported AIDS cases on a ratio scale similar to that on which the Dow-Jones average or the Standard & Poor's index is plotted, over a period of years there will be a sharp rise at first but a clear bending as time goes on. Dr. Langmuir says that the point at which the curve goes flat is the crest of the epidemic. After that point, cases tend to fall off at a rate similar to that at which they increased earlier on. This principle is called "Farr's law," after a British doctor who predicted, fairly accurately, the cresting and ending of the cattle plague of London in 1865–66, on the basis of early reports which nonetheless gave him enough data to plot a graph.

Another system Langmuir uses, which relies on an estimate of the incubation time and on the curve of infections, is based on cohort studies mentioned previously. For example, in the largest San Francisco cohort of homosexuals, which uses blood donated originally to test incidence of hepatitis B, new infections increased from 1.1 percent of the total cohort in 1978 to 11 percent in 1980 to 20.8 percent in 1982, dropping off suddenly to 2.1 percent in 1983.[57] While this cohort does not necessarily reflect the homosexual population of the United States as a whole, it very likely does. None of the other cohorts began as early and, hence when graphed, cannot show an upswing or a peak; but their declines closely match that in the hepatitis-B study. This being the case, the peak in frequency of homosexual infections in major cities in this country was 1982, while 1981 was the point by which one half of all infections had occurred.

If the exact incubation time of all AIDS cases were, say, five years, then AIDS cases would peak about five years after the peaking of infections. Unfortunately, it is not that simple. First, AIDS cases can incubate in anywhere from seven weeks to an estimated thirty years or more. Second, no one knows for sure how many infections will eventually result in AIDS or on average how long that will take. As noted in chapter 2, researchers are moving to a consensus that eventually 99 percent of all persons infected with HIV will eventually get sick, if not succumb to full-blown AIDS.[58]

Langmuir believes that HIV *infections* among all homosexuals—

not just those in major cities—peaked no later than 1982. He predicted that AIDS *cases* among U.S. homosexuals might crest as early as 1989. Since infections in the other risk groups probably peaked later,* this will move the crest for all AIDS cases somewhat later in time. This modification will probably not be substantial, says Langmuir, since homosexuals make up over two thirds of all present cases.

Langmuir is the first to admit that he is an optimist. He also readily admits to having been wrong twice before in prematurely predicting crests in the AIDS epidemic. Yet in neither case was the formula at fault. In one, he underestimated the lag time in reporting (cases are often reported months and occasionally years after diagnosis); and in the other, he underestimated the incubation time—an almost universal mistake. Langmuir could be wrong again, since no one yet knows for sure how accurate the average incubation time estimates are, or exactly when most homosexuals were infected, or exactly what percentage of all infections are homosexual. Finally, the widespread use of AZT in seropositives who have not yet developed symptoms may delay the onset of AIDS, thus significantly extending incubation times.

It is noteworthy that the bottom range of the 68-percent confidence interval figure predicted by the CDC shows the epidemic plateauing in 1988 and starting to fall off in 1989, with total cases for 1992 coming in at 13,000—almost exactly what Langmuir predicted. (See figure 21.4.) This development prompted no small delight on Langmuir's part.

If Langmuir is completely correct, we should expect to see no more than 200,000 AIDS cases among homosexuals—and a correspondingly low number among the other risk groups—by the end of the century. Unfortunately, the lag time in reporting cases to the federal health authorities is so great as to preclude drawing such a conclusion with certainty until long after it has already occurred: that is, it will be hard to get a good fix on how many cases were really diagnosed during 1988 until 1990. Nevertheless, the lag is a fairly consistent one, so if we were to find that this year's level of AIDS cases reported was only slightly higher than that of the year before, it would be a good indicator that by this year the peak had gone flat. In the first six months of 1989 (the latest figures available at this writing) cases were being reported at a rate that, extrapolated over the whole year, would equal 34,344.[59] This

*Hemophiliacs and transfusion victims are thought to have peaked somewhat later. Hemophiliacs appear to have peaked in 1984, as probably also did transfusion victims, since by 1985 hemophiliac clotting factor was being treated for HIV and blood was being effectively screened. No one knows when IVDAs peaked, but they probably did so after homosexuals. The heterosexual category, made up as it is overwhelmingly of partners of IVDAs, will run basically parallel to, but later than, the IVDA curve.

TABLE 21.1

*AIDS Diagnoses by Half Years in San
Francisco, Los Angeles, and New York City**

	San Francisco	Los Angeles	New York City
Pre–Jan 1982	31	23	174
Jan–June 1982	34	19	179
July–Dec 1982	69	56	307
Jan–June 1983	126	110	466
July–Dec 1983	169	147	555
Jan–June 1984	223	196	793
July–Dec 1984	354	267	961
Jan–June 1985	425	406	1233
July–Dec 1985	451	492	1426
Jan–June 1986	583	658	1805
July–Dec 1986	702	753	2091
Jan–June 1987	722	851	2212
July–Dec 1987	740 (666)	794 (715)	2268 (2041)
Jan–June 1988	789 (631)	920 (736)	2290 (1710)

*Figures in parentheses equal estimated number of cases that fit old
(pre-September 1987) AIDS definition only assuming 10 percent of
cases are new definition for July–December 1987, and 20 percent
for January–June 1988. Approximately 10 percent of 1986 and first-
half 1987 figures may also comprise new definition cases added
retroactively.

SOURCE: Health departments of San Francisco, Los Angeles, and
New York.

figure is just a little above the 31,953 cases reported in all of 1988.[60] This
is just about what we would expect if AIDS cases *diagnosed* were
peaking in 1989 or even a bit earlier.

The lag in reporting a diagnosed case is caused by a delay in reporting
from doctors to local public health authorities and local authorities to
state and federal authorities. Thus the lag is much less in reporting to
the cities. Another way, therefore, of checking Langmuir's theory is to
investigate the statistics for the three cities with the most homosexual

FIGURE 21.1

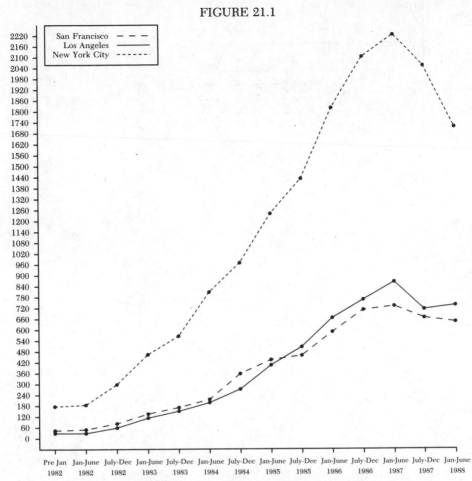

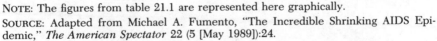

NOTE: The figures from table 21.1 are represented here graphically.

SOURCE: Adapted from Michael A. Fumento, "The Incredible Shrinking AIDS Epidemic," *The American Spectator* 22 (5 [May 1989]):24.

cases. The problem with analyzing the figures is that they are distorted in three ways. First, the reporting time lag (shorter than the federal government's but still considerable) will understate the figures. Conversely, the new case definition will exaggerate the city figures just as they exaggerate the federal figures, by about 20 percent. Finally, there is the problem of underreporting, which is probably far greater for IVDAs than for middle-class white homosexuals but to what extent no one is sure. Thus, it is possible for two epidemiologists to interpret the same figures differently, depending on how they have compensated for these three distortions.

MISINFORMATION IN MICROCOSM

FIGURE 21.2A   New Cases of AIDS, 1979 through 1988,
in the U.S.

FIGURE 21.2B   Development of AIDS cases in the USA.

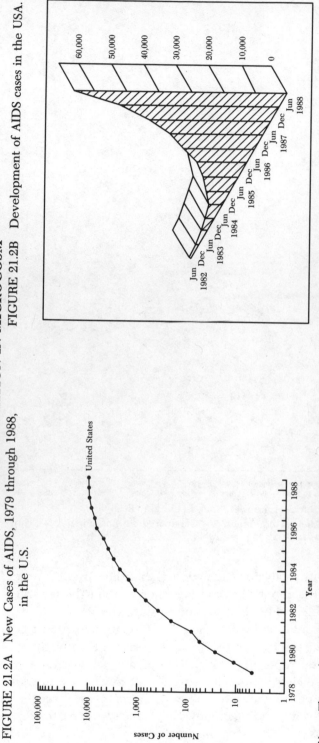

NOTE: The number of new cases is shown on a logarithmic scale according to six-month periods. Because of delayed reporting by many countries, reports for 1988 are not yet final.

SOURCE: Eduardo Cortes et al., "HIV-I, HIV-II, and HTLV-I Infection in High-Risk Groups in Brazil," *NEJM* 320 (15 [13 April 1989]): 1006.

SOURCE: Panos Institute, *AIDS in the Third World*, 3d ed. (Philadelphia: New Society, 1988): 128.

NOTE: The graph on the left is taken from the 13 April 1989 issue of the *New England Journal of Medicine*. The graph shows at a glance the epidemic coming to a crest. Such graphs could be found in medical magazines, but not in the popular press. The graph on the right is from the publication *AIDS in the Third World*, put out in late 1988 by the Panos Institute, an international organization that is alarmist even by the standards of the World Health Organization. Both graphs use the same numbers, but the Panos graph shows cases cumulatively instead of new cases. Further, it has been given a three-dimensional effect and has been turned toward the viewer to allow the illusion of an epidemic that, far from cresting, appears to be accelerating almost to infinity—meaning saturation and death of the entire population.

FIGURE 21.3 AIDS cases, by quarter of report and case definition—
United States, 1981–1988

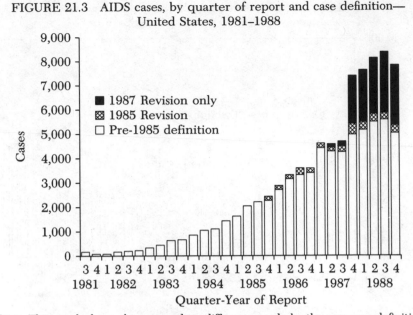

NOTE: This graph shows the tremendous difference made by the new case definition. Since this graph depicts U.S. AIDS cases by the period in which they were reported, not diagnosed, the bars will lag somewhat behind real cases due to the lag time in reporting. Nevertheless, the graph still shows cases possibly approaching a plateau, since the case level in the last quarter of 1988 is actually lower than the previous two quarters.

SOURCE: CDC, "AIDS and Human Immunodeficiency Virus Infection in the United States: 1988 Update," *MMWR* 38 (S-4 [12 May 1989]): 33, fig. 1.

Nevertheless, early figures show that since early 1987 there has been an apparent leveling off in New York City and a decrease in Los Angeles and San Francisco (as in the following table).

To eliminate the reporting–time-lag problem, I use no data later than the first half of 1988 (see figure 21.1). Since at the time this graph was prepared, even the latest reporting period was 14 months old, chances are few new cases will be added to it, much less to the older periods. As the chart reveals, there is—even without factoring in the new case definition—a clear plateau in San Francisco and Los Angeles and a drop in New York. Thus, the peaking in deaths shows that the peak in cases actually occurred some time earlier, since deaths lag about one and a half years behind diagnoses. It was this run-in with reality that led New York City to lower its estimate of seropositivity from 500,000 to 400,000 to a minimum of 142,000, notwithstanding the howls of Mathilde Krim and the homosexual activists. With the epidemic having begun to peak

FIGURE 21.4   Incidence of AIDS, by quarter and year of
diagnosis—United States, pre-1982–1992

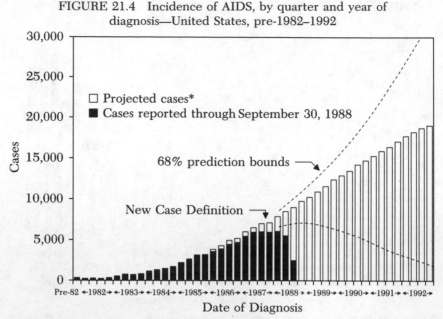

Date of Diagnosis

*Estimated numbers of cases diagnosed through December 1987 are reported cases
adjusted for estimated reporting delays. Estimated numbers of cases for 1988–1992 are
projected from cases diagnosed as of June 30, 1987, and reported as of March 31, 1988.
NOTE: This graph depicts U.S. AIDS cases by the period in which they were diagnosed.
While graphing the figures by diagnosis has the drawback of providing incomplete data
for the later periods (the reason the bar for the first quarter of 1988 is so low is because
at the time the graph was prepared there were still many cases from that period that had
not been reported), it has the advantage of showing cases when they became cases, as
opposed to whenever they happened to get to CDC. While figures for the last few
quarters depicted will end up being somewhat higher as more cases come in, considering
that 30 percent of all the cases during this time frame are new case definition only, this
graph, too, shows a general flattening of the epidemic curve. Contrast this with the empty
bars depicting CDC's "best guess" rate of increase showing 365,000 cases by the end of
1992. The bottom dotted line, CDC's best case scenario, follows approximately the path
predicted by former CDC chief epidemiologist Alexander Langmuir.
SOURCE: CDC, "AIDS and Human Immunodeficiency Virus Infection in the United
States: 1988 Update," *MMWR* 38 (S-4 [12 May 1989]): 36.

after a total of less than 20,000 cases, that figure, too, will come tum-
bling down.

Thus, the good news is that despite all the doomsaying about the
inability of our major cities to cope with the problem of more AIDS
cases, in some ways the worst is behind them. (Although for some time
the number of living AIDS patients will continue to grow and will be
a continual burden.) The even better news is that as New York, Los
Angeles, and San Francisco have gone, so must go the nation. Because
of these declines in diagnoses, these three cities no longer provide a

majority of the nation's new cases. Nevertheless, if the AIDS epidemics in those cities peaked some time ago, and if, as the cohort studies seem to indicate, the epidemic in the nation as a whole does not lag far behind that in the three cities struck first and hardest, it is entirely possible that the entire epidemic is peaking.

In Great Britain, it clearly already has. New diagnoses there peaked in the middle of 1987, thoroughly embarrassing the government's Centre for Disease Surveillance and Control. That agency had predicted 1,837 AIDS cases for 1988, while the nongovernmental Office of Health Economics in 1987 predicted about 3,000 cases for 1988. No statistician predicted fewer than 1,200 cases. In fact, the actual number reported came in at about 755 cases for the year.[61] The death rate in Britain, too, has been dropping.[62]

(Despite this, in an extraordinary act of chutzpa, scientific advisors in November 1988 told the British government to expect between 10,000 and 30,000 more cases by 1992. The report also shamelessly predicted that the epidemic in homosexuals would *begin* to peak in the early 1990s.[63] As with so many of the AIDS alarmists, these scientists were not about to let reality rain on their parade.)

Whether the epidemic is peaking for the entire United States is not yet certain, but one thing is: unless the CDC keeps expanding the definition of AIDS to catch earlier and earlier stages of HIV infection (and Harold Jaffe says there is sentiment in that direction[64]), it is going to start talking less and less about its best guess of 365,000 cases by 1993. And fewer people will be betting against Alexander Langmuir's top-end prediction of 200,000 homosexual cases for the entire epidemic.

The Shrinking Pandemic

If the official U.S., British, and New York City estimates have fallen, what may we expect of the official World Health Organization's (WHO) estimates? In November 1986, Director General Halfdan Mahler, in a fit of handwringing, proclaimed, "Everything is getting worse and worse in AIDS, and all of us have been underestimating it, and I in particular."[65] Underestimation was a mistake he would not make again. Instead, his organization now warned that up to 100,000,000 could be infected worldwide by 1990. Current infections were put at 5,000,000 to 10,000,000, an estimate WHO used as late as the last week in August 1988.[66] So when, in late July, I called James Chin, chief of the AIDS Surveillance Unit, WHO Global AIDS Program in Geneva, Switzerland, I was surprised to be told that "the most reasonable estimate at this time is 5,000,000."[67] Behind the scenes at least, the 10,000,000 top range had been dropped. As with the CDC, rather than showing an increase of infections, the new figures show a dramatic plummet. Dr. Chin, who took great pains to point out that he was not responsible for the 5,000,000-to-10,000,000 figure, said it was proclaimed "before anyone had any data." "Before there was *any* data?" I asked incredulously? Well, "they knew it was clearly not 1,000,000 or 100,000,000; they asked what was reasonable and so they picked a number," said Chin.[68] It is highly doubtful that the reporters and government leaders who quoted the WHO figure as if it were biblical had any idea of the seat-of-the-pants calculating that had produced it.

The 5,000,000 figure was finally mentioned in the October *Scientific American* but was buried so deep in a lengthy article that the media missed it entirely.[69] The article made no mention of the previous 10,000,000 high-end estimate. Months later, the media—including the *New York Times,*[70] the *Washington Post,*[71] and the Reuter news service[72]—were continuing to use the 5,000,000-to-10,000,000 figure; and the January 1989 issue of *WorldAIDS,* put out by the international Panos Institute, displayed a large chart using only the 10,000,000 figure.[73] Thus, WHO could claim to have improved its accuracy, even while gaining the benefit (in attention and funding) of the older, much higher figure. Not incidentally, the title of the *WorldAIDS* piece was "The Dilemma of Resources."

The 100,000,000 by 1990 figure was also dropped, in December of 1988, to 6 to 7 million. Associated Press covered the story,[74] but few papers appeared to carry it.

AIDS, by the way, has been good to WHO's budget. The organization's global AIDS coordinating office grew from a staff of one physician and one secretary with a budget of $580,000 a year in November 1986 to a full-time and part-time staff of almost 100 with a budget of $66,000,000 in 1988.[75]

More than anything else, what forced the estimates of seropositivity down was the growing evidence that everyone with HIV would become sick and perhaps all go on to get AIDS. If, as was originally believed, only about 10 percent of all seropositives would develop AIDS, then it could be said that for every case there is now or will be, there are 9 other seropositives. But as a consensus developed that infections eventually equate to AIDS cases, one could no longer look at the caseloads and estimate levels of seropositivity many times higher. Although the official statisticians have not stated as much, this is assuredly what forced down the WHO figure and edged the CDC figure down slightly.

The Bankrupting of America?

It has probably occurred to the reader by now that the cost estimates of AIDS might have been somewhat exaggerated as well. For the last few years, horrifying figures have been bandied around about the projected exhaustion of financial resources and even of physical space for AIDS victims. Every year we are warned that the health care system is so badly strained that it might not hold up any longer. Indeed, to hear Larry Kramer declare, "Let's talk about hospitals. Everybody's full up, fellows. No room in the inn,"[76] one might think he made the statement this year. In fact, he made it early in 1983 when the hospitals in his city, New York, had a tiny amount of AIDS patients compared with those they would be handling six years later. But if the inn never got full, there were still some saying the till might be empty. A figure oft-repeated by the media was the Rand Corporation's estimate that by 1991 direct medical costs for AIDS (that is, medical expenses only with lost wages not included) could be as high as $133 billion.[77] *U.S. News & World Report* flatly declared, "What is now becoming clear to an array of leaders—in medicine, business, government and academia—is that AIDS not only threatens untold death and suffering but could bankrupt America's health-care system as well."[78]

That the system has not gone bust has been the result of three factors: first, that the scope of the epidemic itself has been grossly exaggerated; second, that the human ingenuity for reducing costs as those costs exert greater pressure was ignored; and third, that once again, the doomsayers insisted upon looking at AIDS in a vacuum, ignoring the myriad other diseases that have been, are, and always will be more expensive to deal with than AIDS.

On the second point, some calculated per-patient medical costs by using the cost of treating such patients during the early years of the epidemic. In doing so, they ignored a standard rule in economics that the higher costs are forced up, the more incentive there will be for alternatives to be developed to drive costs down. One such response was to begin placing patients in hospices, which not only made their remaining days more comfortable but freed up hospital space and reduced per-patient overhead tremendously. The result is that while some were using such figures as almost $150,000 in medical costs per patient,[79] Joel Hay and his co-authors have concluded that, even with a growing number of extremely expensive drugs such as AZT (which originally cost $12,000 a year), the expected average medical cost per patient is only $22,000 at U.S. cost averages (1988 dollars) or at $32,000 for San Francisco area ones.[80] They concluded that far from $133 billion being spent on AIDS patients and others with HIV-related illness by 1991, the actual figure would be in the range of $4 billion to $12 billion.[81]

Much of the panic was caused by the lack of realization that *all* diseases, from colds to cancers, impose both medical costs and costs in lost wages. Doctor Neil Schram of the Los Angeles AIDS Task Force told "Nightline" that "current estimates are that $8–$16 billion in medical costs—this is the U.S. Public Health Service estimate—will be required to care for those AIDS patients that I've talked about [those cases diagnosed from 1981 to 1991]. Life insurance companies will clearly lose money on policies already in effect. . . . We are facing catastrophe."[82] He did not point out that total U.S. medical costs are approximately $550 billion per *year*, with $80 billion a year for heart disease alone.[83] In perspective, it is very difficult to see how $8 billion to $16 billion for the first *decade* of AIDS cases amounts to economic "catastrophe."

Last Refuge of the Scoundrels

Notes Dennis Altman,

> Once a disease becomes "fashionable," it generates its own establishment and vested interests. Aided by politicians, lobbyists and the media, the money and attention focused on AIDS in the United States since mid-1983 have ensured the development of an AIDS industry, involving researchers, doctors, therapists, social workers and administrators, who have taken control of the definition and management of the disease.[84]

For all the talk about wanting nothing more than an end to the sickness and dying, the AIDS industry looks upon a declining epidemic as a whale ship captain might have looked upon an oil derrick. Researchers will face tighter budgets, administrative positions will be axed, celebrities will fade away, lecturers will find their services in less and less demand. The party favors lined up for the day a vaccine is put into mass production will have to be put away. The first reaction of the AIDS industry will be resistance—to downplay, obfuscate, and conceal the new data as well as possible. Indeed, we have already been seeing this for some time. But eventually the writing will be on the wall for all to see.

As it becomes ever more apparent that not only was the risk to heterosexuals overplayed but so, too, was the entire scope of the epidemic, there will be various reactions from the doomsayers. Many will simply slip back into the obscurity whence they came. Some, like Surgeon General Koop, will simply deny their earlier words. Some will attempt to argue that they basically had the right idea but through some form of luck disaster was averted, the corollary being that those who claimed all along that the epidemic was being exaggerated were merely lucky guessers.[85]

But the lowest of the low will claim that there would have been such an epidemic *but for* their doomsaying, which prompted the nation to take decisive action just in time. Health and Human Services Secretary Otis Bowen hinted at this early on when, exactly a year after giving his famous "Black Death" speech, he said that his Black Death allusion had been misinterpreted, and that he had now decided, "We do not expect any explosion into the heterosexual population. But I think it's important . . . that it is still possible, and I'd like to think that in the past two years that our educational efforts have been effective enough to help turn some of those dangers around."[86]

As noted above, blood sampling in major U.S. cities showed that homosexual infections began declining in 1981 and 1982; this was five years *before* the federal government began its national education campaign.[87] The federal government did not get its advertising campaign geared up until October–November 1987 (the release of the Education Department booklet, National AIDS Awareness Month, and the first advertising blitz), by which time federal officials in addition to Harold Jaffe were already beginning to concede privately that the predictions of heterosexual doom no longer appeared to be valid.

Even as the shrill cries of doom from the alarmists reached ever higher levels, the level of AIDS cases in the cities hit first and hardest were starting to flatten. They flattened before massive government education programs, before issuance of the surgeon general's and Education Department's misleading booklets, before teaching children the intricacies of anal intercourse and condom usage, and before the sale of a single book by Masters, Johnson, and Kolodny. They flattened long before the President's AIDS commission issued its final report calling for massive AIDS spending[88] and even longer before the National Academy of Sciences issued its 1989 report calling for a virtual blanketing of the airwaves with explicit warnings and pitches for prophylactics.[89]

It was rather like throwing a party at which the guest of honor failed to arrive. In the 1960s, antiwar activists used the slogan: What if they gave a war and nobody came? In the 1980s we got the answer to: What if they gave an apocalypse and nobody came?

An AIDS researcher writing in *Scientific American* stated,

> Major events in human history tend to spawn their chroniclers: the Trojan
> War inspired Homer, the decadence of the Roman Empire was chronicled
> in the *Satyricon* of Petronius Arbiter and its decline was analyzed by Gibbon.
> The AIDS pandemic also promises to take a major place in the history of the
> species, but it has not yet attracted a recorder of classic stature.[90]

Nor, indeed, will it. For, in retrospect, AIDS will never compare to
these great events, nor to the great epidemics and pandemics of history.
It is only our own historical narcissism that allows us to think otherwise.
While many of us have fancied that history will view us as the brave
combatants of the greatest pestilential scourge in history, in fact histori-
ans, to the extent they cover this aspect of our decade at all, will view
us as the ass of a horse. We laugh or groan in response to some of the
outlandish reactions of societies in response to other diseases—blaming
bad air or Jews poisoning the wells for the Black Death, killing cats
during the plague of London in 1666 to stop a disease that turned out
to be spread by rats, wearing useless masks to prevent the spread of
Spanish Flu. Just so, future generations of high-schoolers will listen with
incredulity as their teachers relate that a world that decades earlier had
put a man on the moon reacted to one of the least transmissible germs
ever discovered by, in some cases, wearing space suits to touch AIDS
victims and by proclaiming that the world's population could be killed
twice over.

It's sad, really. When a member of the president's AIDS commission
proclaims, "The AIDS epidemic is the greatest threat to society, as we
know it, ever faced by civilization—more serious than the plagues of
past centuries"[91] and when the nation's highest health official makes a
similar invocation,[92] we debase everything our poor, suffering ancestors
went through. But at least they are not here to see it. What of those,
however, who are afflicted by AIDS and are here to witness our hysteria
over their disease? Writes *Village Voice* editor Richard Goldstein, "for
heterosexuals to act as if AIDS were a threat to everyone demeans the
anxiety of gay men who really are at risk, and for gay men to act as if
we're all going to die demeans the anguish of those who are actually
ill."[93]

Many aspects of the AIDS crisis brought out the best in many of us,
especially those who tended the sick and dying while oblivious to the
political fights swirling about them. But the hysteria with which we

turned such a limited disease into the coming of the apocalypse displayed the very worst in us, the dark side of a society that is not always as sophisticated and enlightened as it would like to think. Yes, our hysteria demeaned our ancestors, homosexuals in general, and especially those truly at risk. But ultimately those most demeaned were ourselves.

22

The AIDS Lobby: Are We Giving It Too Much Money?

The evidence continues to come in that the scope of the epidemic—including its effect on homosexuals, its effect on sexually active heterosexuals, its effect on persons in neither category, and its effect on the economy—have been grossly overplayed. The time has come to ask whether spiraling increases in AIDS funding are justified.

It would be nice to live in a world where one could simply assign more money, more personnel, more resources in general to any given problem without worrying about any other problem being short-changed. But we live in a world of scarce resources. Money and attention devoted to one cause means resources pulled off another. And there's the rub. Clearly, there is a connection between the perception of AIDS as a world catastrophe and the willingness to fund the campaign against it. It is not the present caseload; there are still fourteen causes of death in America that are ahead of AIDS. It was the predictions of millions or tens of millions or hundreds of millions of future cases that had many of us rating AIDS as the number-one health priority. As AIDS activists are well aware, to challenge those predictions could be tantamount to challenging the pouring of massive amounts of resources into the anti-AIDS fight.

Indeed, rumblings are being heard. Dr. Vincent T. DeVita, Jr., just before stepping down from his position as director of the National Cancer Institute (NCI), bemoaned the loss of resources to the AIDS industry: "[AIDS] has been an extraordinary drain on the energy of the scientific establishment. . . . It's been a big stress. It's taken a lot of intellectual energy away from the cancer program."[1] The American

Heart Association, for its part, in order to trigger more donations for heart research, began running advertisements in early 1989 showing the risk of getting AIDS versus that of getting heart disease.

Despite the far greater health threat posed by cancer, federal AIDS funding allocated to the Public Health Service at $1,300,000,000 (of which about $400,000,000 goes to education, not research) now nearly matches cancer funding. In President Bush's budget proposal for fiscal year 1990, this figure rises to $1,600,000,000. Cancer funding, by contrast, with the AIDS portion pulled out, comes to about $1,450,000,000. Even if the AIDS epidemic kept up with the CDC projection and did not peak until 1993, AIDS cases diagnosed that year would be but a fourth of all 1993 cancer deaths. Each year a million cases of cancer are diagnosed, almost half of which end in death. This will be the case the next year and the year after that, with no peaking or decline anticipated until scientists bring one about. Heart disease kills more people than even cancer, over 750,000 Americans a year; yet funding to fight it is two thirds that of AIDS.[2]

AIDS research has now drained cancer research to a point where the NCI's ability to fund promising new research proposals is less than at any time in the past two decades. During fiscal year 1989, only 25 percent of cancer grant applications approved by review committees will receive funding. During the 1970s, between 43 percent and 60 percent of such approved grants were funded. Two top NCI doctors left the agency in 1988, partly in frustration over this. "They bled cancer to feed AIDS in terms of people's time," complained one.[3]

Perhaps we could just trade funds earmarked for F-16s or MX missiles for AIDS research, as some have suggested, but even this would not alleviate the problem that when it comes to researchers, this is pretty much a zero-sum game. It takes up to a decade to put a high school graduate through medical school. Thus, in the short run, AIDS researchers must come from and have come from other research areas, primarily but not exclusively cancer. In a medical newspaper editorial asking "Are We Spending Too Much Money on AIDS?" two young psychiatric researchers spoke of having to resist the "seduction" of AIDS research money. "Unfortunately," wrote the researchers, "many other young scientists may have no choice but to go into the field that offers the most easily obtained funding. If this happens, other areas of research important to the welfare of the U.S. public will be neglected for years to come."[4] One of the two retiring top NCI officials exclaimed that NCI "is withering away."[5] Further, the 1989 appropriations bill signed into law by President Reagan expressly called for hiring an additional 780 AIDS researchers. Where will they come from? They'll come from where they've *been* coming from. For non-AIDS work, the National Institutes of Health has lost almost 1,100 employees since 1984. At the same time, the number of employees engaged in AIDS work has increased by more than 400 to 580 workers or their full-time equivalents, according to *Science* magazine.[6]

Terrible as it sounds, there will never be enough researchers or money to go around. Hard decisions have to be made about what programs should be emphasized and what ones de-emphasized. AIDS has prompted a general de-emphasis of other medical problems. The blunt fact is that people will die of these other diseases because of the overemphasis on AIDS. We will never know their names, and those names will never be sewn into a giant quilt. We will never know their exact numbers. But they will die nonetheless.

Of course, a comparison of death counts is not the only appropriate factor in allocating funding and researchers. Another argument used to advocate massive AIDS spending is to look at federal spending for patient care; in other words, "pay me now or pay me later." But when the preceding two researchers did just that, they found that in terms of both persons affected and patient costs, direct and indirect, the toll caused by psychiatric disorders swamps that of AIDS. The ratio of AIDS research and development spending to federal patient costs is vastly out of proportion to other deadly diseases. For example, cancer research expenditures will equal about 4.5 percent of cancer patient costs. For heart disease, it is about 2.9 percent; and for Alzheimer's disease, federal research expenditures will equal less than 1 percent of federal patient costs. But with AIDS, using a conservatively high estimate for federal patient costs, federal research expenditures will be an astounding 230 percent greater than federal patient costs for AIDS patients this year.[7]

Aside from death rates and patient costs, there may be some justification to spend more for AIDS. Perhaps AIDS research will lead to new discoveries in other areas. However, direct research is generally more efficient than spinoff research. As it happens, of the only five drugs approved for treatment of AIDS or its conditions, two (AZT and alpha interferon) are spinoffs of *cancer* research. Dr. Robert Gallo, co-discoverer of the AIDS virus, began his research as a cancer specialist. So the "overlap" argument really comes to something of a wash. Further, only about a fourth of the PHS AIDS budget goes for the kind of hard research that could even have the possibility of aiding other research. About $385 million out of the fiscal year 1989 budget of $1.3

billion. Nevertheless, perhaps a breakthrough for AIDS is closer than for other diseases. Perhaps AIDS deserves more money because it is a more horrible way to die. Perhaps it deserves more money because its victims tend to be younger than those of heart disease and cancer. Perhaps. But if the case for disproportionate AIDS spending is to be made, it must be done with realistic numbers, not projections driven by ignorance or political concerns.

Finally, such a massive increase in one area is begging for boondoggles. And while the media, undoubtedly out of a sense of national purpose, has circumspectly avoided reporting on these, they exist nonetheless. In December 1988, the National Institute of Allergies and Infectious Diseases announced two grants totaling $22,800,000 to, as the Associated Press put it, study non-IVDA heterosexuals in order to "prevent a huge new epidemic."[8] Speaking on condition of anonymity, one prominent federal epidemiologist said of the study, "I think it's complete bullshit." He said, "That amount of money is ridiculous. You can do a good study for a tenth of that amount; in fact, PHS already is. Plus, it's an area that's being studied intensively and my sense is they're not asking very good questions." He told me, "My sense was that a huge amount of money got dumped on NIAID and that by the time they got around to awarding the money a lot of good institutions had already been funded and all that was left was schlock." Alas, this "schlock" adds up to one third of the entire yearly federal allocation for Alzheimer's disease, a cruel, debilitating malady that wipes away memory and that, because people are living longer, will continue to take an ever-higher yearly toll unless medical intervention becomes possible. Indeed, if scientists do not find a way to treat Alzheimer's by the middle of the next century, there will be five times as many victims of this disease in the United States as there are now. Up to 6,000,000 older Americans will be living in nursing homes, instead of the 1,000,000 there today.[9] The increased costs, of course, will be tremendous.

While writers like Randy Shilts have made an excellent case that too little was spent on the AIDS epidemic early on because its scope was understated, does that justify too much now being spent because it was subsequently overstated? Should there be an affirmative action program for AIDS spending? Put another way, while it's a tragedy that in the first two years of AIDS appropriations the federal government allocated only $34,000,000 to be spent on the disease, are we going to make amends for that by wasting $22,000,000 on a single project at this much later date?

Homosexuals have learned to use their victim status as a powerful lobbying tool. Their pink triangles are ubiquitous in major cities, slapped on everything from newspaper boxes to telephone booths to stoplights, with superadhesive that will probably keep some of the stickers stuck for longer than the AIDS epidemic will last. In the 1940s, the pink triangle was used to send homosexuals to German concentration camps, and often to their deaths. In the 1970s, the pink triangle became a symbol of Gay Liberation, of a demand to be treated with the same rights and respect given to heterosexuals. By the late 1980s, the pink triangle was used like an American Express Platinum Card, as a means of getting special privileges available only to the bearer. AIDS victims began the 1980s by asking to be treated no worse than victims of other fatal diseases. But within a few years they were demanding funding and other treatment far superior to that received by sufferers of any other disease.

Likewise, the problems AIDS victims had with the Food and Drug Administration were no different from the problems other disease sufferers have had for decades. The FDA has established testing procedures for all food additives and drugs. These procedures, which have been developed to ensure that these products are both safe and effective, are controversial because they can substantially delay the marketing of an important product. Nobody has established that the FDA slowed AIDS drug development any more than it had slowed up everything from life-saving beta blockers for heart disease to fat substitutes for food to a formula for growing hair. AIDS victims demanded preferential treatment. Like all special interests, the AIDS victims and their fellows wanted us to believe theirs was especially special. Yet why did the government have "blood on its hands" for AIDS, as some of the stickers claim, but for no other cause of death? It might have been because AIDS did not receive as much funding early on as it is now agreed it should have gotten. This was a strong theme in Randy Shilts's book. In hindsight, it is easy to see that much more money should have been spent much more quickly on AIDS than was the case. For that matter, though, hindsight also tells us that those same public health authorities strongly overreacted to the swine-flu scare in the mid-1970s. But would funding have been substantially different if the afflicted had been, to use one congressman's comparison, tennis players instead of homosexuals?[10] This is something that Shilts's exhaustive research and his memos obtained under the Freedom of Information Act did not reveal. The conclusion is left more to conjecture and occasional conversational tidbits than anything else. If early funding had been made available, how greatly would this have affected the course of the epidemic? Again, this is a matter of conjecture.

AIDS advocates have said it is wrong to treat victims of this disease differently from victims of other diseases. After all, heart disease and cancer, especially lung cancer, are often behaviorally-linked as well. Nobody lectures the dying cigarette smoker, we are reminded. Fair enough. But nobody exalts him, either. If AIDS victims want to be treated as well as victims of other diseases, that is their right. But they have no right to be treated any better, either. There is no national guilt for AIDS, and there is no excuse for condescending to AIDS activists as if there were.

AIDS is a terrible disease that, even though the worst will soon be over, is not going to go away on its own. But there are many other terrible diseases that will not go away. All deserve our attention, and all their victims deserve our compassion. But compassion begins with allocating resources on the basis of where they can do the most good, not on the basis of oiling the wheel that squeaks the loudest. It is not fair to penalize victims of cancer and other life-threatening illnesses because they do not knit quilts or blockade the Golden Gate Bridge or picket magazines that say things they don't believe should be allowed in print. And lest they forget, homosexuals get cancer, too.

Dennis Altman, chronicler of the Gay Liberation movement, wrote in *AIDS in the Mind of America,*

> The real test posed by AIDS was expressed by Jesse Jackson in a speech to the Human Rights Campaign Fund dinner in New York in 1983 when he said: "Gay health issues, such as a cure for AIDS, *are* important. But I suggest to you this night that when you give life you gain life. If there is a commitment to health care for *whatever* the disease, based upon need and not based upon wealth or class—then within health care is encompassed the issue of AIDS. AIDS is not the only disease in the nation tonight. Be concerned about AIDS but also sickle cell. Never let it be said that you are a one-agenda, self-centered, narcissistic movement."[11]

If that was the test of AIDS, then clearly the test was failed. AIDS activists, homosexual and otherwise, have become exactly what the Reverend Jackson warned against.

23

Alarmism
for Fun and Profit

If there is one thing to be said for alarmism it is that it is ephemeral. The pit bull terrier terror came and went, as did the millions of missing children. The "population bomb" has been replaced by the efforts of Western nations to encourage more births. Of the AIDS hysteria it can also be said: This too shall pass.

Alarmism in general, however, is here to stay. It's just too damned profitable. As a society we encourage alarmists; they seem so concerned and compassionate as they talk about the lives that are endangered and that they are trying to save. We march them before congressional committees and presidential committees. We award them fat book contracts and government grants. We give them jobs in the White House. Then, after the panic has died away, we almost forget the alarm ever occurred and completely forget the names of the individual alarmists.

By contrast, we discourage those who dare challenge the prevailing hysteria. Their coolness is taken to be coldness and indifference. They are "irresponsible" and "uncompassionate," "lulling us into a false sense of security." If you insisted that the world's population was not outstripping food production, you were said to favor starvation. If you said the missing children numbers were vastly overstated, you obviously didn't care about those poor little waifs wandering by the millions in the countryside or tied up in the basement of some thin-mustached child molester. If you said that the AIDS threat was overblown, you must have had some evil motive; why else would you lead millions of heterosexuals down the path of disease and death?

Alarmists have plied their wares throughout history, and there's no reason to think the human race is going to catch on now, since the alarmists keep coming up with new alarms. Yet, there is a possibility that the public can develop an immunity to a certain type of alarm. The AIDS crisis marks the second time in a decade that the federal government and, specifically, the Public Health Service, has made dire predictions of epidemic only to be proven wrong. Never mind that the first, the swine-flu fiasco in 1976, had better grounds than the AIDS terror. What the public will remember is that they have been deceived, whether intentionally or otherwise.

One reader, in responding to an article of mine, declared that even if I were right about *this* epidemic, we should still endeavor to permanently change heterosexual sex habits in case another dangerous disease comes along. This makes as much sense as stockpiling gas masks in anticipation of a new, deadly airborne germ. Nevertheless, it is fair to ask, what *would* happen if a new virus came along that fulfilled the alarmists' promise of what AIDS was supposed to do? After all the cries of wolf about AIDS, it is possible that no amount of screaming and crying and presentations of true statistics could convince heterosexuals that they were truly at risk this time.

And what if AIDS *had* become a heterosexual epidemic? Between a bewildered surgeon general, a media more interested in sales and social consciousness than facts, and a whole panoply of special interests from democratizing liberals to moralistic conservatives, and from those merely seeking fifteen minutes of fame to those who weren't beyond terrorizing the public to achieve it—if the epidemic had been real, God help us.

24

The 1989
Montreal Conference
on AIDS

Eleven hundred eighty participants convened in Montreal, Canada, for the Fifth International Conference on Acquired Immune Deficiency Syndrome from June 12 through June 16, 1989—more than one for each three Americans who would be reported to have AIDS in the course of the year. The line between science and politics, always a thin one with this disease, crumbled as AIDS activists delayed opening ceremonies for over an hour, and thereafter continued to heckle speakers such as Canadian Prime Minister Brian Mulrōney and a Third World woman diplomat, who dared make reference to persons suffering from AIDS as "victims."[1] Reported the *Wall Street Journal*'s Marilyn Chase,

> Scientific jargon mingled with chants and slang. Demonstrations by gay men, lesbians and prostitutes vied for attention with reports on drugs and vaccines. Poster presentations on autoeroticism [masturbation] and a video called "Safe Sex Slut" competed with lectures on virology and epidemiology.[2]

Both Dr. Robert Gallo and Luc Montagnier, co-discoverers of the virus and key players in the search for the cure that the demonstrators were demanding, complained of the disruptions. "Many of us would wish there were more time for scientific discussion."[3]

On the whole, news coverage was down dramatically from that of the previous conferences in Washington, D.C., and Stockholm. This was due in part to unrest in China and the massacre there of pro-democracy students, but it also reflected a lack of exciting new developments and the fact that as more and more research is done on AIDS, be it virological or epidemiological, truly new revelations come farther and farther apart.

The conference did, however, signal a fundamental change in media reporting. Originally, most of this was geared toward overplaying the epidemic, although some of it was in the form of exaggerating the impending possibility of a cure or vaccine. The coverage of the Montreal Conference made it clear that the media were finally growing tired of the former and beginning to put their emphasis on the new treatment or drug that is always "just around the corner." "About half" of the articles on AIDS, says CDC public information officer Don Berreth, "are about 'medical breakthroughs' that never amount to anything."[4] It is telling that the two most talked-about drugs at Montreal, AZT and aerosolized pentamidine, far from being new, have been used successfully for the last few years in AIDS patients. The shift also is apparent in the rhetoric of the AIDS industry. Having already established the need for a burgeoning institution through predictions of millions, tens of millions, or hundreds of millions of American deaths, the industry now feels it must justify its existence through a steady display of progress.

In raising both false fears and false hopes, the AIDS industry demonstrates that despite its endless entreaties to show "compassion" regarding AIDS, it does not understand the meaning of the word. Indeed, one paper presented at Montreal reported that one category of homosexual and bisexual men who "continue sexual risk taking despite basic safe-sex counseling" includes "those who believe a cure for AIDS will soon be found."[5] Thus we see again how by providing false information, media sensationalism may go beyond mere infliction of mental trauma to the point of actually endangering lives. AIDS still should be considered a death sentence, and it will be sad indeed if a person engages in high-risk activity and finds this out the hard way after having been convinced otherwise.

BILLIONS FOR TREATMENT

One development at Montreal that eventually should be among the most controversial was Assistant Secretary of Health and Human Services James Mason's announcement that CDC, the Food and Drug

Administration, and the National Institutes of Health were drafting a recommendation for spending $2 to $3 billion a year to provide free immune system testing facilities for persons who already have tested positive for HIV. If their immune systems were sufficiently weakened to put them at risk for developing *pneumocystis carinii* pneumonia (PCP), the biggest killer of AIDS victims, they would be given regular doses of aerosolized pentamidine, which has been shown to be effective in preventing the onset of PCP.[6] It is difficult to see such a proposal as anything other than a highly cynical attempt to placate the AIDS lobby. To comprehend why, it is necessary to understand that for all of its cost, the proposed system will have no direct effect in either saving lives or hurrying the end of the epidemic. Aerosolized pentamidine has been shown to be highly effective in staving off PCP, but PCP is only one of the many opportunistic infections that afflict persons suffering from AIDS or other HIV-related disease. Despite the application of pentamidine, the patient's immune system will continue to decline just as quickly, and the patient will simply succumb to some other disease. The only way in which pentamidine can be seen as a life saver for AIDS patients is that marginal victims, by virtue of living a few months or a year longer, may live long enough to use a drug that really is effective against the entire syndrome. By contrast, there are any number of applications for which a similar amount of money actually could save— not merely extend slightly—large numbers of lives. For example, in 1988 there were about 130,000 breast cancer cases (all but 900 in women), of which approximately 43,000 will result in death.[7] Yet the cure rate for breast cancer is virtually 100 percent if caught before it becomes invasive.[8] Combined with physical exams, regular x-rays (called mammograms) could prevent almost all of those deaths. Unfortunately, they are not cheap, perhaps costing $100 apiece, depending on the geographic area. Yet if that same $3 billion were put toward providing free mammograms for women 55 years of age and older, we could screen all of them, preventing over 30,000 breast cancer deaths a year. Tens of thousands of others could avoid traumatic radical breast removals, instead undergoing less disfiguring lumpectomies. (This assumes, of course, that the women testing positive seek treatment.) Why are we willing to spend those billions to extend some lives but not to save tens of thousands of others? Why is the life of an HIV victim inherently worth so much more than that of a breast cancer victim?

One possibility that should be excluded is that such a program will help slow the epidemic. While it is entirely possible that persons receiving anti-virals such as AZT are less infectious to their sexual or needle-sharing partners, persons receiving pentamidine are as infectious as ever. Theoretically, Mason's proposed program *could* result in more persons submitting to HIV testing and those persons testing positive *might* then refrain from high-risk activities. Yet while there is substantial evidence that persons testing positive do subsequently reduce their high-risk behavior, this is among a group of persons who have been tested purely for the sake of finding out their status. Presumably the reason many want to know is so they can take actions to keep from infecting others if need be. It does not follow that persons submitting to testing to avail themselves of pentamidine or other treatment necessarily will be as altruistic.[9] Also, it might be possible to turn such a system of monitoring infected persons into one used to identify potentially infected partners through contact tracing, which in some areas has been found to be useful. But Mason disavowed any attempt to use the immune system monitoring for this purpose.[10]

MORE OF THE NUMBERS GAME

One item that caught more immediate press attention was CDC's chief of AIDS surveillance and evaluation Timothy Dondero's reevaluation of the number of Americans infected with the AIDS virus. Dondero's abstract at the conference concluded, "Our evaluation method suggests that U.S. estimates in the vicinity of 1,000,000 are currently most plausible."[11] Yet what *USA Today* readers saw when they looked at the front page of their newspaper was a headline declaring "Best Guess at AIDS in USA: 1.5M."[12]

The ostensible purpose of the paper was to evaluate three estimates of existing U.S. seroprevalence: the Masters, Johnson, and Kolodny and Hudson Institute figure of 3,000,000, the Joel Hay bottom-range figure of 500,000, and the bottom-range CDC figure of 1,000,000. The actual purpose was to refute both the 500,000 and 3,000,000 figures. Hay strongly disputes Dondero's methodology which, he says, included such things as extrapolating from test results of federal prisoners.[13] Further, Hay notes that at a government-sponsored AIDS research conference in May of 1989 he presented his estimate of 500,000 to 800,000 infections, and CDC chief statistician W. Meade Morgan commented in writing that "the 500,000 to 800,000 figure is indeed reasonable in light of data now available on the extent of the epidemic."[14] At any rate, the Dondero figure clearly represented a lowering of the CDC estimate, the middle point of which in 1987 had been 1.25 million and in 1988 had been 1.2 million. Thus the incredible shrinking epidemic continued to shrink even further.

One news item that coincided with the Montreal conference was a survey which, according to the sponsors, indicated that cases were being understated in the Midwest and among whites. Underreporting of AIDS cases is nothing new, but any mention of whites and AIDS always grabs press attention, and this was no exception.[15] However, the method of conducting the survey was a bit strange, to say the least. Most evaluations of underreporting consist of looking at death certificates and comparing them to AIDS reports, searching for clues on the certificates that might indicate death due to immune deficiency. This one, however, relied on asking respondents how many AIDS victims they knew personally and asking them to provide age, race, and other characteristics.[16] Any number of variables, such as the white people surveyed simply having more friends and acquaintances than blacks, would completely throw the survey off. The authors hypothesized that underreporting of whites could occur because more often they tend to have personal physicians who could keep their conditions secret.[17] They did not seem to realize that it is precisely because whites tend to have better access to health care that they probably tend to be reported more than minorities, who often die in the gutter without ever being diagnosed. In fact, a study published six months earlier by Rand Stoneburner and others found that deaths due to AIDS among intravenous drug users (the vast majority of whom are minorities) have been substantially underreported;[18] the result would show whites and the middle class greatly overrepresented in the city with more AIDS cases than any other class. Similarly, a paper presented at Montreal also found that in San Francisco, "Minority AIDS deaths may be substantially underreported, even from an area considered to have a good AIDS reporting system."[19] The only other Montreal paper that addressed this subject found no statistically significant difference in underreporting between black and white populations in South Carolina.[20]

Another study that got swept up with the Montreal coverage concerned what the media has dubbed "silent infections." It involves a testing system that, rather than seeking antibodies to HIV, is supposed to detect part of the virus itself. Thus it has been touted by some as more likely to detect the virus early on than the antibody test, since antibodies are a reaction to the virus and thus necessarily develop after a delayed time period. The test used to detect the DNA is called Polymerase Chain Reaction (PCR). A study performed at UCLA appearing in the *New England Journal of Medicine* immediately before the Montreal conference found that 23 percent of men in an extremely high-risk group (men who continued to engage in unprotected anal intercourse) were negative to the HIV antibody test, but positive using PCR or virus cultivation. Some men seroconverted (became antibody positive) as much as 35 months after becoming positive for virus detection, while others had yet to seroconvert after 36 months.[21] Another study, presented in a paper at Montreal, found that a substantial number of sex partners of hemophiliacs who were negative for HIV antibodies were nonetheless positive by the PCR test.[22]

The implications of such silent infections are obvious. First, it could mean the blood supply is not as safe as was once thought. Second, it could mean that there are more infected persons than was once thought. In fact, regardless of the validity of the silent infection tests, there are already mitigating factors; as even the authors of the UCLA study pointed out, one cannot extrapolate from such a high-risk group to the general population.[23] Just as false positives are far more likely in a low-risk population because there are so few truly infected persons in that population (this is one argument against mandatory testing of such groups as marriage license applicants), so, too, will false negatives be exaggerated in a high-risk population. Thus, no one is arguing that we should simply slap on an extra 23 percent to all estimates of the numbers of infections. As for the blood supply, great efforts are already being made to screen out high-risk donors.

Yet, it is by no means clear that the studies that seek to detect the virus itself are in fact legitimate. Harold Jaffe told me, "We have done similar studies using PCR at CDC, including gay men at high risk and steady female partners of men with hemophilia, and we don't find this. We found small numbers of people [in the homosexual cohort] who were PCR positive shortly before seroconverting. We don't find any steady sex partners [of hemophiliacs] who are PCR positive."[24] Another study conducted by CDC's John Ward and others using PCR also found "HIV-seronegative partners had no evidence of occult infections."[25] Thus CDC's studies all directly contradict the findings of the UCLA researchers and the Montreal hemophiliac partner abstract.

"There are other data besides ours that argues against what UCLA reported," said Jaffe. He cited one study published in *Transfusion* in 1989, which also found not a single hemophiliac sex partner who was antibody negative but positive by PCR or other viral tests, leading the researchers to conclude, "HIV-I infection in antibody-negative sexual partners of HIV-I infected individuals is probably very low."[26] A study by Jerome Groopman and others of 37 homosexual or bisexual partners of men with AIDS or ARC also found no evidence of prolonged HIV infection that did not show up in antibody tests.[27] A team of French scientists, including HIV co-discoverer Luc Montagnier, presented a paper at Montreal showing no one in their studied cohort to be antibody negative who still tested positive for the virus, leading them to conclude "This study indicates that latent HIV-I infection in seronegative high-risk subjects is not a frequent event."[28] Another Montreal paper found that PCR testing, rather than finding more infections than did antibody testing, in fact failed to find the virus in 50 percent of hemophiliacs shown to be infected through antibody testing.[29]

"Some studies [relying on virus culture] I know are wrong," said Jaffe, making specific reference to an earlier study by Jerome Groopman, in which Groopman originally announced that a woman with an impotent hemophiliac husband had tested positive for virus culture. The study was seized upon by those seeking to sound the alarm about the dangerousness of kissing but, said Jaffe, Groopman "has told me that he has gone back to that wife several times and found her culture and antibody negative."[30]

Stoneburner, in an interview after the Montreal conference, told me that "an entire section at Montreal did not support" the UCLA study or the alarming hemophiliac partner study.[31] Dennis Osmond, a research epidemiologist in the Department of Epidemiology and International Health at the University of California, San Francisco, who also attended the Montreal conference, confirmed that "there was a lot of skepticism about those results." According to Osmond, the PCR test is unusually sensitive, and therefore susceptible to improper decontamination, which can result in a slew of false positives. He added:

It's certainly possible that DNA being detected is not from a viable organism. It may be a defective virus or part of a virus, and may not be a real infection capable of spreading itself. It may not be a competent form or able to replicate; that's very possible. That raises questions as to whether it [a positive PCR reading] means very much. No one knows whether a person who tests positive [under the PCR test] is infectious. I don't think any of that is known. It's clear that most individuals infected get a clear antibody response. If they don't get one, it's clear that there's something atypical about them already.[32]

All three researchers, Jaffe, Stoneburner, and Osmond, expressed their belief that the "silent infection," to the extent that it may exist at all, is probably a very rare occurrence, although only Osmond works directly with the process in question.

One method of evaluating the possibility (other than the aforementioned studies that actually attempted the process) is to simply monitor antibody-negative persons who were once at high risk to see if eventually they become seropositive despite discontinuation of risk behavior. A German study presented at the Montreal conference found that of a group of 320 hemophiliacs who had been taking clotting factor prior to the development of heat treatment and who were hence at risk for HIV infection, none developed HIV antibodies any later than a year after the last year in which the factor was still contaminated, 1984. Thus, the study concluded, "the lack of any seroconversion after a 5 years' observation period suggests that late seroconversion might not be of great epidemiologic significance."[33]

From what one reads or hears from the media, however, one might never guess that these other countervailing studies or opinions exist. Thus the *New York Times* quoted Jaffe talking about his CDC studies, but omitted reference to all others that had appeared. It also quoted Jaffe as saying, "If it's correct, it's very concerning," without telling the reader that Jaffe doesn't believe it is.[34] Yet, as Jaffe told me, "In my heart of hearts I think it's wrong."[35] *Newsweek*, the only one of the three major newsmagazines to cover the "silent infection" story, only included two confusing sentences making reference to one CDC study.[36] *USA Today*, in what was by that paper's standard a long article, made no mention whatever of other countervailing studies or opinions.[37] Once again the media, either out of sheer laziness or a desire to pump up fear, omitted vital data. The real infection was in their silence.

GAO AND "NEW EVIDENCE"

As new data continues to refute alarmist predictions, we will see a drift away from facts and figures and toward non-arguments and non-falsifiable arguments. Examples of non-arguments are portrayals of select heterosexual AIDS victims, which actually tells us nothing more than that there is at least one heterosexual victim of AIDS, and personal attacks aimed at the motivations of non-alarmists. A non-falsifiable argument is one that cannot logically be disproved. One such line of reasoning that will be directed against this book will be something like, "While the argument may have been valid at the time the book was written, since then a new study has been released that shows . . . " Then a recent study, *any study,* will be proffered and interpreted so as to refute what I have written. Obviously, I cannot put out a new edition each time someone puts forth a new study. By addressing the Montreal abstracts I have made some headway against such a tactic, since many of the articles that will appear in the medical journals over the next year from the time of this writing will be based on those abstracts. But the best thing I can do for the reader is to point out that this book is replete with examples of people claiming that "it looked for a while as though we could breathe easier, but now . . . " after which it turned out that the new evidence was the same old nonsense. From an epidemiological perspective, so many studies have been done that there probably is very little room for truly new material. Blood testing—be it in hospitals, prisons, marriage applicants, STD clinics, alternate test sites, blood banks, or military applicants—has become so widespread as to leave very few relevant groups whose blood is not now being sampled. Most of the alarmists' "new" material will come from old news that already has been addressed. For example, consider the Government Accounting Office report released shortly after the Montreal conference. Entitled "Undercount of Cases and Lack of Key Data Weaken Existing Estimates," the reaction the media gave it was typified by the *USA Today* headline that stated flatly without qualification, "AIDS Forecasts Are Too Small."[38] Surgeon General Koop immediately embraced the report even though it challenged the Public Health Service figures, the second time, at least, that he willingly tossed away the material of his own lieutenants when he found something more extreme to go with. Said Koop in a fit of democratization, "It means that . . . this epidemic will eventually affect everyone."[39] The report stated that there would probably be 300,000 to 480,000 AIDS cases by the end of 1991,[40] as opposed to the CDC's range of 185,000 to 320,000, and CDC's "best guess" of 285,000. It also stated that the potential number of heterosexual cases may have been greatly understated.[41]

But among the many problems with the report is that it is highly selective. For example, it evaluates thirteen different models forecasting AIDS cases through 1991, including several that never appeared in medical journals. Yet Alexander Langmuir's model, which did appear in a medical journal[42] and was presented at hearings before both the U.S. Commission on Civil Rights and the President's Commission on the Human Immunodeficiency Virus Epidemic, was absent. The GAO report addresses, with alarm, the increase in the percentage of cases attributable to heterosexual transmission among native-born Americans. While most of this increase is due to the "pie chart phenomenon" discussed in chapter 17 (that it isn't so much the heterosexual slice increasing as it is the homosexual slice decreasing), part of it is also attributable to the new CDC case definition.[43] Indeed, GAO finally does make reference to this when it states in tiny type at the bottom of a chart, "A recent report by the U.S. Public Health Service indicates that because of the definition change, it is not possible to conclude whether there has been a real increase in heterosexual cases."[44] GAO's writers understood that even conscientious reporters don't read agate type when they're on a deadline.

GAO scrapes for every heterosexual transmission case it can find, while omitting cases that might have been inaccurately listed as heterosexual transmission. The report is critical of CDC's policy of putting persons with multiple risks including heterosexual transmission into some category other than that. Thus, for example, a bisexual with AIDS always is put into the homosexual/bisexual category, even though by definition he also has had sex with women and it is theoretically possible that he contracted the virus not through a male partner but through a female one. Possibly somewhere out there is a bisexual who did in fact get AIDS from a woman. More probably there are women who both shared needles and had intercourse with infected men and who contracted the virus through intercourse, but were listed as having gotten it through needle sharing. But the CDC system makes sense because needle sharing and anal intercourse are known to be so much more efficient in transmitting HIV that the overwhelming probability is that indeed the patient did contract the virus through the means listed, even though there were other risk factors. Whatever undercount does exist is no doubt readily made up for and then some by the overcount resulting from people lying about their risks. Nowhere in the entire GAO report is this possibility mentioned. As noted earlier in this book, if a woman who shares needles has sex with a needle sharer, she will quite possibly attribute her infection to coitus alone and deny narcotics abuse. Likewise a man will tell investigators he had intercourse with a drug-abusing prostitute. Whether these stories are investigated at all depends entirely on the city or state where the case is reported. As I noted in chapter 2, lying on the part of female IVDA alone, as indicated by the disparity in New York City's female IVDA to heterosexual transmission category versus that of the rest of the United States, could grossly overstate female heterosexual transmission cases in the nation.

The GAO thesis is basically straightforward—much more so than it might seem from reading it in detail. It says that AIDS cases in the past have been significantly underreported and that, since models predicting future cases have been based on past caseloads, those models are therefore seriously underestimating the number of future cases. Thus its model basically consists of shifting the other models to reflect this under-reporting. But whatever the true rate of past underreporting—a highly debatable subject—the biggest problem with GAO's predictions is that, like so many we have seen so far, they simply are divorced from reality. Again, it is like the weatherman who proclaims nothing but sunny weather for the next two days even as raindrops are pattering against the window. Even as GAO was proclaiming the CDC projections to be too low, the cases coming in were demonstrating those projections to be hopelessly overstated. In mid-1989, CDC stated that "The number of cases is expected to increase by about 10,000 per year."[45] Yet case reports coming in even then were showing less than a 3,000 increase over the previous year.[46] For the GAO projections to be accurate, the trend of cases coming in at ever slower rates would have to suddenly reverse itself and there would have to be an explosion of new cases. But nothing in the GAO report argues that any such explosion would or could occur. Thus, just as the CDC estimate of 285,000 cases by 1992 is being thrown off even without factoring in a peaking, the GAO figures are being thrown off each month by that much more.

Much of the most important information to come out of Montreal did not get reported by the media. Perhaps the single most important paper of the conference, indeed of the last several conferences, from an epidemiological perspective, was provocatively entitled "Are AIDS Cases Among Homosexual Males Leveling?" Authored by researchers from CDC and the departments of health of major U.S. cities, the paper looked at AIDS caseloads in New York, San Francisco, and Los Angeles of non-drug using homosexuals. The striking conclusion: "Reported AIDS cases among [homosexual/bisexual] males are leveling across the U.S., noted earlier in selected metropolitan areas."[47] It should have been great news, not just for Dr. Langmuir's reputation but for the nation as a whole. Yet it was not news at all, in the sense that it was not reported anywhere. Similarly, a paper authored by Rand Stoneburner and others in New York found a plateau of AIDS cases among homosexual men in that city.[48] A paper by the San Francisco Department of Public Health concluded that homosexual and bisexual cases in that city had plateaued, even without taking into account the new case definition.[49] (Since about 98 percent of San Francisco's cases come from homosexuals and bisexuals, a plateau in this category equals a plateau for all categories combined.) This revelation is really more of an admission considering that in a paper presented by the San Francisco Department of Health just a year earlier at the Stockholm conference, the city predicted no plateau in AIDS cases until at least 1993.[50]

One paper out of Norway also had great importance in determining the future of the epidemic. Researchers there applied the rule that 100 infections must give rise to at least 101 more to create an expanding epidemic (see chapter 2). The paper stated that "The epidemic is not self-sustained in the heterosexual population when the average transmission probability is below 1 percent per intercourse, and there is not input of infection from other groups." Since, the paper said, empirical studies indicate that 1 percent is too high, the conclusion was that "With current behavior the Norwegian heterosexual population is not likely to sustain the HIV epidemic in isolation."[51] There is no reason to think that this does not apply to the middle-class population in the United States or to the rest of Western Europe as well.

TRANSMISSION INCREASERS AND DECREASERS

Two papers provided evidence that practices long theorized to be associated with increased HIV transmission may in fact be just that. The first looked at the use of amyl and butyl nitrites by homosexual males. The practice of inhaling such substances, which come in capsule form and once were readily available at sex shops and adult book stores or from dealers (amyl required a prescription, butyl did not), was ubiquitous among male homosexuals, who believe they intensify the pleasure of intercourse and orgasm. In the Montreal paper, 80 percent of the 329 men studied had a history of nitrite use. The study found that "Those who practiced receptive anal intercourse while simultaneously using nitrites were significantly more likely to be infected than individuals who practiced receptive anal intercourse without simultaneous use of nitrites," and that this was true even taking into account the differences in numbers of sexual partners and exposures of the two groups.[52] This, then, could be yet another factor explaining why homosexual intercourse is so much riskier than heterosexual intercourse, perhaps even heterosexual anal intercourse.

The second paper looked at risk factors in female-to-male intercourse. It found that "A signficiant increase in transmission risk was found when couples had sexual contacts during menses" and that the "presence of HIV-infected blood cells in the vagina could explain the increase of risk observed in couples having contacts during menses."[53] Again, it has long been theorized that intercourse during menses could increase the man's risk since, other than the woman having a vaginal infection, there is otherwise little opportunity for a significant number of white blood cells that carry HIV to be present in vaginal and cervical fluids.

A National Institutes of Health study reaffirmed an earlier study (reported in chapter 3) that saliva inhibits HIV activity and may reduce the risks of oral sex and wet kissing. It found that "HIV-I infection was completely inhibited in all salivas from women and children. Salivas from 6 of the healthy males completely inhibited infectivity and partial inhibition was found in the remaining 3 samples."[54]

More information came in linking lack of circumcision to the African epidemic. One study attempted to match up circumcision practices of various tribes with HIV infectivity among those same groups, concluding "The correlation between these two variables in 37 African countries was high. . . . This finding is consistent with existing clinic based studies that indicate a lower risk of HIV infection among circumcised males."[55] A New York City study found chancroid "strongly associated with . . . lack of circumcision."[56] Chancroid and other ulcerating STDs (as noted earlier in chapter 4) have themselves been strongly associated with increased risk of transmission, an association confirmed by several studies presented at Montreal.[57]

MARRIAGE LICENSE APPLICANTS

In Alabama, marriage license applicant seropositivity declined from 21 per 10,000 in the first year of testing to 11 per 10,000 in the second year, ending 31 January 1989, although the numbers were so small in the first place that the decline may not be statistically significant.[58] Only Alabama presented comparative figures. A few other states and smaller areas presented premarital testing figures, which ranged from zero in Mississippi and Long Beach, California, to 66 per 10,000 in Alameda County, California (includes Oakland), which has very high rates of intravenous drug usage and a large percentage of blacks.[59]

Meanwhile, the Illinois Department of Public Health submitted a

paper finding that each seropositive individual identified under the
mandatory premarital testing program was costing $217,641, even
while it was costing $770 per seropositive through the state's anony-
mous voluntary testing service. Even among the few seropositives identified through the mandatory premarital testing, most belonged to the
traditional risk groups.[60] Shortly thereafter, the Illinois House voted to
repeal premarital testing, along with syphilis testing. The Illinois Senate
had previously done so, and the governor signed the bill into law.

Blood Sampling Elsewhere

Among 9,400 consecutive placental cord blood specimens obtained
from four County Hospitals in Los Angeles County, only 4 per 10,000
proved positive. This even though Hispanics and blacks were vastly
overrepresented in the cohort, with 38 percent of all Hispanic births in
Los Angeles County during the sampling period being represented and
23 percent of all the black births, but only 8 percent of white births.[61]

Denver, which has been sampling STD patients since 1985, has found
that while homosexual seropositivity remains alarmingly high at almost
50 percent of applicants, for IV drug users the figure remains low and
for non-IVDA heterosexuals remains near zero. The paper concluded,
"By 1988, at least 10 years after the first HIV infection in Denver, there
is no evidence that the HIV epidemic is advancing beyond gay men,
IVDA, and their sexual contacts."[62] Similarly, testing in a London STD
clinic of 4,261 heterosexuals found 8 positives. Five were from the
central African or Caribbean areas, 2 had sexual contact with IVDA,
and only one so much as claimed to have no risk factors. The report
concluded, "This sexually active population with a higher than average
prevalence of gonorrhea, chlamydia and other STDs has low HIV seropositivity in spite of the potential for importing cases from endemic
areas [Africa and the Caribbean]."[63]

A broad study of 8 women's health clinics across the country found
that "HIV seroprevalence rates in women attending family planning,
prenatal, and abortion clinics vary, but are generally low. Rates are
higher in black women and in more populated areas."[64]

Among minorities in some areas, seroprevalence remains alarmingly
high. One study of newborns in New York City's South Bronx found that
the incidence of infection in children born of mothers claiming to have
no history of drug abuse was 6 percent.[65]

If AIDS were to begin "breaking out" into the general heterosexual population it would almost certainly do so first in New York because of that city's high number of intravenous drug abusers and comparatively high number of infected heterosexuals. However, a comparative survey of attendees at an STD clinic in 1987 and in 1988 found that while 7.5 percent were positive the first year, only 4.9 percent were positive in 1988. Although the sample sizes were too small to represent a statistically significant drop, nevertheless they did indicate stability in infections over an 18-month period.[66] Similarly, a survey of 3,556 women giving birth or having induced abortions in New York City found that "HIV-I seroprevalence among pregnant women remained stable."[67]

If seropositivity were increasing among any group in New York, it would be among crack users, as Dr. Stoneburner warned (see chapter 10). One STD clinic study in that city found a significant number of heterosexually transmitted infections (albeit no more than the year before) and found a connection with crack cocaine use.[68] A second study, this one of 61 steady heterosexual partners of infected persons, found that the chance of the partner becoming infected was "related most strongly to crack use and to anal intercourse."[69] (A San Francisco study also found crack use associated with syphilis infection, which may aid in the spread of HIV, albeit not with HIV infection directly.[70])

AFRICA

The day before the Montreal conference, I was on a radio talk show with AIDS activist Robert Kunst (see chapter 14) who declared that studies out of Africa presented at the conference were showing 50 percent rates of infection.[71] He should have said "study," singular. The highest rate by far in any paper was from high STD areas in part of Angola. Among nine groups tested, HIV-I and HIV-II rates were found from 10.8 percent to 46.0 percent.[72] Happily, no other study had figures anywhere near these, and the Angola one is probably best viewed as demonstrating yet again the vital importance of STDs in spreading HIV in Africa. One study of 8,000 blood samples in Kinshasa, Zaire, found only 2.44 percent infected,[73] while a study of 508 pregnant women in that country found a 3.76 percent infection rate.[74] Another study found a 2.9 percent infection rate in pregnant women in a rural area of Zaire, with a 2.1 percent rate in blood donors.[75] A third study, testing samples in both Kinshasa and rural Zaire over the period 1986–89, appeared to confirm the belief of some researchers that HIV infection in epidemic areas of Africa has leveled off. With the caveat that "Our data reflect HIV infection in only the populations we sampled [blood donors, pregnant women, female prostitutes, general population, factory workers, and hospital workers] and should not be used to assess the overall HIV situation in Zaire," the report stated:

> Except for a progressive increase in seroprevalence in [Kinshasa] prostitutes, the continuing occurrence of incident cases of infection in the face of a relatively stable seroprevalence suggests the possible emergence of a steady state of HIV infection in the groups studied.[76]

Some parts of Africa still appear to have little or no HIV infection, either of HIV-I or HIV-II.[77] Clearly rates of 2 to 3 percent are still a cause of concern, but they are comparable to estimates of seropositivity in New York and San Francisco. Just as clearly, reports of the death of African civilization have been greatly exaggerated.

Ultimately, nothing in this appendix can preclude the argument that "something new" has come along to change everything. The best advice I can proffer is: be skeptical in all things related to AIDS. Keep in mind that while your goal may be to learn as much about the epidemic in the time you have allotted, the media's goal is to entertain you, terrify you, get you to buy their product, and raise your level of "social consciousness." The goal of the AIDS industry in general is sheer self-perpetuation. Those seeking the truth about the spread of AIDS would be well advised to seek elsewhere.

APPENDIX A

An Update: Still Waiting for the "AIDS Disaster"

The AIDS Disaster. That was the ominous title of one of the last books published in 1990 on AIDS—the same year the first edition of *The Myth of Heterosexual AIDS* appeared. It called for massive, no-holds-barred spending on AIDS at levels the authors admitted guaranteed a great deal of waste.[1] And truly, for many, AIDS has been a disaster. For homosexual males and for intravenous drug abusers in America's larger cities, AIDS is exacting a toll greater than did the first and most awful sweep of the Black Death through Europe in the mid-1300s. But on a national scale, by 1990 it was clear that the estimates and projections about AIDS had been grossly overstated.

Nineteen-ninety was a banner year for AIDS predictions. Oprah Winfrey declared that one-fifth of all heterosexuals would be dead (*Myth*, page 3); Gene Antonio said 64 million Americans would be dead or dying of AIDS (*Myth*, page 184). What proved to be dead, however, were those scary predictions—both dead wrong. AIDS diagnoses by the end of 1992 were at about one-quarter of a million,[2] and the one-fifth of the heterosexual population that was supposed to have died of AIDS is alive and well. But as silly as those numbers seem to us now, back when they were asserted (Winfrey's in 1987, Antonio's in 1985), they convinced and terrified many people.

Oprah and Gene Antonio are one thing, but even the authorities issued vastly overblown predictions. In 1989, the U.S. General Accounting Office projected from 300,000 to 480,000 cases of AIDS in the country by the end of 1991 (*Myth*, page 343). The media immediately converted this to "as many as 480,000 cases,"[3] a spin which Surgeon General Koop uncritically accepted (*Myth*, page 343). But even by the end of the next year, 1992, with 206,000 cumulative cases reported the country was nowhere near even the bottom of the GAO's estimate for 1991. As I noted in this book, "For the GAO projections to be accurate, the trend of cases coming in at ever slower rates would have to suddenly reverse itself and there would have to be an explosion of new cases. But nothing in the GAO report argues that any such explosion would or could take place" (*Myth*, page 345).

In 1986 the World Health Organization (WHO), with Dr. Jonathan Mann as the director of its Global Program on AIDS, predicted as many as 100 million worldwide infections by 1990, yet by 1990 they were admitting to only 8–10 million.[4] Even this figure was grossly inflated, since it contained dubious subestimates such as that one in seventy-five males was currently infected in North America. Applied to the U.S., this would mean 1.66 million infected males.[5] Yet, the CDC total estimate for both United States males and females was one million.[6] If WHO were fudging the figures from the part of the world where the best information is available, it seems likely they might be doing so also from those parts of the world where information is far more sketchy. Yet just as WHO's old faulty estimate was taken as gospel, so too are today's new faulty estimates.

When virologist William Haseltine, now on leave from Harvard and one of the AIDS alarmists singled out for special attention in *Myth*, testified before Congress in 1992 that a fifth of the earth's population would have the AIDS virus early in the next century, Reuters reported the claim uncritically.[7] If they had inquired into the source of his information, however, they would have found he had simply made it up, just as he had made up numbers in his 1985 congressional testimony, which the media also dutifully reported (*Myth*, pages 251–52). Reuters did not quote anyone who contested the figure, nor did it supply the much-lower estimate of the World Health Organization.

The AIDS alarmist motto is: "Never apologize; never explain." Gene Antonio now denies (on CNN's "Crossfire"), that he ever made the 64 million prediction, over 200,000 copies of his book notwithstanding. Yet in 1993 he published a new book, *AIDS: Rage and Reality*, declaring that *100 million* Americans will be dead or dying of the disease by the end of the century.[8] In 1985, Walter Reed Hospital infectious disease specialist Dr. Robert Redfield told eager reporters, "This is a general disease now. Get rid of the high risk groups, anyone can get it" (*Myth*, page 16). Five years later, with the risk groups the same as ever, as indeed they are now, Redfield was still being quoted by eager reporters, including *Newsweek*'s.[9]

No More Sex Scare, Please, We're British

In the United Kingdom too, the epidemic has proved a gross disappointment to the doomsayers. In 1985 and 1986 the British were told:

- "A million people in Britain—one in fifty—will have AIDS in six years (1991) unless the killer disease is checked, the Royal College of Nursing claims today."[10]
- (Quoting Chief Medical Officer of Health Donald Acheson): "For planning purposes we are assuming that between 1,000 and 2,000 new cases of AIDS will occur in the U.K. in 1988."[11]
- "Between 20,000 and 40,000 people will die of AIDS each year by the turn of the century, according to official estimates from the government's Communicable Diseases Surveillance Centre."[12]

But when 1991 rolled around, there were only slightly more than four thousand cases reported in all of the UK, the total number after ten years of epidemic; with 755 diagnosed in 1988.[13] Acheson, incidentally, had some nasty things to say about how terribly wrong *Myth* was when it came out. To quote the London *Daily Telegraph*, Acheson "argues that Fumento and other critics of the present campaign are expressing 'denial.' 'Psychiatrists know this mechanism well,'" said Acheson. "'If we do not want to believe something may affect us, we try to think it is something to do with people who are different from us and of whom we may not approve.'"[14]

Alarmists commonly denigrate nonalarmists by the ad hominem technique of accusing them of being in denial—a form of mental illness. But it is they who, year after year, deny the statistics, as often as not compiled by their own offices. The ad hominem jibe allows them simply to sidestep arguments on the facts, much like saying, "you can't trust my opponent because he's a communist," or "because he's a racist."

In the United States, with the media so thoroughly on the side of the AIDS alarmists, such epithets go a long way. Yet "over there," the British, benefiting from a more politically diverse media than exists here, are beginning to catch on. For some time after several major British papers began questioning the government's "everybody is at risk" campaign, the government refused to budge. But by 1992, it began to grow uneasy. That year it slashed its expenditures for local authorities on AIDS by 20 percent. The subtitle of a London *Sunday Telegraph* article summed up the situation: "Ministers [of the government] lose interest in the apocalypse that never happened."[15]

By June of 1993, even the alarmist British newspaper *The Independent*, which had blamed me just weeks earlier for launching the anti-alarmist backlash with my book excerpt in the *Sunday Times*,[16] reported, "The spread of AIDS among heterosexuals in England and Wales will be slower than predicted, the Public Health Laboratory Service said yesterday. Figures to be published later this month will show that the projected number of cases has fallen by two-thirds in two years, as data from anonymous blood screening of the population has become available."[17]

Contrast that with Health and Human Services Secretary Donna Shalala's statement before Congress in early 1993, reported by at least one national news service: "We could spend our energy on research and immunization and education and still not have any Americans left unless we're prepared to confront the crisis of AIDS."[18] That's right, *not any*. Did the news service give space to any contradictory remark? No; this is the objective American media.

THE DECLINE OF THE ESTIMATES

But what of the U.S. Centers for Disease Control (CDC) estimates? To my knowledge, I was the only journalist in the nation, with the exception of columnist Patrick J. Buchanan, who asserted that the CDC's estimates of total current HIV infections and of future cases would both prove wrong (*Myth*, pages 307–319). This is not to boast, but to show the slavishness of the American media. Indeed, to the extent any reporters ever challenged the CDC data it was to present the even higher estimates of a report issued by a conservative think tank the Hudson Institute (*Myth*, pages 19, 22, 56, 95, and 305) and by the U.S. General Accounting Office (*Myth*, pages 342–45). Ironically, just as *Myth* was hitting the stores, the CDC lowered first its estimate of future cases and then its estimate of current infections.

In January 1990, CDC announced it was lowering its projections of new AIDS cases over the next few years by about 15 percent.[19] The next month it lowered its estimate of current HIV infections from a range of about 1–1.5 million to 1 million.[20] Still, many alarmists remained undaunted. Thus a month after the CDC knocked down its infection figure, Hudson Institute author Kevin R. Hopkins wrote an op-ed for *USA Today* claiming, "Each day, 500 people contract the AIDS virus through sexual intercourse and illicit drug injections."[21] That adds up to 182,500 new infections a year.

Just as the downward revision in the estimate of current infections didn't prove adequate, so too the CDC's downward revision in projected AIDS cases fell short. In December of 1992 the CDC had to lower them again. The projected minimum of 61,000 diagnoses of AIDS in the year 1994 dropped to 43,000.[22] The CDC also admitted that the epidemic was leveling off.[23] You probably didn't hear about it. Major newspapers like the *Los Angeles Times* completely ignored the downward revision. But it happened all the same.

CREDIT WHERE NO CREDIT IS DUE

As one might expect, those whose predictions were grossly in error downplayed the importance of the revision and dredged up far-fetched excuses for their mistakes.

Thus, James Hyman, head of the mathematical modeling group at the Los Alamos National Laboratory in New Mexico, told the *Wall Street Journal*, "The number of cases is still increasing, but the rate of increase has slowed," and the title of an article in the December 1989 issue of *Science* read, "Is the AIDS Epidemic Slowing?"[24] In fact, Hyman and *Science*'s headline would have been out of date as far back as 1983. From 1982 to 1983, reported AIDS cases increased 163 percent. From 1983 to 1984, they increased 146 percent, from 1984 to 1985, 86 percent, and so forth.[25] Far from resulting from medical intervention or behavior modification, this trend is common to all epidemics, from the Black Death (bubonic plague) to polio to the flu. All epidemics follow a curve which is never linear, never truly exponential. Even as they grow larger they grow more slowly, until eventually they level and drop off (*Myth*, pages 311–12).

The Public Health Service (the parent of the CDC), and others, for their part, turned what might have seemed a mistake into a victory. Dr. Sten Vermund, chief of the epidemiology branch of the division of

AIDS at the National Institute of Allergies and Infectious Diseases, was reported by *Science* to have said, "We have seen what we had always hoped we would see: Some kind of measurable public health benefit from these huge investments that we are making."[26] The miscalculation was generally attributed to new developments, either prophylactic drug therapy involving use of AZT, or inhaled pentamidine to stave off a particular AIDS-associated pneumonia in those yet to be diagnosed with AIDS, or to "prophylactics," meaning use of condoms, abstinence, or other risk reduction activity.

I argued strenuously in print that there was no evidence of this,[27] relying in part on the work of Dr. Joel Hay of the University of Southern California. Hay's research showed that medical intervention could not have explained the flattening curve. Still, the "new developments" theory quickly became the general line. As one commentator put it, "It is widely known and accepted that the leveling off in new AIDS cases among homosexual men . . . was the direct result of therapy with AZT."[28]

Finally, the cover blew off in 1993 when a group of British researchers decided to carry out to the end a study looking at the effect of AZT in delaying the progression of HIV to full-blown AIDS. The American studies had never been completed since it was decided that ethically it would be wrong to continue once it had been established that those using AZT were faring better than those using placebos. The problem was that it hadn't been established at all. Rather, the American researchers had simply seen an increase in the CD4 (a type of white blood cell) count of patients and assumed this translated into better health and longer life. The British researchers also saw this increase but carried the experiment out long enough to find there was no relationship between CD4 counts and developing AIDS, at least among those using AZT. Indeed, they found that those using AZT as prophylaxis developed full-blown AIDS just as soon as those who did not use it.[29]

The real reason for the epidemic going flat is that data collected by CDC and others indicate that despite the years of hype over an epidemic supposedly growing by leaps and bounds, HIV in terms of infection had done most of its dirty work by 1985—the year of the first big media scare. In fact, it would seem to have leveled off in homosexual populations in some major U.S. cities by 1982 and probably in all of them by 1984.[30] Since infections begin manifesting themselves as AIDS cases in as little as two to three years, the peak in infections would begin to manifest itself as a sudden slowing in the case diagnosis rate in two to three years, or by 1987 for the nation as a whole. And since the national government AIDS education campaign didn't even begin until November 1987, three years after the infections had leveled, it is hard to argue that education had anything to do with the leveling—not that it wasn't asserted just the same.

While the AIDS establishment has eagerly remarked on the flattening of the epidemic among homosexuals, it has been loathe to discuss the flattening among IV drug abusers (IVDAs). This is probably because the IVDA data contradict the claim of homosexual groups and AIDS educators that their "safe-sex" campaigns are responsible for fewer cases being reported. That's why one representative of Gay Men's Health Crisis with whom I appeared on TV became enraged when I mentioned the IVDA figures.[31]

Over and over again we were told that "good progress has been made among homosexuals, but the rest of the epidemic continues out of control." In January of 1991, U.S. Surgeon General Novella amended her statement to say that "In the original target population of homosexual men, AIDS might be leveling . . ."[32] In another instance, the front-page story in the *Los Angeles Times* concerning the first (1990) CDC announcement that it was lowering its projections was entitled "Slower Spread of AIDS in Gays Seen Nationally,"[33] even though the estimates dropped for the epidemic as a whole, not just homosexuals. And again, Dr. Roy Anderson of Imperial College in the UK, who wrote off *Myth* as simply wishful thinking,[34] said in the April 1990 *JAIDS* that while homosexual male cases were flattening in the Western countries, there was a "continued and rapid rise among IV drug users."[35] He cited no statistics and indeed could not have, since there were none for him to cite.

THE *STILL* ONCE AND FUTURE HETEROSEXUAL NONEPIDEMIC

According to the most recent data from the federal Centers for Disease Control and Prevention (CDC), overall, AIDS cases increased only 3.5 percent in 1992 from the year before,[36] while cases increased only 5 percent from 1990 to 1991.[37] This notwithstanding, when I debated Public Health Service Director James Mason on the "Today Show" in January of 1992, he disputed my claim that the epidemic was leveling, citing a thirty-three percent rise in AIDS cases from the previous year.[38] Meanwhile, Surgeon General Novella told journalist Gregg Easterbrook in 1992, "Don't, don't believe that AIDS has leveled off."[39]

Similarly, on a June 1993 CBS Evening News broadcast Dan Rather warned of "sharply-growing heterosexual AIDS in this country," while CBS health correspondent Dr. Bob Arnot told viewers, "Heterosexual AIDS among Americans is growing faster than any other risk group, up 30 percent in 1992 alone. The CDC says this is a frightening trend."[40] What the CDC really said, through its figures, was that cases attributed to heterosexuals increased 17 percent in 1992,[41] down from a 21 percent increase in 1991.[42] The increase in female cases declined from 17 percent in 1991[43] to 9 percent by 1992.[44]

Nonintravenous, non-drug-abusing heterosexuals comprise 95.5 percent of the population, but only 6 percent of all AIDS cases. This is the figure if you use the CDC classification that includes Haitians and Africans diagnosed in the United States in the heterosexual category. Excluding the Haitians and Africans, the figure is 5 percent.[45]

More heterosexuals died of cancer by the third day of this year than will die of sexually-transmitted AIDS during the rest of the year.[46] By the end of January, more women died of breast cancer alone than will die of sexually-transmitted AIDS during the entire year.[47]

In an accompanying press release to the third National Commission on AIDS report, released in August of 1990, NCA Chairman Dr. June Osborn stated that "many parts of rural America are about to be blindsided by the epidemic."[48] Three years later, in arguing against aiming AIDS education at those at highest risk for the disease, she said the epidemic "is very rapidly spreading throughout smaller and smaller communities each year."[49] Yet, since the government began collecting case data on this in 1990, the figure for nonmetropolitan areas has remained stable at about 5 percent of the total of AIDS cases.[50]

Yes, but what of infections? In 1992, the CDC released its second report of infection data gathered from a variety of sources across the country. Although the media virtually ignored it, the report was packed with information about the size and shape of the epidemic.

One key paragraph summarized the report. It noted that "high rates of seroprevalence [infection]" were found among homosexual males, with an average infection rate of 32 percent. "By contrast, considerably lower prevalences" were found among intravenous drug abusers, with an average infection rate of about 4 percent, and "almost all other groups." These other groups included persons at sexually transmitted disease (STD) clinics who claimed no homosexual or drug-injecting activity. The average infection rate for males was 1.1 percent and for females 0.7 percent. Since women are far more likely to become infected by a man than vice-versa, this figure undoubtedly includes a number of men who had other risk factors but would not admit to them. Women seeking reproductive health services had a mere 0.2 percent rate of infection while those tested at a number of select hospitals around the nation (usually in major cities where infection rates are higher) called "sentinel hospitals" had an average infection rate of slightly less than 1 percent. Job Corps applicants, who are primarily male, black, or Hispanic, had an infection rate of much less than 1 percent, while the rate for military applicants was only 0.12 percent.[51]

If women have an average rate of infection of from 0.2 to 1 percent compared to an average of 32 percent for homosexual males, how can one conceivably conclude that the AIDS virus does not discriminate?

Despite desperate efforts on the part of former Health and Human Services Director Louis Sullivan (more on this below) and of the National Commission on AIDS to convince rural America that it is now at terrible risk of getting the disease, the CDC report found that "for the broader populations surveyed across the country, analysis of local patterns indicated generally that urban populations continued to have much higher prevalences than rural populations." It did go on to say that some childbearing women in small town and rural areas in the southeastern states had high infection rates,[52] but "southeastern states" appears essentially to mean Florida,[53] where Haitians and a terrible drug problem have contributed to a high overall AIDS rate and infection rate, as well as a high rate of infection for childbearing women. Both for overall AIDS incidence and incidence of children with AIDS, Florida has the second-highest rate of any state (next to New York) in the country.[54]

The two largest bodies of infection data, military applicants and first-time blood donors, "have shown progressive declines in HIV since 1985," when testing began, according to the report.[55] It warns that these two categories do not mirror averages of infection in the general population since persons who suspect they are infected often don't get tested. But this doesn't explain why after, say, 1987, rates within these categories continued to drop. Male infection rates from first-time blood donors dropped from 7 out of 10,000 in 1985 to about 3 in 10,000 in 1990, while female ones dropped from about 2 per 1,000 in 1985 to half that in 1990.[56] Male infection rates for civilian applicants to military service dropped from 18 per 10,000 in 1985 to 10 per 10,000 in 1990, while for females the drop was from about 7 to 3 per 10,000.[57]

Looking at the epidemic as a whole, the June 1992 CDC report concluded, "Thus, serosurveillance overall has indicated relative stability rather than a clear increase or decrease in HIV prevalence."[58] Since the CDC has never been known for its optimism when it comes to AIDS, this must be seen as a worse-case scenario, yet it is rosy compared to the claims of 95 percent of the nation's AIDS commentators. The continued decline in the two largest-sample areas of testing, military applicants and first-time blood donors, quite strongly supports the case that the overall HIV rate is declining. However, decreases in these categories, which are heavily weighted toward heterosexuals, may be offset by a relatively large number of new homosexual infections (discussed below).

Nonautomatic Transmission

One question left begging in the research available at the time of the first edition of *Myth* was the rate of transmission efficiency of HIV from female-to-male. It has been well established that the transmission rate is considerably less than male-to-female, which hovers around 20 percent for a relationship of several years (*Myth*, pages 27–28). We now have the results of one partner study in which women were originally infected and men were not.

Conducted by Dr. Nancy Padian of Berkeley, the most recognized name in the AIDS partner studies, this study showed that of forty-one originally uninfected men, over a period of years, only one became positive and that relationship involved "over 100 episodes of vaginal and penile bleeding."[59] Most couples, it is safe to say, do not have intercourse under such conditions. At any rate, the only study we now have quantifying female-to-male transmission has put it at one-tenth the rate of male-to-female. Obviously one study is just that—one study. But such a rate of transmission seems to jibe with what epidemiologists had expected to find. For a disease to sustain itself in a population each old case must equal one new case. A male-to-female rate of one new case for five old ones could not fulfill this rule, much less a female-to-male transmission rate of fifty old cases to one new case.

SEX, LIES, AND FLORIDA HETEROSEXUALS

Chapter seven of *Myth* deals with the problem that when a disease is contracted under embarrassing circumstances, some persons will falsely deny those circumstances. Since virtually no one who is not an intravenous drug abuser or homosexual will claim to be one, and since those who are intravenous drug abusers or homosexuals may deny it, the portion of the epidemic assigned to heterosexual transmission will be exaggerated. This is especially so given the common practice of health authorities simply to accept the patient's word for it that they are neither an IV drug abuser nor homosexual. A Florida study published in the *American Journal of Public Health* in 1993 provides further evidence that the number of AIDS cases assigned to the heterosexual category is greatly exaggerated.

CDC researchers analyzed the cases categorized as "heterosexual transmission" in two southeastern Florida counties and found, just by going through their files, that about a fifth had been misclassified.[60] For example, a diagnosis of anal gonorrhea or anal syphilis in a man would be a clear indicator of homosexual activity.[61] Some of these were also reclassified based on their own late admissions. Ultimately, of the non-Haitians, slightly over half of the presumed heterosexual men were reclassified, as were over 10 percent of the women. An additional third of the men reinterviewed but not reclassified had evidence of anal disease (such as a loose sphincter muscle) that may or may not have been caused by sex with another man.[62] Thus, it appears that the great majority of the non-Haitian men originally classified as heterosexual transmission cases, as well as a sizeable number of non-Haitian women, were not heterosexual transmission at all. There is no reason to believe that if the CDC looked closely at cases categorized as heterosexual transmission in the other forty-nine states it wouldn't come up with similar findings, which might subtract by half or more in men, and by many in women, from the overall U.S. heterosexual transmission category. A major lowering of the male figure along with a lesser lowering of the female figure would be more consistent with the evidence from Nancy Padian's female-to-male partner study, as well as explaining why, when a heterosexual woman's sex partner is so much more likely to be infected than a heterosexual man's, the heterosexual transmission category is only about three-fifths female.[63] It's very easy for a man with AIDS simply to say a woman gave him the virus, especially when he claims he doesn't know which woman. It gets even easier when the AIDS establishment is eager to trumpet women as a likely source of infection, as witness the basketball star Earvin "Magic" Johnson.

Do You Believe In Magic?

Every year, the alarmists find something on which to hang their heterosexual AIDS message—that *this year* the wolf really has appeared. Every year the media use AIDS to sell magazines, newspapers, and TV shows, and find ways to sell us on the idea that AIDS is a democratic disease that doesn't single out homosexuals because of their sex practices, and that an ever greater infusion of federal research funds is needed.

In 1991, the new message on the AIDS front was Magic Johnson's revelation that he had been infected with HIV. CNN jumped on the Johnson story to tell us that now "anyone can get AIDS."[64] *Time*'s article on Johnson's revelation was titled, "It Can Happen to Anybody. Even Magic Johnson,"[65] while *Newsday*'s story was titled, "Heterosexual AIDS Risk; Magic Johnson's Infection Spreads the Word: Everyone's in Danger." Michael Merson, who succeeded Jonathan Mann as the director of the World Health Organization Global Program on AIDS, said that "you're up to over 10 percent heterosexual cases in the U.S. now, and it's climbing."[66] A simple call to the CDC would have informed *Newsday*'s reporter that U.S. heterosexual transmission cases, even counting all diagnosed Haitians and Africans, was 6 percent. Not counting foreign-acquired infections, it was 4.5 percent.[67] *Newsweek* declared, "The gist of Johnson's initial message has been that if *I* got it, everyone must worry about the AIDS virus. No reputable researcher would argue with such a position."[68] (An accompanying article, however, pointed out that very few men get the disease the way Johnson said he did, and that "if Johnson indeed contracted the disease from a woman, he was very unlucky . . .")[69]

In other instances, Marilyn Chase, the AIDS reporter-crusader at the *Wall Street Journal*, ran a story entitled, "Johnson Disclosure Underscores Facts of AIDS in Heterosexual Population."[70] And one Los Angeles TV station ran five straight nights of special broadcasts about the alleged heterosexual AIDS epidemic. Predictably, AIDS testing centers were swamped. "I think every man in New York City who's ever had unprotected sex is calling about getting tested,"[71] said one director of an AIDS facility in New York.

In the wake of his revelation, Johnson found himself in the position of Tom Sawyer—he heard his own eulogy, and not once but dozens of times. "In Magic Johnson," editorialized the *Chicago Tribune*, "the war against AIDS has a new volunteer, a superb spokesperson, a fresh hope, a peerless teacher, an almost mystic symbol."[72] To hear the media tell it, thirty years from now people will be remembering where they were when they heard Johnson's announcement, as with the assassination of JFK.[73]

Johnson himself gladly assumed the role of Nathan Hale of the basketball court: he all but regretted that he had but one immune system to give for his country. "Sure, I was convinced that I would never catch the AIDS virus," he told *Sports Illustrated*, "but if it was going to happen to someone, I'm actually glad it happened to me. I think I can spread the message concerning AIDS better than almost anyone."[74]

And now for the facts: what we knew about AIDS on the day of Johnson's press conference was the same as what we had known the day before. Johnson's having HIV changed none of the statistics collected over the last decade. The virus had not suddenly mutated.

Let us say that the media, rather than concentrating on spreading AIDS hysteria (with occasional time-outs for Alar, asbestos, cellular phones, and a few other scares), decided to terrorize Americans into believing that shark attacks were rampant and escalating, in complete contradiction of all the statistical evidence. Now let's say that one day a famous athlete or movie star gets bitten by a shark and states as much on national TV. Would this prove that the media had been right all along?

For all the talk about Johnson having gotten the disease from a woman, and the ramifications thereof for society, few have noted that the evidence for this is based on one thing only—his word. That's it. Even this story had only gradually evolved. At the press conference itself a reporter asked how he got it. Johnson bounced the question to the team physician, Michael Mellman, as if Mellman would know who infected Johnson. Mellman bounced the question back to Johnson, noting that this was something the player would have to explain. But Johnson just took another question. Later, Mellman stated to the *Orange County Register*, "This is a heterosexual individual who was infected through heterosexual activity."[75]

Of course, Mellman knows nothing of the sort—the only way anyone could possibly know how Johnson got HIV for sure would have been by having followed him from bed to bed for about, oh, say the last ten years. Before we blithely accept the media's version of what happened all those years beneath Magic Johnson's rumpled sheets, we should note that not telling the truth about risk factors is common among men diagnosed with AIDS. Entertainer Liberace denied both his homosexuality and his sickness until he died of AIDS—his manager blamed the pianist's illness on pernicious anemia induced by a watermelon-only diet for weight reduction. Indeed, in 1959 Liberace sued a British newspaper for implying that he was a homosexual—and won.[76] Johnson also threatened to file suit against persons who might write that he was a bisexual, saying of one such, "He won't be writing for nobody else no more."[77]

But in Johnson's case, the impetus to lie would be far greater than with other men. By one estimate, he stood to lose more than $25 million in endorsement fees.[78] He was also, it seems, poised to receive some several million dollars for a second autobiography. "The money is already on the table and the pot will probably grow," reported the *Washington Post* two weeks after the fateful press conference.[79] If HIV were going to kill Johnson, then Johnson was going to make a killing off HIV. There's nothing wrong with that. But for Johnson to admit to either bisexuality or drug abuse would have wiped out the big money in his being "a spokesman for the HIV virus"[80] (to use his curious locution), destroyed the groundswell of sympathy he has received, and canceled his endorsements and book deals. Lesbian tennis player Martina Navratilova made a rather bitter comment concerning this.[81] Most people would, after all, be sorely tempted to lie for $25 million and save their reputation to boot.

While no one doubts Johnson's statement that he has slept with many people, there have been rumors for years that he, as Woody Allen has put it, has twice the chance of having a date on Saturday night. The prevalence of this rumor has been such that persons in Florida's homosexual enclave of Key West have been spotted wearing T-shirts saying, "I love basketball; I had a Magic Johnson." The sports-page editor at the *Los Angeles Times*, Paul Kupper, confirmed that such rumors were circulating long before his announcement that he was infected. When I asked if the *Times* were going to investigate these rumors, he said he didn't think so. "I don't know what difference it makes. He has it [HIV] and that's all there is to it. What does it matter?" *What does it matter?* It matters because the media have gone ballistic over a possible false premise since Johnson announced he contracted the disease through heterosexual sex. Because HIV testing clinics were splitting at the seams with terrified heterosexuals. "Doesn't the truth have an intrinsic value to it?" I asked Kupper.

"Yes," he answered thoughtfully, but he didn't see how that was relevant to Magic Johnson. After all, "heterosexuals do get AIDS; I think that's more important than how he got it."

After Congressman Stewart McKinney died of AIDS, purportedly from a blood transfusion, both the *Washington Post*[82] and the *New York Times*[83] launched an investigative probe to find if this were true. (It wasn't.) Similarly, when a Texas minister died of AIDS and his family claimed it was from apparent casual contact in his ministry to AIDS victims, a reporter from the *Washington Times* went into the local gay bars and dug up the same story on the preacher (*Myth*, page 91). Will we see the same done with Johnson? Not while he's alive. So much as suggesting that Johnson may be bisexual is considered heresy most foul. Donald Drake, the medical reporter for the *Philadelphia Inquirer*, once tried to write a piece which, to the best of his recollection, began, "If Magic Johnson got HIV through heterosexual sex, he either had to have had a lot of partners or he was very unlucky, because it's unusual for heterosexuals to get AIDS that way." *Inquirer* editors ordered the line stricken for so much as hinting that Johnson might have contracted HIV through homosexual intercourse.[84]

The media weren't about to let a little thing like the possibility of bisexuality stand in the way of their scare about heterosexual contagion. After all, if Johnson didn't get AIDS the way he said he did then he *should have*. Woe unto the reporter who challenged that.

How many times have we heard what a hero Magic Johnson was just for announcing that he was infected? Even Vice President Dan Quayle called him a "true champion" for publicly disclosing his condition.[85] Yet by his own admission in the *Sports Illustrated* article, his teammates were beginning to catch on.[86] Even *Newsweek*, which lauded him as a hero, noted that the story had already leaked.[87] By holding his press conference, Johnson probably beat the news coming down the pipeline by a day, maybe two.

The standards for being a hero today are somewhat different from the days when heroes were expected to storm a machine gun nest or save babies from burning buildings. The media called Johnson a hero by virtue of his being famous and beloved, and mostly for having contracted the virus and saying he got it heterosexually. (Quayle, for his part, was engaged in his ongoing and unsuccessful campaign to placate the media.) For years, AIDS activists had been praying for a famous heterosexual to get AIDS and now many of them could scarcely conceal their glee. *U.S. News & World Report* said that the AIDS establishment cheered Johnson's announcement.[88] And so it did. A letter to the *Los Angeles Times* read simply, "November 7, 1991: On this date in history, AIDS became a heterosexual disease."[89]

After giving stunning performances at the 1992 Olympics and the NBA All-Star game, Johnson announced he would be playing again for the Lakers. The entire sports world was overjoyed. Yet his return and downfall would come back-to-back. In February of 1992 I wrote an article for the *American Spectator*. I noted that the assumption that Johnson got the disease from a woman was just that, that he had reason not to tell the truth, that the numbers indicated that he probably hadn't—though I had no personal evidence to that effect—that the rumors about him had begun long before his HIV announcement, and that the media were refusing to follow up on those rumors.[90] The article received a fair amount of attention but nothing compared to the firestorm that would be generated when *Sporting News* writer David Kindred, a former columnist for the *Washington Post*, penned a column in which he called for Johnson to come clean about how he really got the disease, citing statistics from and quoting the *American Spectator* article. "Now [Johnson] should do one thing," wrote Kindred. "Tell the whole truth about how he acquired the AIDS virus."[91]

Johnson disingenuously attempted to blame all of the rumors on a single player, whom he later identified as Detroit Pistons star Isaiah Thomas,[92] and for the most part the media went along with it. "Magic Slam Dunks Rumors," read the headline of a *New York Post* article, subtitled, "Laker Star Confronts Source of Story."[93] But at least one other national columnist wrote, "What I do know for sure is more than one marquee player has indicated to me during the last year his belief that Magic isn't straight, and Isaiah wasn't one [of them]."[94] I myself was swamped with people calling and writing me to relate stories of Magic consorting with men. I can vouch for none of them and none of them may have been true, but I started hearing of them long before Johnson fingered Thomas. Adding to the pressure on Johnson was the discomfort that some NBA players said they felt playing with an HIV-infected competitor, though none refused to do so.

Finally, Johnson once again stunned the sports world by quitting. Many simply could not understand his action. "There is something going on here," said one sports psychologist. "After listening to things

Johnson said about how he seeks basketball, how he missed the big games, he missed going one on one with all those talented people. Something is happening here behind the scenes leading to the second retirement."[95] I would suggest that Johnson knew that at some point the papers would no longer be able to cover for him, that the rumors would no longer be just that. Only by quitting could he head this off, and indeed the talk stopped right along with his career. I think that someday when he is gone—and may that be a long time from now—the truth will come out.

Not content with one heterosexual poster boy, members of the media revealed the illness of tennis star Arthur Ashe, since deceased, who said he contracted the virus from a transfusion during open heart surgery. Ashe felt compelled to call a press conference after a *USA Today* reporter called him up to verify a tip he had received.[96] Ashe said he had desperately tried to keep his condition a secret not only to protect his own privacy but that of his five-year-old daughter, who may now have to face "new, different, and sometimes cruel comments."[97]

Such concerns were not shared by *USA Today*. To quote the *New York Times*, *USA Today* managing editor John M. Simpson said Ashe's forced sacrifice was worth "'the good that may come out of the process,' as AIDS loses its stigma."[98] And the *Times* itself, in an editorial, seemed to back that sentiment, saying, "A few well-placed smashes from Mr. Ashe might well energize the nation's response to AIDS—and could help change the ignorant attitudes that forced him underground."[99] Apparently, not only is the truth expendable in a good cause, the privacy and wishes of a good and decent dying man don't merit any consideration either.

THE NEW CASE DEFINITION—THE CDC MOVES THE GOALPOSTS

Beginning in January 1993, the CDC, which acquired the lofty new name of Centers for Disease Control and Prevention (though retaining the familiar CDC initials), began using an expanded definition of what constitutes AIDS. It was the fourth time the CDC would do so, though this was by far the most expansive—and the most cynical. In addition to keeping the old criteria, which comprised a finding of HIV positivity plus any two of a number of life-threatening diseases such as Kaposi's sarcoma or Pneumocystis Carinii Pneumonia, the new definition defines an AIDS case as anyone with HIV whose CD4 count falls below 200 per microliter of blood. Most healthy people have about 800 per microliter.

One problem with this is that CD4 testing is notoriously inaccurate, varying from laboratory to laboratory and from day to day, much as blood pressure readings vary each time you take them. One study of San Francisco homosexual males who originally tested below 200 CD4 cells found that fully three-fourths of them, in a subsequent test, had levels above the 200 threshold.[100] If you don't like your CD4 results on Tuesday you can always go back on Wednesday for another count. Another is that AIDS will lose all its meaning as the end-stage of HIV disease, because while there is a rough correlation between deletion of CD4 cells and the onset of illness, it is very rough. There will be people walking around with AIDS diagnoses that have never shown a single sign of illness, and may not for years. Magic Johnson could win his next Olympic gold medal after a diagnosis of AIDS under the new definition.

AIDS now also includes three new definitional diseases: pulmonary tuberculosis, recurrent pneumonia, and invasive cervical cancer. All three of these are associated with nonhomosexual victims of HIV, most especially cervical cancer.

The bottom line is that, temporarily at least, there has been—as predicted—an explosion in new cases under the new, expansive definition. The CDC predicted a 75 increase for 1993 as a whole.[101] The first three months of the year showed approximately a 200 percent increase, with almost 36,000 cases diagnosed in the first quarter of 1993 versus about 12,000 the year before,[102] although that will almost certainly not be sustained during the rest of the year. Further, by diagnosing people much earlier than before, the new definition will make it seem as if people are living much longer with AIDS than formerly, for which, given previous experience, the medical sector of the AIDS industry will almost certainly take a deep bow.

In explaining its new definition—the implementation of which was delayed for some time because of bitter opposition by epidemiologists and others—the CDC cited the recommendation of the Council of State and Territorial Epidemiologists.[103] It did not cite pressure from AIDS activists. Yet it was commonly believed that activists were behind it, so much so that when the new definition was announced, the title of the Associated Press story was, "CDC Bows to Activists, Adds New Diseases to Proposed AIDS Definition."[104] In his internationally distributed 1992 pamphlet "ACT-UP, the AIDS War & Activism," ACT-UP member George M. Carter wrote, "ACT-UP and many public health professionals realized that [the then-] definition was too narrow and pressured the CDC to change it. CDC officials are reluctant . . ." Nevertheless, he noted, "Under activist pressure, CDC announced a proposed expansion of the AIDS definition in the summer of 1991."[105]

The new definition is in large part simply another effort in the AIDS industry's crusade to expand both the perceived size and scope of the epidemic. Since the three new diseases affected primarily intravenous drug abusers, the percentage of homosexuals on the AIDS rolls is guaranteed to decrease. The cervical cancer definition, moreover, helps accomplish the goal of portraying women as being at greater risk.

Ultimately, however, the change in definition will only provide a temporary fix. If we can assume that all persons with severely depleted CD4 counts would eventually have qualified as having AIDS under the older definition, then all the new definition does is to create a spike in the chart which will be matched later on by a dip at that point in time when those persons would have been diagnosed anyway. By and large, the media did report that the huge new jump was attributable to the change of definition, to its credit. Still, as surely as these words are set into type, we will hear talk about how women and nonhomosexuals are suddenly comprising a bigger portion of the epidemic, without any reference to the change in definition.

WOMEN AND CHILDREN FIRST

There is an apocryphal *Washington Post* headline that reads, more or less: "World to be Destroyed Tomorrow; Women and Children to Suffer Most." Portraying women and children as victims sells newspapers, magazines, and TV shows. It democratizes the epidemic by casting it as not only pertinent to adult males; and it appeals to society's sentimental and protective instincts. A disease that harms women and children is much more apt to draw sympathy for all its victims, and money for its research.

Children are certainly the most pathetic of AIDS victims for being truly innocent and for losing so many years of life, but this does not justify exaggerating their numbers. Nevertheless, in 1992, Surgeon General Novella told interviewer Gregg Easterbrook that "there is a new means of transmission now—from women with HIV to their children as they are born. That was not an issue 10 years ago when the epidemic started, but it is an issue now."[106] And on 20 April 1992 the CBS Evening News reported, "It's no secret that AIDS is ravaging the nation's very young. Up to 20,000 children have AIDS." This though the actual number at the end of that year was a little more than four thousand.[107]

Exactly ten years before Novella's statement, the CDC published its first report on AIDS in babies who had apparently received the virus from their mothers (*Myth*, page 36). New York City later found evidence of children being infected from their intravenous drug-abusing mothers as early as 1977 (*Myth*, page 36). But the epidemic of AIDS babies failed to materialize. In 1991, the year before Novella's statement, incidence of pediatric AIDS overall and those who specifically got the disease from their mothers dropped for the first time,[108] though both went up again slightly the next year.[109] In 1992, children with AIDS who got the disease through their mothers comprised 697 cases, or 1.5 percent of all AIDS cases reported that year.

Though male cases outnumber female ones by eight to one according to the CDC,[110] Surgeon General Novello told readers of the *Los Angeles Times* in June of 1993: "Sad to say, women are bearing the brunt of infection."[111] The *Washington Post* told its readers in a front page story in July, 1993 titled "AIDS Spreads Fastest Among Young Women," that "Last week the Centers for Disease Control and Prevention reported that American women of all ages were coming down with AIDS four times as fast as men."[112] *USA Today* informed readers in 1991 that "women are 12 times more likely to get AIDS . . ." The newspaper's source: a Yale *psychologist*.[113] At about the same time, a letter to the *New York Times* from the director of the AIDS resource Network in Hermosa Beach, California, began, "Statistically, women represent the highest risk group in the United States for contracting AIDS." The *Times* ran the letter at the top of the section under the title, "Women Become Top U.S. AIDS Risk Group."[114] The next year, the *Times* featured an article on AIDS and women, with an accompanying chart showing that AIDS cases in women in the last year had increased 37 percent, along with seven photos of women afflicted with AIDS or HIV, all of them white.[115] In fact, AIDS cases among women had increased only 14 percent the year before, down from 17 percent the prior year. White females make up about 80 percent of the nation's female population, but just a fourth of U.S. AIDS cases.[116]

TEEN ANGST

But nothing grabs the media's and thus the public's attention like AIDS and teenagers. Within a period of a few months, *U.S. News and World Report* warned that "the AIDS epidemic has taken an ominous turn toward America's youth," and that "AIDS and HIV infection are rising fastest among teens and college-age kids."[117] Newspapers sported headlines like "AIDS Runs Wild Among Teenagers,"[118] and *Newsweek* carried a cover story on the exploding new epidemic.[119]

In officialdom, in a March 1992 press conference, Health and Human Services Secretary Louis Sullivan, accompanied by top officials from the Public Health Service and the CDC, announced a $1.5 million ad campaign targeting the area where "the epidemic is spreading most rapidly today . . . among heterosexuals, among teens and young adults, and in areas outside the big cities." He showed reporters a chart depicting among thirteen- to nineteen-year-olds a "rate of increase [that has] been quite rapid. For those age 13 to 19, we see a continuing increase in cases."[120]

The next month, the House Select Committee on Children, Youth, and Families, chaired by Rep. Pat Schroeder of Colorado, issued a report entitled: "A Decade of Denial: Teens and AIDS in America." In a swipe clearly aimed at the Bush and Reagan administrations, the report called the federal response to teen AIDS a "national disgrace,"[121] and claimed that the virus was "spreading unchecked"[122] among teens and that every day it "gain[ed] ground and threaten[ed] the loss of another generation."[123] The "another" implied that a generation had already been lost, but was not explained. Another scaremonger, Judith Stoia, executive producer of a horrifying 1991 PBS-ABC special, "AIDS in the Shadow of Love: A Teen AIDS Story," declared, "American teen-agers sit directly in the path of the worst epidemic of the century."[124] More recently, in June of 1993, the National Commission on AIDS warned that AIDS "threatens a new generation of Americans," with Vice Chairman David Rogers declaring, "We will never break the back of the epidemic without a tough, explicit, culturally appropriate delivery of facts to our teen-agers."[125]

The only problem with all this was that it wasn't true. In 1990, a grand total of 170 teenage AIDS cases had been diagnosed, a number that dropped to 159 in 1991, the year before the Schroeder report and the Sullivan press conference.[126] In 1992 that figure remained even.[127] Cases among college-age kids showed a similar drop, from 1,626 in 1990 to 1,485 in 1991,[128] and a further slight drop to 1,446 in 1992.[129] By comparison, some 5,000 youths, 15 to 24 years old, commit suicide[130] and 12,000 die in auto accidents per year.[131] About half these auto fatalities could have been prevented if the victims had been persuaded to wear their seat belts rather than condoms.

While a late 1991 *Time* magazine article entitled "Teens: The Rising Risk of AIDS" told its readers in bold letters, "Although the incidence of AIDS among teenagers is still low, it is doubling every 14 months,"[132] the actual doubling time—1990 to 1992—was every forty-eight months and steadily increasing.[133] Teenagers constitute far less than 1 percent of all AIDS cases, and twenty to twenty-four year olds make up only 3 percent of the total. Both categories are actually declining as a percent of the overall total.[134]

And while the CDC's top AIDS person, James Curran, told the listeners of CBS News that heterosexual transmission "already accounts for 25 percent of the cases in adolescents," the actual figure was 12 percent counting foreign-born individuals, 11 percent without.[135]

The implicit message sent by virtually all of the fright articles and government reports on teens is that the allegedly exploding number of teen cases is due to heterosexual intercourse. Homosexuals, drug abuse, and other factors are rarely mentioned. Yet, the largest cause of teen AIDS cases is blood or blood products, as was the case with Ryan White, who was a hemophiliac. While teenagers are more likely than adults to claim heterosexual transmission as their only risk factor, the huge total of these cases in 1992 was forty-one.[136]

As with AIDS in general, the focus with teen AIDS isn't just on heterosexuals but on white ones, especially white females. *Newsweek*'s cover story featured the face of a white girl. But as with AIDS in general, the disease among teens is disproportionately black, and Hispanic, and male. Black teen AIDS cases outnumber white ones.[137]

As for HIV infections, testing of teenage applicants to the military have shown a steady overall decline. In the last year of testing which has been reported in a medical journal, the infection rate was found to be less than one in four thousand.[138] The majority of these infections were in blacks.[139] This compares to the estimated national figure of *one in 250* (250 million Americans divided by one million infections). In some ways, military applicants are not representative of the population as a whole. In some ways, they very likely understate infections, but in two major ways—in being disproportionately black and from urban areas—they overstate infections. In any case, surely an infection rate less than one-tenth that of the nation as a whole is not cause for alarm and belies any claim to high numbers of teenage infections. Indeed, the aforementioned June 1992 CDC "National HIV Surveillance Summary" found that, "For both men and women, infection is most prevalent in persons in their late twenties and early thirties."[140]

But the media will stop at nothing to depict an AIDS crisis among America's heterosexual youth. *Myth* (pages 266–67) relates the cries of panic over the 1988 college study of infections which commentators like Barbara Walters on ABC's "²⁰/₂₀" claimed to be heterosexual. This even though the study actually found an infection rate about half that which the CDC had estimated for the country as a whole, and even though of the total of thirty infections found, twenty-eight were in men.

Then, in 1990, Cable News Network informed its viewers, "A new report from CDC indicates that AIDS is on the rise on college campuses."[141] The message, of course, was that this study had shown an increase over the 1988 study. But, in fact, this *was* the 1988 study[142]— it had taken a medical journal two years to print an article on it, and it was on this that CNN built its story. Only with AIDS can an old study be declared an alarming increase over itself.

In the minds of the media, the cause of democratizing AIDS to include youth is so just and so great that none of the usual, more basic, ethical rules apply. "In the Shadow of Love: A Teen AIDS Story,"[143] uniquely broadcast on consecutive days by PBS and ABC and later nominated for an Emmy, depicted HIV as nearly more common than acne among teenagers. It starred playwright Harvey Fierstein, outspoken AIDS activist. In it, one of the characters informs the others that a single condom can save "hundreds of lives." In case one wonders how a single condom can do all that, by amazing coincidence, the show was underwritten by Carter-Wallace, the manufacturer of several lines of prophylactics.

Surgeon General Novella endorsed the show.[144] Virtually every major newspaper and wire service heaped praise it. AP said, "There's more than enough reason to drag your teen-agers to the television set, kicking and screaming if need be";[145] the *Boston Globe* called it "an hour of incalculable value";[146] the *Los Angeles Times* said it was a "first-class survival resource for adolescents";[147] the *New York Times* declared, "Television is finally working up enough courage to state the obvious";[148] United Press International opined that it "should be seen by every teenager";[149] and the *Washington Post* proclaimed that, "in communicating some harsh facts about AIDS to teenagers . . . it may be unparalleled."[150] Only the *Los Angeles Times* mentioned the Carter-Wallace connection, and then only in passing.[151]

STAND BY YOUR MANN

Shortly after *Myth* came out, A. M. Rosenthal, in his *New York Times* column, blamed "some journalists" attacking "AIDS specialists who are worried about the spread of heterosexual transmission" for the forced departure of Jonathan Mann from his position as director of its Global Program on AIDS. Rosenthal specifically cited me and *Myth*.[152] I would gladly take credit were it true. And just in case Mann thought so, when a short while later I found myself seated next to him at lunch during an AIDS conference, I yanked off my name tag, believing discretion to be the better part of valor. But in all humility, I must report that Mann hanged himself. Indeed, any public health official who relays so huge a misstatement—that there would be as many as 100 million HIV infections worldwide by 1990, off by over 90 million by his organization's own admission—is guilty of gross incompetence or willful deceit.

Mann's crusade was by no means finished, however. He was immediately hired by the Harvard School of Public Health, where he established the Global AIDS Coalition, which lists June Osborn as the sole American on its steering committee.[153] The name of the coalition doesn't exactly lend itself to medical disinterestedness, nor does Mann's title as "Professor of Health and Human Rights."

At Harvard, Mann produced a study which Osborn called "an extraordinarily useful resource"[154] and which the media so readily embraced that it reported some of the results long before the study was completed and released in 1992 as *AIDS in the World*. As one might expect, Mann's findings were utterly horrifying. The German newsweekly *Der Spiegel* ran a cover article and a two-page map depicting the predicted devastation.[155] The worst aspect was Mann's speculation that a slow upward creep in the numbers of AIDS would suddenly culminate in a terrible explosion of infections between the years 1995 and 2000. Thus, for example, while the CDC estimate for adult HIV infections at the end of 1992 was 1,000,000 and Mann's estimate was just a little higher, Mann's best estimate for 1995 was about 1.5 million, to reach as high as 8 million by the year 2000.[156]

Such a development, of course, flies completely in the face of what we know about AIDS and what we know about epidemics in general. Epidemics follow the pattern of a bell curve, with a sudden increase at the beginning which slows gradually then flattens off before beginning to fall (*Myth*, pages 311–312). The AIDS epidemic in the U.S. has fit that pattern exactly. Mann, however, would have us believe that far from continuing its flattening course, HIV will suddenly explode. Moreover, we know that AIDS cases lag by about eight to ten years behind HIV infections. If AIDS cases are flattening out now, then infections must have flattened out long ago. Finally, as noted, data continuously being collected from all over the country show no increase in the level of infections. If Mann's estimates for the United States are so clearly wrong, it's that much harder to credit his estimates for the rest of the world.

Where, then, do all these new infections come from? Ultimately, from the fertile imagination of Jonathan Mann. Not that he did anything so crude as simply to write down numbers—though other AIDS alarmists have done just that. Instead, he solicited estimates from a number of people, some of whom he doesn't even name and others whom he only describes by name and occupation.[157] Not one of the Americans listed is considered a leader in the field. The list, in fact, is a loaded deck. Indeed, among the few recognizable names are those recognizable as AIDS alarmists, such as Thomas Quinn, whose cries are described repeatedly in *Myth* (pages 92–93, 95, 107, 117, 274). Nowhere does *AIDS in the World* even pretend to show the methodology of any of his handpicked consultants. We are completely at the mercy of the book's conclusions.

Not that any of this bothered the media, which gave Mann tremendous play in articles with titles like "Spread of AIDS May Now be Beyond Control,"[158] "Leading Authority Says Fight Against AIDS has Stalled,"[159] and "World AIDS Experts Fear Disease Out of Control."[160] Nor, presumably, would it bother the media that in a 1993 article in *Issues in Science and Technology*, Mann and the coauthor of *AIDS in the World* wrote, "The factor most closely linked to an increased risk of exposure to HIV is discrimination."[161] No, not anal sex, not sharing needles, but discrimination. The point cannot be emphasized too strongly: Not all truth-be-damned AIDS activists wear black T-shirts with pink triangles and scream at television cameras. All too many speak in soft voices and wear white jackets and spectacles.

THE NON-"BIG CHILL"

In *Myth* I argued that there was little evidence that, despite the fear campaign, efforts to get heterosexuals to reduce their sexual activity were having much effect. Lip service is given, of course. In England, before taping a debate with an AIDS activist, I met a young woman journalist who said that she was quite worried about AIDS and therefore took great precautions. Upon inquiry it proved that these great precautions consisted of having her latest lover wear a condom for the first six weeks of sex. I did not ask the obvious question: How did that protect her for the subsequent portion of their sexual relationship? Talismanic actions such as these appear to be far more common among heterosexuals than actual changes in lifestyle.

That has been borne out in studies since the first edition of *Myth*. Despite the special targeting of teenagers, a study released in the 4 January 1991 CDC *Morbidity and Mortality Weekly Report* found that the number of teenagers (those aged 15–19) engaging in sexual intercourse increased steadily from 1970 to 1985, and continued to increase from 1985 to 1988. In fact, the rate of increase *accelerated* in those last three years. The increase applied to both blacks and whites.[162]

Another study reported in the *New England Journal of Medicine*, "Sexual Behavior of College Women in 1975, 1986, and 1989," concluded that "sexual practices among these college women did not change markedly in 14 years with respect to the number of sexual partners or specific sexual acts, although it did find that there had been some increase in condom usage."[163] Similarly, a study of Canadian college students released in 1990 found that almost 75 percent of the men and 70 percent of the women were sexually active but that only about 25 percent of the men and 16 percent of the women claimed consistently to use condoms. Condom usage was even lower among those with ten or more sexual partners.[164] And at the June 1993 Berlin conference, the CDC released a survey of 12,000 students at 137 high schools which found that slightly over half were having intercourse and that while many used condoms for birth control, of those who used birth control pills, only 19 percent used condoms.[165]

All of these data refute the contention of AIDS alarmists that the only reason the heterosexual epidemic never appeared is because people heeded their warnings.

The media and AIDS activists have looked upon such data with great alarm, and some conservatives might argue that from a moral perspective it is sad that heterosexuals have not shifted more towards monogamy. But such moral or political concerns have little to do with the facts about AIDS.

Now, as much as ever, our concern should be focused on those groups that really suffer from the AIDS epidemic: racial minorities, especially blacks—which very much includes heterosexuals—and homosexual men.

HOMOSEXUAL RECIDIVISM

Even before the 1993 International AIDS Conference in Berlin, evidence was growing that male homosexuals, especially younger ones, were beginning to relapse from earlier efforts at preventing infection. In one study presented at the International AIDS Conference in San Francisco in 1990, 19 percent of such men reported that they had relapsed,[166] and King County, Washington, reported a sharp upturn in gonorrhea in homosexual males and suggested that the number might triple from 1988 to 1989.[167] The same practices that spread gonorrhea are spreading AIDS.

At the Berlin conference, a study of San Francisco male homosexuals showed that 38 percent of them had engaged in unprotected receptive anal intercourse with at least two different sexual partners within the last year, while 64 percent had done so with one partner. Fifteen percent reported five or more of these partners. Of the total, about 17 percent were infected with HIV. Among those reporting ten or more partners, the infection rate was nearly 56 percent.[168]

As *Newsweek* put it even before this study came out, "It seems clear that the safe-sex message is not getting through effectively to younger gays."[169] Unfortunately, it did not go the next step to say that part of this was due to the continuing efforts of *Newsweek* and other periodicals to hyperbolize about AIDS to a low-risk audience, while missing the target of high-risk groups.

In all fairness, it must be noted that San Francisco gay men are as educated about AIDS and how it is transmitted as anyone in the world. They have freely chosen to engage in activity that they know puts them at extremely high risk of getting the disease. That may sound surprising to some, but should not be in light of history.

By the early 1930s, according to Allan Brandt in his book *No Magic Bullet*, the most frequently cited figures suggested that approximately one out of every ten Americans suffered from syphilis. Each year, citizens in the United States contracted almost half a million new infections: gonorrhea, according to statistics, proved to be even more extensive, with almost 700,000 new infections annually. As for syphilis: according to one study, 18 percent of all deaths from organic heart disease could be attributed to the disease; if it reached the nervous system, syphilis could cause insanity, paralysis, or blindness; as many as 20 percent of mental institution inmates suffered the consequences of tertiary (advanced) syphilis: 9,000 of the deaths in these hospitals alone each year were tied to syphilis; syphilis was a leading cause of miscarriages, congenital defects, and sterilization; each year, 60,000 children were born with congenital syphilis in the United States.[170]

Yet, people continued to have unprotected intercourse. All this occurred in a population that was half the size it is now, so double the figures to get a comparable picture today. And the same picture emerges. Homosexuals continue to have "unsafe sex" and intravenous drug abusers continue to share needles and new HIV infections and AIDS cases continue to occur. How many, nobody knows.

What the AIDS educators will have to realize is that there is not a thing they or anyone else can do about individuals who insist on engaging in high risk behavior. AIDS cannot be socially engineered out of existence, any more than poverty or war can. The best they can do is what I have tried to do—and what they have been trying desperately to stop me from doing—tell people exactly how the disease is transmitted and who is at greatest risk. This allows individuals to protect themselves if they so wish. That is all we can accomplish. Only a vaccine will bring new AIDS infections to a level anywhere near zero, and that would take massive inoculations of a highly effective vaccine over a period of years. In the meantime, as the AIDS educators say, "Education is our only weapon," and yet no one has campaigned against effective AIDS education more than those who style themselves AIDS educators.

STILL IN THE BACK OF THE BUS

Just as political correctness discourages us from saying that homosexuals have a higher chance of getting AIDS than heterosexuals, we are not allowed to say that whites have less chance of getting the disease than blacks (although, interestingly, we can say that blacks have a higher chance of getting it than whites). To point out how much higher black sexually transmitted disease rates are than white rates is to court charges of racism. Nonetheless, while white syphilis is virtually nonexistent, it is a veritable plague among inner-city blacks.

Whites in 1991 had a syphilis rate of two per hundred thousand, much of that from homosexual activity as evidenced by the rate for men being 2.4 while that for women is 1.6. But for blacks the overall rate that year was a shocking 122.0. (Hispanics had an overall rate of 12.6, putting them between whites and blacks, though much closer to whites.) The disparity is all the more upsetting when one looks at the highest prevalence by age category. For the twenty- to twenty-four-year-old whites, the rate was 4.9 per hundred thousand. For blacks, 382.2 per hundred thousand.[171]

The disparity has always existed, but as the graph below shows it began to grow tremendously in 1985, increasing dramatically to a peak in 1990. One reason for this may be an increase in the use of crack cocaine (*Myth*, pages 137–38), but another surely is that, as some health educators warned and *Myth* so strongly stressed (pages 138–40), funds for AIDS campaigns were stripping away funds and workers from traditional STD programs. The great irony is that, as *Myth* also pointed out, a strong connection exists between infection with such STDs as syphilis and the ability either to transmit or receive HIV (*Myth*, pages 54–55).

At the time *Myth* came out, blacks, although only 11.5 percent of the U.S. population, represented about 25 percent of all reported adult AIDS cases overall, and over 50 percent of all women with AIDS. Today, that has risen slightly to 30 percent of all reported adult AIDS cases and 53 percent of all women with AIDS.[172] Back then, Hispanics, at 6 percent of the population, represented 15 percent of adult U.S. AIDS cases, and 20 percent of all the women's cases. They have essentially held even at that high rate, with 16 percent and 20 percent respectively.[173] At the time of *Myth*, black and Hispanic women made up about 70 percent of all female AIDS cases. Now it's 74

Syphilis (primary and secondary)—by race and ethnicity, United States, 1981–1991

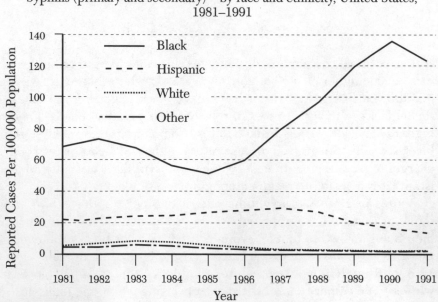

SOURCE: tk

percent. Seventy-six percent of female cases attributed to heterosexual transmission are blacks or Hispanics.[174]

Testing for the virus has shown similar disparities. While Pat Schroeder, *Newsweek*, and others spreading the myth of the teenage AIDS epidemic have tried desperately to present teen AIDS as everybody's problem, the opposite is true. HIV testing of white teenage military applicants has showed a significant decrease from an already low number in 1985 to an even lower number in 1989. Among Hispanics the trend was also down. But among black teenagers, the already relatively high number increased over the four-year period. Among black recruits as a whole, the number dropped slightly in the first years of testing but then held even.[175]

AIDS babies, considered by many the saddest victims of the epidemic, are often portrayed by the media and AIDS activist foundations such as the American Foundation for AIDS Research as white, but that is rarely the case. Black babies infected by their mothers outnumber white ones by four-to-one while Hispanic babies outnumber whites by almost two-to-one.[176]

After *Myth* came out, one Chinese-American columnist, while highly praising the book as a whole,[177] said that I was wrong in lumping all nonwhites into the "minority" category. It was a good point. Asian-American AIDS is practically nonexistent. At 2.9 percent of the population, the "Asian/Pacific Islander" category comprises about half of 1 percent of the epidemic.[178] Not that this stopped an Asian-American homosexual group from staging a noisy demonstration at a Washington, D.C., conference I attended in 1988. Apparently, like some lesbian groups, they were angry at being denied AIDS victim status.

The point isn't that whites are better than blacks and Hispanics, or that Asian-Americans are better than whites. Nor is it that heterosexuals are better than homosexuals. When health officials in early 1993 announced an outbreak of severe food poisoning from E. Coli bacteria resulted from undercooked Jack in the Box hamburgers, they were not saying that Jack in the Box hamburgers were inferior to McDonalds or Burger King hamburgers; they were, rather, giving people specific health-preserving information.

Different cultures have different habits, different preferences, and different access to medical care and education. Clearly the virus discriminates among these. To the extent we do not act accordingly, we do a tremendous disservice. Thus, while we were taking money to tell Biff and Buffy at Valley High that they were at great risk of getting AIDS when they were not, Jamal and Latoya at Booker T. Washington High were being denied the education and health facilities they so desperately needed. The same distortions apply to the miscomparisons between males and females, adults and children, homosexuals and heterosexuals.

None of this seems to bother the AIDS establishment, a broad term I use to describe the government leaders, activists, AIDS educators, and media commentators who have lied so repeatedly and so profusely to the American public as surely to make heterosexual AIDS the single greatest hoax of the last half of the twentieth century.

A GAY BACKLASH AGAINST THE TERROR?

Yet there may be a backlash developing in the gay population itself. Early in 1993, a reporter at a gay San Franscisco newspaper, the *Bay Area Reporter*, became the first person that I know of finally to take me up on my challenge to investigate AIDS spending for fraud and abuse. He quickly found it, and broke the story. What was probably the nation's best-known AIDS hospice had mismanaged at least $2.7

million worth of government contracts, in part by billing the city's AIDS office for services that either didn't exist or weren't being performed. In other words, doing—as is so often the case with AIDS—very bad things in the name of a very good cause.[179]

At around this same time, James Gliden, a freelance writer and playwright, wrote an article for the gay *Washington Blade* of Washington, D.C., which began, "I've had it up to the top of my well-above-ground ears with the leaders of the AIDS community who insist that the only way to get the attention of the power establishment is to convince them that this disease is going to infect those in power or people just like them."

Continued Gliden, "I do not care if this disease ever infects another heterosexual. In fact, I hope it never does. There is a cruel perversity in praying for another group of individuals to be affected by this disease just so something will be done about it."

Gliden then discussed why AIDS is primarily a homosexual disease, accurately describing the combined effects of anal sex and having large numbers of partners who themselves have anal sex with large numbers of partners. He suggested that the "AIDS doesn't discriminate message" had not only been largely ineffectual, but perhaps even counterproductive, causing people to ignore the real victims of the disease. "If we insist that nobody need pay attention to 100,000 dead faggots, then, indeed nobody will."

Wrote Gliden, "We are sending the wrong message and it is killing us. It is time to adopt a radically different tack. No more trying to scare the hets into action. No more angrily denouncing people who think that this is only affecting gay men. It is time we own the disease."[180]

A few people cannot establish a trend. Before I wrote my first word about AIDS, a prominent homosexual, Randy Shilts, who himself carried HIV, bravely criticized those who were saying that AIDS had become or was about to become everybody's epidemic (*Myth*, pages 210–211). He was decidedly not a trendsetter. Given the current climate, it is hard to envision the day when it will become politically correct to say that AIDS does discriminate. But perhaps the way is being paved. Perhaps honest homosexuals will eventually take the lead in denouncing the AIDS propaganda machine.

For it is to their greater benefit. To the extent that AIDS has proved a disaster, much of the responsibility lies with the AIDS establishment portraying it as everybody's problem in a personal sense, rather than in the noble and very real sense that we should all care about our fellow man and his troubles regardless of whether they are our own.

Aside from distracting attention from the real problem spots—homosexual males, blacks, and Hispanics—people entirely outside of the AIDS sphere are suffering because of the flagrant distortions of the AIDS establishment.

In 1991, a consortium of ad agencies announced that it was seeking $30 million in donated air time and space for advertisements targeted, as the *Wall Street Journal* put it, "at people who still think AIDS is someone else's problem."[181] In other words, aimed at white, middle-class heterosexuals. Two years later, an article in that same newspaper noted that anti-drug abuse TV advertisements were being shown less and less because more and more AIDS ads were taking up the air time, noting simultaneously that a recent study showed that after years of decline, student use of drugs was beginning to rise again. "I certainly don't want to criticize the AIDS effort," said one man whose job was to solicit air-time and ad space from media companies, "but it became more difficult to get our spots on the air with as much frequency as we were used to once Magic Johnson announced he was HIV-positive."[182]

This, mind you, was in addition to the aforementioned effort announced in 1992 to spend $1.5 million of our tax dollars for a campaign aimed at those least at risk for getting AIDS. That they *are* least at risk was quite beside the point. Big Brother decided there were higher reasons for concerning the public that up is down, white is black, and pigs can fly.

On the research spending front, AIDS continues to receive about twenty times as much per death as cancer in federal research and education dollars. Ironically, the same day the *Los Angeles Times*'s front-page story told about Magic Johnson and his efforts at AIDS fund-raising,[183] it carried several stories describing promising advances in cancer therapy that had been held up for lack of funds.[184] In real terms, it reported, cancer spending in 1991 was well below its level in 1980,[185] not pointing out that this *included* the fourth of the cancer budget that actually went to AIDS research (*Myth*, pages 328–29). The Clinton administration, in keeping with a campaign promise, has increased the AIDS budget by a massive 28 percent,[186] even while reducing funds for nearly all other disease-research programs.[187]

But while the AIDS disinformation campaign cripples efforts against other diseases, its biggest victim is the fight against AIDS itself. If the Jack in the Box food poisonings were handled the same way AIDS has been handled, the articles, TV news, and commentators would have eschewed any mention of Jack in the Box, the northwest

United States (where the meat had been shipped), or even hamburgers. Instead, we would have been told that "food" was the culprit and that since we all eat, we are all at risk. We would be admonished that "bacteria don't discriminate." Persons who tried to be specific about the mode of infection would be accused of being insensitive and hateful. And people would have continued to sicken and die.

The purpose of the AIDS establishment is to create the impression that the epidemic is much more widespread than it really is. "I think we are still at an impasse with the American public," said National Commission on AIDS Chairwoman June Osborn in September of 1991. "Particularly in the center of this country, if you ask, 'Who does AIDS impact?' you still get the 1982 answer of 'gay men, intravenous drug addicts and not me.'"[188] On a later occasion she said, "This has permitted too many to detach from the fray . . . and retreat to indifference."[189]

Members of the AIDS establishment have different motivations, to be sure, but they are united in the effort to keep the public from "detaching from the fray." Research scientists are trying to pump up their funding. Homosexual activists are doing the same while destigmatizing homosexual activity. Bureaucrats are trying to expand their bureaucratic turf and inflate their reputations. Politicians are trying to score points with the folks back home and against their political enemies. Population control groups are trying to sell the idea of using condoms while condom manufacturers are simply trying to sell them. The media are trying to sell their newspapers, magazines, and TV shows.

And in each case, the effort involves exaggerating those sectors of the epidemic that are the tiniest. Heterosexual AIDS is emphasized because heterosexuals make up the vast majority of the population. White heterosexuals are emphasized because they hold the purse strings and the political power and buy the most magazines. Women are emphasized because you can't have 51 percent of the population thinking it's getting by. Children are emphasized because they tear at our heartstrings, and teenagers are emphasized because it's the best way to bring their parents around.

All this emphasizing of the wrong thing has had a real measure of success. Research budgets have been pumped up, reputations have been inflated, and lots and lots of condoms have been sold. But it has also put the AIDS establishment at complete loggerheads with the entire purpose of the science of epidemiology, which is to identify where a disease *is* occurring and how it is spreading in order to reduce its incidence. To the extent we continue to concentrate on where the epidemic is not, we ignore where it is. To the extent we squander resources to prevent infections that are never going to happen, we lack the resources needed to keep persons truly at risk from sickening and dying. By pretending that the epidemic is widespread in the sense of plague or influenza, we have foregone the use of techniques such as partner tracing, which can have a tremendous effect with hard-to-get diseases like AIDS but are useless with those easily spread.

We need to decide which is more important: Advancing individual agendas and special interests, or waging a campaign against AIDS which has as its first, last, and only purpose the prevention of further infections and further horrible deaths from a disease for which there is no cure in sight.

APPENDIX B

AIDS:
Falsehoods and Facts

I. The party line continues to be, as *USA Today's* Kim Painter put it, "After nine years, AIDS remains a non-discriminating killer."[1] But . . .

FIGURE I.1A As a Percentage of the Population

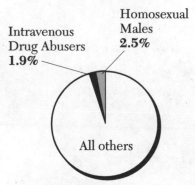

Intravenous Drug Abusers **1.9%**

Homosexual Males **2.5%**

All others

SOURCE: National Institute of Drug Abuse, National Opinion Research Center.

FIGURE I.1B As a Percentage of AIDS Cases

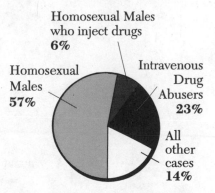

Homosexual Males who inject drugs **6%**

Homosexual Males **57%**

Intravenous Drug Abusers **23%**

All other cases **14%**

SOURCE: Centers for Disease Control and Prevention.

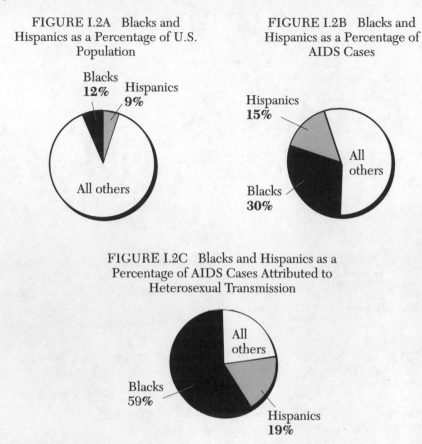

FIGURE I.2A Blacks and
Hispanics as a Percentage of U.S.
Population

Blacks
12% Hispanics
         9%

All others

FIGURE I.2B Blacks and
Hispanics as a Percentage of
AIDS Cases

Hispanics
15%

All
others

Blacks
30%

FIGURE I.2C   Blacks and Hispanics as a
Percentage of AIDS Cases Attributed to
Heterosexual Transmission

All
others

Blacks
59%

Hispanics
19%

SOURCE: Centers for Disease Control and Prevention, U.S. Bureau of the Census.

FIGURE I.3   Women as a Percentage of AIDS Cases

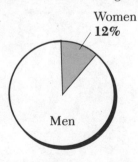

Women
12%

Men

SOURCE: Centers for Disease Control and Prevention.

FIGURE I.4   AIDS Cases by Age

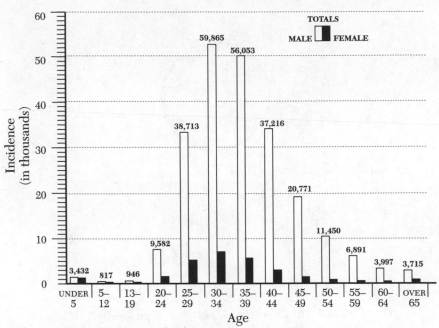

SOURCE: Centers for Disease Control and Prevention.

At 4.4 percent of the population, homosexual males and intravenous drug abusers comprise 80 percent of all AIDS cases.[2] At 12 percent and 9 percent of the population, respectively, blacks and Hispanics comprise 30 percent and 15 percent of all AIDS cases. Male AIDS cases outnumber female cases almost nine to one.[3] AIDS is also overwhelmingly a disease of the middle age of the population, leaving the very old and very young practically unscathed.

II. The media and the AIDS establishment in general have depicted the female proportion of the epidemic as growing by leaps and bounds. *USA Today* informed readers in 1991 that "Women are 12 times more likely to get AIDS,"[4] and the *New York Times* letters page gave top billing to an AIDS activist group that declared, "Statistically, women represent the highest risk group in the United States for contracting AIDS." The *Times* ran the letter at the top of the section under the title, "Women Become Top U.S. AIDS Risk Group."[5] But . . .

FIGURE II.1   Women as a Percentage of AIDS Cases

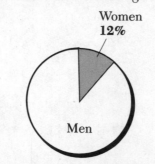

SOURCE: Centers for Disease Control and Prevention.

FIGURE II.2   Female AIDS Cases Reported by Year

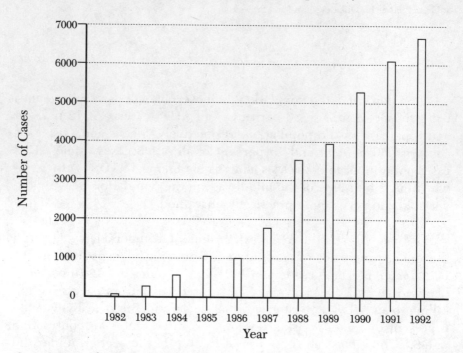

SOURCE: Centers for Disease Control and Prevention.

Male cases outnumber female cases by almost nine to one, and like all sectors of the epidemic, female cases are leveling off.

III. We are continually being told that the epidemic is only leveling among homosexuals. The front page of the *Los Angeles Times* announced in 1990, "Slower Spread of AIDS in Gays Seen Nationally,"[6] and Dr. Roy Anderson of Imperial College in Great Britain wrote in the April 1990 *Journal of Acquired Immune Deficiency Syndromes* that while homosexual male cases were flattening in the Western countries, there was a "continued and rapid rise among IV drug users."[7] But . . .

FIGURE III.1 Cases by Risk Group

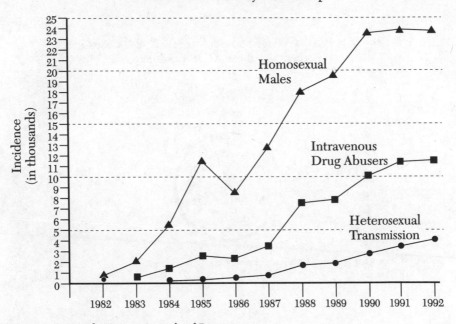

SOURCE: Centers for Disease Control and Prevention.

Reported IV drug abuse cases began flattening out in 1990 at the same time homosexual male ones did. In 1992 the IV drug abuse category grew only one percent. Cases attributed to heterosexual contact are also flattening, with a 17 percent increase from 1991 to 1992 compared to 21 percent increase the year before.

IV. Teens and adolescents are constantly referred to as the greatest AIDS risk group. *U.S. News & World Report* warned that "the AIDS epidemic has taken an ominous turn toward America's youth," and that "AIDS and HIV infection are rising fastest among teens and college-age kids."[8] Newspapers carried headlines like "AIDS Runs Wild Among Teenagers,"[9] *Newsweek* carried a cover story in 1992 on this allegedly exploding new epidemic,[10] and the House Select Committee on Children, Youth, and Families, chaired by Rep. Pat Schroeder, Democrat of Colorado, issued a report entitled, "A Decade of Denial: Teens and AIDS in America" which called the federal response to teen AIDS a "national disgrace," claimed that the virus was "spreading unchecked"[11] among teens, and declared that every day it "gains ground and threatens the loss of another generation."[12] But . . .

FIGURE IV.1   Teenage and Adolescent (20-24) Cases as a
Percentage of the AIDS Epidemic

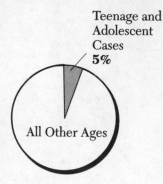

SOURCE: Centers for Disease Control and Prevention.

FIGURE IV.2   Infections Among Teenage Military Applicants

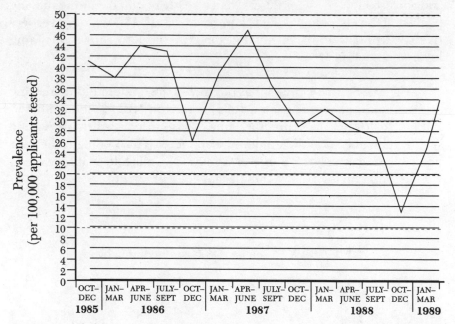

SOURCE: Journal of the American Medical Association.

FIGURE IV.3   HIV Infection Rates

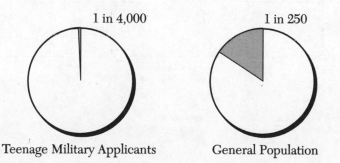

SOURCE: Journal of the American Medical Association, Centers for Disease Control and Prevention.

At the time all of these dire predictions were being made, teenage and adolescent cases (ages 20–24) had already begun declining, having peaked at levels below 1 and 4 percent of all AIDS cases, respectively.[13] Military applicant testing for HIV has also shown declining levels of infection.[14]

V. The AIDS establishment has portrayed the epidemic as increasing by leaps and bounds. During a 1992 debate on NBC's "Today Show," Public Health Service Director James Mason declared there was no such leveling because the epidemic had increased 33 percent the year before.[15] That same year, Surgeon General Novella told an interviewer, "Don't, don't believe that AIDS has leveled off."[16] But . . .

FIGURE V.1 Total AIDS Cases Reported by Year

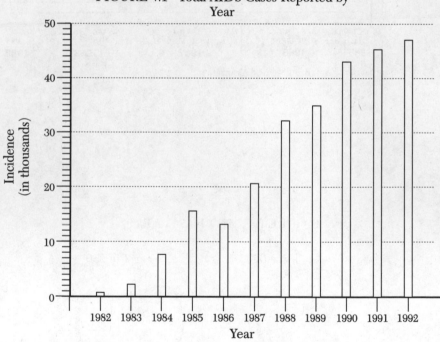

SOURCE: Centers for Disease Control and Prevention.

Reported cases increased only 3.5 percent in 1992 from the year before,[17] even while cases increased only 5 percent from 1990 to 1991.[18] Since reported cases lag behind diagnosed cases, this would indicate a complete flattening.

VI. Pediatric cases receive tremendous attention and are often referred to as a new phase of the epidemic. Surgeon General Novella said in 1992, "There is a new means of transmission now—from women with HIV to their children as they are born. That was not an issue 10 years ago when the epidemic started, but it is an issue now."[19] The CBS Evening News in early 1992 stated, "It's no secret that AIDS is ravaging the nation's very young. Up to 20,000 children have AIDS."[20] The American Foundation for AIDS Research has depicted cute bouncy little white babies in their ads. But . . .

FIGURE VI.1   AIDS Cases Among Children
Infected by Their Mothers

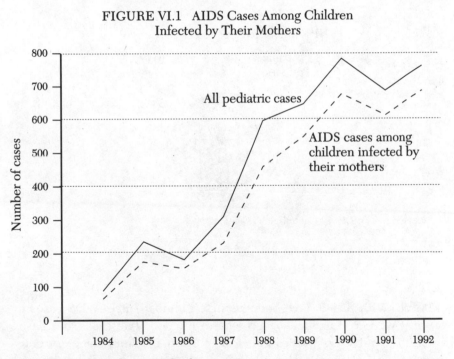

SOURCE: Centers for Disease Control and Prevention.

FIGURE VI.2   Pediatric Cases as a Percentage of the Total

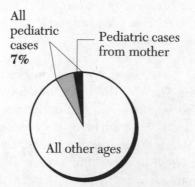

SOURCE: Centers for Disease Control and Prevention.

FIGURE VI.3   Pediatric AIDS Cases by Race

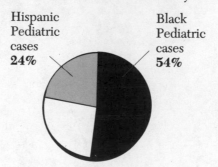

SOURCE: Centers for Disease Control and Prevention.

Babies with AIDS have been reported almost since AIDS cases in general were reported. The growth in all pediatric cases and cases among the subset of babies infected by their mothers has essentially flattened out.[21] By the end of 1992, 4,249 pediatric AIDS cases had been reported in the United States.[22] Children with AIDS who got the disease through their mothers comprise about 1.4 percent of all AIDS cases.[23] Most AIDS babies, like most heterosexual transmission cases, are blacks, with a disproportionate share Hispanics.[24]

NOTES

Note: All references to *Lancet* are for the North American edition. Full article medical references will include all the pages of the article, as is standard in medical texts. For nonmedical articles, reference to the full article will include only the first page number of that article.

Abbreviations

AJE American Journal of Epidemiology
AJPH American Journal of Public Health
AP Associated Press
CDC Centers for Disease Control
JAMA Journal of the American Medical Association

MMWR Morbidity and Mortality Weekly Report
NEJM New England Journal of Medicine
UPI United Press International
U.S. News U.S. News & World Report

Introduction

1. Gina Kolata, "Targeting Urged in Attack on AIDS," *New York Times*, 8 March 1993, p. 1.

2. Michael A. Fumento, "The Political Uses of an Epidemic," *The New Republic*, 199 (6 and 7, iss. 3,839 [August 8 and 15, 1988]): 19.

3. *See* "Deviationism," *The New Republic*, 199 (15, iss. 3,847 [17 October 1988]): 10; Eleanor Randolph, "Rights Panel Reassigns Attorney Who Criticized Administration on AIDS, *Washington Post*, 23 September 1988, p. A19; "Rights Commission AIDS Project Head Reassigned After Critical News Article," Bureau of National Affairs *Daily Labor Report*, (182), 20 September 1988, p. 2.

4. Personal written communication with A. Tony Castiglie, 22 March 1993.

5. Personal communication with Julie Blacklow, KING-TV, 1990.

6. Arthur Hu, "How Much AIDS," *Asian Week*, 19 April 1991, p. 10.

7. Michael Fumento, "The Risks of AIDS, *Westword* 14 (4 [26 September-2 October 1990]): 23.

8. Angel Hernandez, "Libraries, Bookstores Put Spotlight on Censorship," *Rocky Mountain News*, 27 September 1990, p. 20.

9. Mandrake, "Mitterand Gives His People's Opera a Miss," *Sunday Telegraph*, 25 March 1990.

10. Maurice Chittenden, "AIDS Author Claims British Blacklist," *Sunday Times* (London), 11 February 1990.

11. Donna Minkowitz, "Death Sentences," *Village Voice*, 5(35[30 January 1990]): 61.

12. Robert F. Gentry, "New AIDS Denial Promoted," *Orange County Register*, 19 March 1990, p. E1.

13. Minkowitz, p. 61.

14. Duncan Campbell, "Beyond the Evidence," *Nature* 343 (6256 [25 January 1990]):322.

15. Campbell, p. 321.

16. Ibid.

17. Ibid.

18. Personal written communication to the author from Maxine Clarke, 11 April 1990.

19. Cheris Kramarae and Paula A Treichler, *A Feminist Dictionary* (Boston: Pandora Press, 1985).

20. Douglas Crimp, "An Epidemic of Signification," *October*, 43 (Winter 1987): 260–63.

21. Paula A. Treichler, "An Epidemic of Signification," *October*, 43 (Winter 1987): 49.

22. Paula A. Treichler, "Uncertainties and Excesses," *Science* 248 (232[13 April 1990]): 233.

23. Treichler, "Uncertainties," p. 233.

24. Joe Queenan, "Straight Talk about AIDS," *Forbes* 143 (13 [26 June 1989]): 41

25. Personal communication with Joe Queenan, 20 June 1989; David Klinghoffer, "Random Notes," *National Review* 41 (14 [4 August 1989]): 40.

26. Ibid. p. 21.

27. Malcolm S. Forbes, Sr., "Why Did *Forbes* Run Fumento's Fulminations on AIDS" *Forbes* 143 (14 [10 July 1989]): 20.

28. Anne L. Adams, "Applesauce," *New York Daily News*, 22 June 1989, p. 6.

29. "Forbes Apologizes for June AIDS Story," *USA Today*, 28 June 1989, 2B.

30. John Lauritsen, untitled (letter), *Heterodoxy* 1 (12 [May–June]): 2.

31. Michelangelo Signorile, "The Other Side of Malcolm," *Outweek*, 18 March 1990, p. 40.

32. Christopher Winans, *Malcolm Forbes: The Man Who Had Everything* (New York: St. Martin's Press, 1990).

33. Winans, pp. 152–159.

34. Cliff Kincaid, "When *Forbes* Magazine didn't Have any Guts," *Human Events* 50 (47 [24 November 1990]): 18.

35. Michael Fumento, "Exacerbating the AIDS Panic," *Newsday*, 20 November 1990, part II, p. 8.

36. Personal communication with Jack Schwartz.

37. Michelangelo Signorile, "Gossip Watch," *Outweek*, 5 December 1990, p. 45.

38. Leslie Kaufman, "Beat the Press," *Washington Monthly* 25 (3 [March 1993]): 36.

39. Ibid.

40. Personal telephone communication from Joel Hay.

41. Ibid.

42. Ibid.

43. Ibid.

44. Virginia M. Anderson, "The Myth of Heterosexual AIDS," *JAMA* 263 (21 [6 June 1990]): 2949.

45. Andrew M. Wiesenthal, "The Myth of Heterosexual AIDS: How a Tragedy Has Been Distorted by the Media and Partisan Politics," *New England Journal of Medicine* 323 (15 [11 October 1990]): 1078.

46. Jefferson P. Selth, *Ambition, Discrimination, and Censorship in Libraries* (Jefferson, N. C.: McFarland and Co., 1993), pp. 124–25.

47. Mary Ann Porucznik, "Buckling Under to Thugs" (letter), *Crain's Chicago Business*, 6 March 1989, p. 13; Sheryl Dworkin, "Bad Precedent," *Chicago Tribune*, 3 March 1989, p. 20.

48. Tony Mauro, *USA Today*, "First Amendment had a Tumultuous 1990," Gannett News Service, 28 December 1990.

49. Gerald Olivier, "Le Fleau Circonscrit?" ("The Conscripted Plague?") *Valeurs Actuelles* 2797 (15 July 1990): 27.

50. Elio Gaspari, "A Falsa Epidemia," *Veja* (17 January 1990): 52.

51. Markus Krischr, "Wer Hat Angst Vor HIV?" ("Who Worries about HIV?"), *Esquire*, 91 (2 [February 1990]): 38.

52. Michael Fumento, "AIDS: False Alarm for Heterosexuals," Chicago *Sun-Times*, 14 January 1990, p. 41.

53. Michael Fumento, "The Political Uses of an Epidemic," *New Republic* 199 (6 & 7 [8 and 15 August 1988]): 19.

54. *The Bulletin* (Australia): (6 March 1990) cover and p. 44.

55. *Sunday Times* 18 March 1990, p. C1; *Sunday Times* 25 March 1990, p. C1.

56. *Sunday Times*, 18 March 1990, p. C1.

57. Kaufman, p. 38.

Chapter 1. The Reign of Terror

1. "Women Living with AIDS," "Oprah Winfrey Show," transcript of 18 February 1987, p. 2.

2. "AIDS May Dwarf the Plague," *New York Times*, 30 January 1987, p. A24.

3. "Widespread Heterosexual Epidemic Not Foreseen by Secretary of HHS," *AIDS Policy and Law* 3 (1 [27 January 1988]): 2.

4. "America's Number One Health Threat (Interview with C. Everett Koop)," *American Legion Magazine,* 123 (2 [August 1987]): 40.

5. *Life* 8 (8 [July 1985]): cover.

6. Kathleen McAuliffe et al., "AIDS: At the Dawn of Fear," *U.S. News & World Report,* 102 (2 [12 January 1987]): 60.

7. "Spread of AIDS May Send Sex Mores Back to the '50s," *Washington Times,* UPI, 21 April 1986, p. A4.

8. Tom Kelly, "For Many Singles, the Party Is Over," *Washington Times,* 7 October 1987, p. E1.

9. Ed Foster-Simeon, "Looking for Love in the Era of AIDS," *Washington Times,* 7 October 1987, p. E1.

10. Caryl S. Avery, "The Love or Life Choice," *Self* 9 (8 [August 1987]): 122.

11. Lucy Schulte, "The New Dating Game," *New York* 19 (9 [March 1986]): 94.

12. William K. Stevens, "Fear of AIDS Brings Explicit Advice to Campus, Caution to Singles Bar," *New York Times,* 17 February 1987, p. A21.

13. Lewis J. Lord et al., "Sex, with Care," *U.S. News* 100 (21 [2 June 1986]): 56.

14. Thomas B. Allen, "AIDS: We Need a National Survey," (letter) *Washington Post,* 12 May 1987, p. H4.

15. Stevens, "Fear of AIDS," *New York Times,* p. A21.

16. Kevin T. McGee, "AIDS Book Hits Home; Hot Lines Hot," *USA Today,* 6 June 1988, p. A1.

17. See Susan Milligan and Heidi Evans, "AIDS Test Sites Get Busier Here," *New York Daily News,* 11 February 1988, p. 21.

18. Niki Cervantes, "Women Stampeding AIDS-testing Clinics," UPI, 13 March 1987.

19. Chris Norwood, *Advice for Life: A Woman's Guide to AIDS Risks and Prevention* (New York: Pantheon, 1987), p. 8.

20. Niki Cervantes, "County Agrees to Open Two More AIDS Testing Centers," UPI, 17 March 1987.

21. Donald C. Drake, "Who Is at Risk? Variables Complicate the Picture," *Philadelphia Inquirer,* 21 June 1987, p. A18.

22. Cervantes, "Women Stampeding."

23. Advertisement for Blood-Check, Inc., *Washington Times,* 13 November 1987, p. A5.

24. "Dear Playmates," *Playboy* 36 (2 [February 1988]): 38.

25. Carol Innerst, "AU Students to Hear Blunt Talk About AIDS: Safe Sex Is No Sex," *Washington Times,* 19 August 1987, p. A1.

26. For a critical appraisal, see Jeffrey Hart, " 'Safe Sex' and the Presence of the Absence," *National Review* 39 (8 [8 May 1987]): 43. Hart is a professor of English at Dartmouth and a nationally syndicated columnist.

27. Innerst, "AU Students," p. A1.

28. " 'AIDS Road Show' Stoking a Feud," *New York Times,* 16 March 1988, p. A14.

29. John A. Fall, "Pace Closes Student Newspaper for Printing High-Risk Sex Article," *New York Native* 6 (6, iss. 142 [6–12 January 1986]): 11.

30. Mark Mooney, "State May Teach Tots About AIDS," *New York Post,* 20 July 1987, p. 21.

31. A copy of this material is on file in the office of U.S. Senator Jesse Helms (R.-N.C.).

32. "AIDS: A Pop Quiz," *Fairfax Journal,* 3 June 1987, p. A4.

33. Jeff Baron, "AIDS Has Kids' Fearful Respect," *Fairfax Journal,* 3 June 1987, p. A1.

34. David Streitfeld, "Putting Your AIDS Cards on the Table," *Washington Post,* 14 May 1987, p. C5.

35. Foster-Simeon, "Looking for Love," p. E1.

36. Tom Morganthau et al., "Future Shock," *Newsweek* 108 (21 [24 November 1986]): 33.

37. Hilary Stout, "40% of Americans Fear They Will Contract AIDS, a Poll Indicates," *New York Times,* 29 November 1987, p. 26. Figures on heart disease and cancer are from the National Institutes of Health.

38. *Miami News,* 16 March 1987, p. 6A.

39. American Association of Blood Banks poll of 15 June 1988, p. 9.

40. Suzanne O'Shea, "Woman Behind 'Sexy' AIDS Advert," *Daily Mail* (London), 19 February 1988, p. 5.

41. Feona McEwan, "Early and Not So Early Warnings," *Financial Times,* 5 March 1987, p. 20.

42. *Lancet*-I (8533 [14 March 1987]): 641.

43. Peter Almond, "British Approve AIDS Drug, Wage Giant Media Campaign," *Washington Times,* 6 March 1987, p. A9.

44. William Safire, "Failing the Tests," *New York Times,* 4 June 1987, p. A27.

45. David A. Noebel, Paul Cameron, and Wayne C. Lutton, "AIDS Warning," *New American* 3 (2 [19 January 1987]): 20.

46. Paul Cameron, "AIDS Free Zones: Recommendations to Contain the Spread of AIDS," *Family Research* 2 (September–October 1987): 3.

47. These examples are from Joseph P. Frolkis, "AIDS Anxiety," *Postgraduate Medicine* 79 (6 [1 May 1986]): 265–69.

48. Sandy Rovner, "Can AIDS Travel from Women to Men?" *Washington Post,* 8 January 1986, p. 11.

49. Joyce Price, "Fear of Fatal Illness Stifles 'AIDSophobics,' " *Washington Times,* 26 November 1987, p. A1.

50. Michael A. Jenike, "Coping with Fear-Reactions to AIDS," *Medical Aspects of Human Sexuality* 21 (11 [November 1987]): 22.

51. Price, "AIDSophobics," p. A11.

52. Ibid.

53. Ibid.

54. Ibid.

55. "Heterosexual AIDS: Horror or Hoax," "Geraldo," transcript of 1 December 1987, p. 7.

56. Ibid., p. 8.

57. Ibid.

58. Ibid., p. 9.

Chapter 2. The Once and Future Heterosexual Non-Epidemic

1. Kathleen McAuliffe et al., "AIDS: At the Dawn of Fear," *U.S. News & World Report* 102 (2 [12 January 1987]): 60.

2. Paul Raeburn, "AIDS Shows Signs of Spreading to General Population, Researchers Say," AP, 17 April 1985.

3. See United States Public Health Service, "Report of the Second Public Health Service AIDS Prevention and Control Conference," *Public Health Reports* 103 (supp. no. 1 [1988]): 11.

4. Personal communication with Don Des Jarlais, director of medical research, Beth Israel Medical Center. May 1989.

5. New York City Department of Health AIDS Surveillance Unit, "AIDS Surveillance Update," 25 January 1989, p. 4.

6. CDC, "HIV/AIDS Surveillance," February 1989, p. 10.

7. Chris Norwood, *Advice for Life: A Woman's Guide to AIDS Risks and Prevention* (New York: Pantheon, 1987), p. 41.

8. Personal communication, 6 February 1989.

9. John Tierney, "Straight Talk," *Rolling Stone* (17 November 1988), p. 126.

10. *Accident Facts* (Chicago: National Safety Council, 1988), p. 20.

11. Ibid., calculated from data on p. 48.

12. *Accident Facts,* p. 52.

13. Ibid.

14. National Center for Health Statistics, Public Health Service.

15. *Accident Facts,* p. 13.

16. Ibid. p. 12.

17. Ibid. p. 13.
18. See the editors of Heron House, *The Odds on Virtually Everything* (New York: G. P. Putnam, 1980), p. 180.
19. *Accident Facts,* p. 8.
20. William H. Masters, Virginia E. Johnson, and Robert C. Kolodny, *Crisis: Heterosexual Behavior in the Age of AIDS* (New York: Grove, 1988), pp. 4, 7, respectively.
21. Kevin R. Hopkins and William B. Johnston, *The Incidence of HIV Infection in the United States* (Indianapolis, Ind.: Hudson Institute, 19 August 1988), p. 55.
22. CDC, "Human T-Lymphotropic Virus Type III/Lymphadenopathy–Associated Virus Antibody Prevalence in U.S. Military Recruit Personnel," *MMWR* 35 (26 [4 July 1986]): 421.
23. Donald S. Burke et al., "Demography of HIV Infections Among Civilian Applicants for Military Service in Four Counties in New York City," *New York State Journal of Medicine* 87 (5 [May 1987]): 262–63.
24. Robert Bazell, "Surviving AIDS," *New Republic* 195 (21, iss. 3749 [24 November 1986]): 20.
25. Ann Guidici Fettner, "Is the CDC Dying of AIDS?" *Village Voice* 31 (39 [30 September 1986]): 14.
26. Paul D. Cleary et al., "Compulsory Premarital Screening for the Human Immunodeficiency Virus" (letter), *JAMA* 259 (7 [19 February 1988]): 1014.
27. Ann Fettner, "HTLV-III Disease, Not AIDS: An Interview with Major Robert Redfield," *New York Native* 5 (12, iss. 118 [17–30 June 1985]): 23.
28. Personal communication with Robert Redfield.
29. CDC, "Trends in Human Immunodeficiency Virus Infection Among Civilian Applicants for Military Service—United States, October 1985—March 1988," *MMWR* 37 (44 [11 November 1988]): 678.
30. Rand L. Stoneburner et al., "Risk Factors in Military Recruits Positive for HIV Antibody," *NEJM* 315 (21 [20 November 1986]): 1355.
31. Philip Renzullo et al., "Epidemiology of HIV Infection in Male Soldiers Reporting No Identifiable Risk (NIR)," IV International Conference on AIDS (Stockholm, Sweden) 12–16 June 1988, abstract 4002.
32. Norman Hearst and Stephen B. Hulley, "Preventing the Heterosexual Spread of AIDS," *JAMA* 259 (16 [22–29 April 1988]): 2428, citing CDC, "Human Immunodeficiency Virus Infection in the United States," *MMWR*, 36 (5–6 [18 December 1987]).
33. CDC, "Trends in Human Immunodeficiency Virus," p. 677.
34. CDC, "HIV Infection in the United States," p. 4.
35. Personal communication with Dr. Paul Cummings, director of American Red Cross, 6 February 1989.
36. CDC, "HIV Infection in the United States," p. 5.
37. Kevin R. Hopkins and William B. Johnston, "AIDS Battle, Round 38 (letter)," *National Review* 40 (25 [30 December 1988]): 6.
38. Norwood, *Advice for Life,* p. 5.
39. James W. Curran et al., "Epidemiology of HIV Infection and AIDS in the United States," *Science* 239 (4840 [5 February 1988]): 613.
40. H. Hunter Handsfield, "Heterosexual Transmission of Human Immunodeficiency Virus," *JAMA* 260 (13 [7 October 1988]): 1943.
41. See, for example, CDC, "Quarterly Report to the Domestic Policy Council on the Prevalence and Rate of Spread of HIV and AIDS—United States," *MMWR* 37 (36 [16 September 1988]): 551.
42. California Department of Health Services, "State Health Director Announces Details of Study of HIV Infection," 9 February 1989.
43. Masters, Johnson, and Kolodny, *Crisis,* p. 7.
44. Hopkins and Johnston, "AIDS Battle," p. 6.
45. CDC, "Human Plague—United States, 1988," *MMWR* 37 (42 [28 October 1988]): 653–56.
46. Andrew R. Moss et al., "Seropositivity for HIV and the Development of AIDS or AIDS Related Conditions: Three Year Follow Up of the San Francisco General Hospital Cohort," *British Medical Journal* (Clinical Research) 296 (6624 [12 March 1988]): 745–50.

47. "50% of Carriers to Get AIDS, Study Reports," *Los Angeles Times*, 13 March 1988, p. I-3 (home ed.).

48. H. R. Brodt et al., "Spontanverlauf der LAV/HTLV-III-Infektion," *Deutsche Medizinische Wochenscrift* 111 (31–32 [1 August 1985]): 1175–80.

49. Testimony before Presidential Committee on HIV, quoted in "From Infection to Illness: A Virus's Advancing Toll," *New York Times*, 15 February 1988, p. A14.

50. Nancy A. Hessol et al., "The Natural History of HIV Infection in a Cohort of Homosexual and Bisexual Men: A Decade of Follow-up," IV Intl. Conf. on AIDS, abstract 4096.

51. Alan R. Lifson, George W. Rutherford, and Harold W. Jaffe, "The Natural History of Human Immunodeficiency Virus Infection," *Journal of Infectious Diseases* 158 (6 [December 1988]): 1362.

52. Ibid.

53. Ibid.

54. J. Giesecke et al., "Incidence of Symptoms and AIDS in 146 Swedish Haemophiliacs and Blood Transfusion Recipients Infected with Human Immunodeficiency Virus," *British Medical Journal* (Clinical Research) 297 (6641 [9 July 1988]): 99–102.

55. Lifson et al., "Natural History," p. 1362.

56. Hearst and Hulley, "Preventing the Heterosexual Spread of AIDS," p. 2430, citing Harold W. Jaffe et al., "The Acquired Immunodeficiency Syndrome in Gay Men," *Annals of Internal Medicine* 103 (5 [November 1985]): 662–64; and Nancy A. Hessol et al., "The Natural History of Human Immunodeficiency Virus Infection in a Cohort of Homosexual and Bisexual Men: A Seven Year Prospective Study," III International Conference on AIDS (Washington, D.C.), 1–5 June 1987, abstract M.3.1.

57. James A. Wiley, Nancy Padian, and Warren Winkelstein, "Male-to-Female Transmission of Human Immunodeficiency Virus (HIV): Current Results and Infectivity Estimates" (henceforth "Current Results"), unpublished report (unnumbered).

58. Thomas A. Peterman et al., "Risk of Human Immunodeficiency Virus Transmission from Heterosexual Adults with Transfusion-Associated Infections," *JAMA* 259 (1 [January 1988]): 55–58.

59. Steven Findlay, "AIDS Is Rising Among Heterosexuals," *USA Today*, 3 June 1987, p. D6.

60. CDC, "HIV Infection in the United States," p. 28.

61. James W. Curran et al., "Epidemiology of HIV Infection and AIDS in the United States," *Science* 239 (4840 [5 February 1988]): 613.

62. Norwood, *Advice for Life*, p. 33.

63. Personal communication with Harold Jaffe, 3 February 1989.

64. B. D. Colen, "AIDS: A View Above the Fray," *Newsday*, 13 October 1987, p. 8.

65. CDC, "HIV/AIDS Surveillance," p. 8.

66. CDC, "Human Immunodeficiency Virus Infection in the United States: A Review of Current Knowledge," *MMWR* 36 (5–6 [18 December 1987]): 40.

67. Alan P. Bell and Martin S. Weinberg, *Homosexualities* (New York: Simon & Schuster, 1978), p. 308.

68. Harold Jaffe et al., "National Case Control Study of Kaposi's Sarcoma and *Pneumocystis Carinii* Pneumonia in Homosexual Men: Part 1, Epidemiological Results," *Annals of Internal Medicine* 99 (2 [August 1983]): 146.

69. Warren Winkelstein, Jr. et al., "Selected Sexual Practices of San Francisco Heterosexual Men and Risk of Infection by the Human Immunodeficiency Virus (letter)," *JAMA* 257 (11 [20 March 1987]): 1471.

70. Colen, "AIDS: A View Above the Fray," p. 8.

71. Rand L. Stoneburner et al., "HIV-1 Infection in Persons Attending a Sexually Transmitted Disease Clinic in New York City," IV Intl. Conf. on AIDS, abstract 6094.

72. Personal communication with Rand Stoneburner.

Chapter 3. A Primer on a Pestilence

1. Peter Duesberg, "HIV Is Not the Cause of AIDS," *Science* 241 (4865 [29 July 1988]): 514, and rebuttal, W. Blattner, R. C. Gallo, and H. M. Temin, "HIV Causes AIDS," p. 515.

2. See Katie Leishman, "The AIDS Debate that Isn't," *Wall Street Journal,* 26 February 1988, p. 14; and Katie Leishman, "AIDS and Syphilis," *Atlantic* 261 (1 [January 1988]): 17.

3. This explanation is taken from Paula A. Treichler, "AIDS, Homophobia, and Biomedical Discourse: An Epidemic of Signification," *October* 43 (Winter 1987), n. 65, citing June E. Osborne, "The AIDS Epidemic: An Overview of the Science," *Issues in Science and Technology* 2 (2 [Winter 1986]): 47.

4. See John Langone, *AIDS: The Facts* (Boston: Little, Brown, 1988), p. 37.

5. Randy Shilts, *And the Band Played On* (New York: St. Martin's Press, 1987).

6. "The Man Who Gave Us AIDS," *New York Post,* 6 October 1987, p. 1.

7. Personal communication with Randy Shilts, 3 May 1989.

8. Personal communication with Harold Jaffe, 4 May 1989.

9. James I. Slaff and John K. Brubaker, *The AIDS Epidemic* (New York: Warner, 1985), p. 25.

10. *Newsweek* 108 (21 [24 November 1986]): cover.

11. Paul Raeburn, "Spread in Africa Provides Glimpse Into Future," AP, 30 December 1985.

12. CDC, *"Pneumocystis* Pneumonia—Los Angeles," *MMWR* 30 (21 [5 June 1981]): 250–52.

13. Michael Gottlieb et al., *"Pneumocystis Carinii* Pneumonia and Mucosal Candidiasis in Previously Healthy Homosexual Men," *NEJM* 305 (24 [10 December 1981]): 1425–31.

14. B. Lamey and N. Malemeka, *Médicine Tropicale* 42 (5 [September–October 1982]): 507–11, as cited in the Panos Institute, *AIDS in the Third World,* 3d ed. (Philadelphia: New Society, 1989) p. 72.

15. Anne C. Bayley, "Aggressive Kaposi's Sarcoma in Zambia," *Lancet*-I (8390 [16 June 1984]): 1318–20.

16. Robert J. Biggar et al., "The Epidemiology of AIDS in Europe" (editorial), *European Journal of Cancer and Clinical Oncology* 20 (2 [February 1984]): 157–73; N. Clumeck et al., "Acquired Immune Deficiency Syndrome in Black Africans" (letter), *Lancet*-I (8325 [19 March 1983]): 642; J. B. Brunet and R. A. Ancelle, "The International Occurrence of the Acquired Immunodeficiency Syndrome," *Annals of Internal Medicine* 103 (5 [November 1985]): 670–74.

17. CDC, "Update on Kaposi's Sarcoma and Opportunistic Infections in Previously Healthy Persons," *MMWR* 31 (22 [11 June 1982]): 294–301.

18. CDC, "Opportunistic Infections and Kaposi's Sarcoma among Haitians in the United States," *MMWR* 31 (26 [9 July 1982]): 353–61.

19. CDC, *"Pneumocystis Carinii* Pneumonia Among Persons with Hemophilia A," *MMWR* 31 (27 [16 July 1982]): 365–67.

20. CDC, "Possible Transfusion-Associated Acquired Immune Deficiency Syndrome (AIDS)—California," *MMWR* 31 (48 [10 December 1982]): 652–54.

21. CDC, "Unexplained Immunodeficiency and Opportunistic Infections in Infants—New York, New Jersey, California," *MMWR* 31 (49 [17 December 1982]): 665–67.

22. Ibid.

23. CDC, "Immunodeficiency Among Female Sexual Partners of Males with Acquired Immune Deficiency Syndrome (AIDS)—New York," *MMWR* 31 (52 [7 January 1983]): 697–98.

24. Pauline Thomas et al., "HIV Infection in Heterosexual Female Intravenous Drug Users in New York City, 1977–1980 (letter)," *NEJM* 319 (6 [11 August 1988]): 374.

25. Don C. Des Jarlais et al., "HIV-I Infection Among Intravenous Drug Users in Manhattan, New York City, From 1977 Through 1987," *JAMA* 261 (7 [17 February 1989]): 1010.

26. Shilts, *And the Band Played On,* pp. 3–7, 35, 116, 117, 118, 193, 277, 458, 566.

27. In some of those cases, such as that of the St. Louis boy, the retrospective diagnoses of AIDS are now supported by positive blood tests for HIV. These are taken from Renée Sabatier, Panos Institute, *AIDS in the Third World* (Philadelphia: New Society Publishers, 1988), p. 73.

28. Personal communication with Dr. Allan Brandt, 9 January 1989.

29. See Paul M. Sharp and Wen-Hsiung Li, "Understanding the Origins of AIDS Viruses" (letter), *Nature* 336 (6197 [24 November 1988]): 315.

30. A. J. Nahmias et al., "Evidence for Human Infection with an HTLV-III/LAV-like Virus in Central Africa, 1959," *Lancet*-I (8492 [31 May 1986]): pp. 1279–80.

31. W. Carl Saxinger, "Evidence for Exposure to HTLV-III in Uganda Before 1973," *Science* 227 (4690 [1 March 1985]): 1036–38.

32. Langone, *AIDS: The Facts*, p. 39.

33. J. W. Carswell, "How Long Has the AIDS Virus Been in Uganda?" *Lancet*-I (8491 [24 May 1986]): 1217.

34. Robert J. Biggar et al., "Non-Specificity of HTLV-III Reaction in Sera from Rural Kenya," *East African Medical Journal* 63 (10 [October 1985]): 683. See also Thomas L. Kuhls, "Analysis of False Positive HIV-1 Serological Testing in Kenya," *Diagnostic Microbiology and Infectious Diseases* 9 (3 [September 1988]): 183–84.

35. Panos Institute, *AIDS in the Third World*, p. 71, citing, as examples, J. A. Levy et al., "Absence of Antibodies to the Human Immune Deficiency Virus in Sera from Africa Prior to 1975," *Proceedings of the National Academy of the Sciences* 83 (20 [October 1986]): 7, 935–37; S. F. Lyons et al., "Lack of Evidence of HTLV-III Endemicity in Southern Africa," *NEJM* 312 (19 [9 May 1985]): 1257–58; anonymous, *AIDS Forschung* 1 (January 1987): 5–25.

36. Nancy A. Hessol et al., "Seroconversion to HIV Among Homosexual and Bisexual Men Who Participated in Hepatitis B Vaccine Trials," IV International Conference on AIDS (Stockholm, Sweden) 12–16 June 1988, abstract 4614.

37. Personal communication with Thomas Shinnick, Leprosy Branch, CDC.

38. Gene Antonio, *The AIDS Cover-up?* (San Francisco: Ignatius Press, 1986), p. 119.

39. Ibid., p. 106; Katie Leishman, "AIDS and Insects," *Atlantic* 260 (3 [September 1987]): 56; David A. Noebel, Paul Cameron, and Wayne C. Lutton, "AIDS Warning," *New American* 3 (2 [19 January 1987, special reprint]): 11.

40. Chris Norwood, *Advice for Life: A Woman's Guide to AIDS Risks and Prevention* (New York: Pantheon, 1987), p. 17.

41. James W. Curran et al., "Epidemiology of HIV Infection and AIDS in the United States," *Science* 239 (4840 [5 February 1988]): 615.

42. Ibid.

43. "AIDS Strategies," *Wall Street Journal*, 4 June 1987, p. 30.

44. Margie Alfonso, "Report on AIDS to Support Mandatory Testing," Conference Sponsored for Members of the U.S. Congress by Congressman Dan Burton, 6th District—Indiana, 18 March 1987, p. 2.

45. Robert S. Gottfried, *The Black Death* (New York: Free Press, 1983), p. 57.

46. See Max (Myron) Essex and Phyllis J. Kanki, "The Origins of the AIDS Virus," *Scientific American* 259 (4 [October 1988]): 68–69.

47. Michael Crichton, *The Andromeda Strain* (New York: Alfred A. Knopf, 1974).

48. Gary P. Wormser, Charles S. Rabkin, and Carol Joline, "Frequency of Nosocomial Transmission of HIV Infection Among Health Care Workers" (letter), *NEJM* 319 (5 [4 August 1988]): 307.

49. L.B. Seeff et al., "Type B Hepatitis after Needle-Stick Exposure: Prevention with Hepatitis B Immune Globulin," *Annals of Internal Medicine* 88 (3 [March 1978]): 290; Barbara G. Werner and George F. Grady, "Accidental Hepatitis B Surface-Antigen-Positive Inoculations," *Annals of Internal Medicine* 97 (3 [September 1982]): 368.

50. Janine Jagger, "Rates of Needle-Stick Injury Caused by Various Devices in a University Hospital," *NEJM* 319 (5 [4 August 1988]): 284.

51. Personal communication with Chuck Fallis, CDC director of public affairs.

52. Lawrence A. Kingsley, "The Relative Sexual Transmission Efficiency of HIV and HBV in Homosexual Men," IV Intl. Conf. on AIDS, abstract 4578.

53. Langone, *AIDS: The Facts*, p. 54.

54. Alan R. Lifson, "Do Alternate Modes for Transmission of HIV Exist?" *JAMA* 259 (9 [4 March 1988]): 1354.

55. Ibid., pp. 1353–54.

56. Curran et al., "Epidemiology of HIV," p. 615.

57. Volker Wahn et al., "Horizontal Transmission of HIV Infection," *Lancet*-II (8508 [20 September 1986]): 694.

58. Curran et al., "Epidemiology of HIV," p. 615.

59. Philip C. Fox et al., "Saliva Inhibits HIV-1 Infectivity," *Journal of the American Dental Association* 116 (6 [May 1988]): 636.

60. Gerald H. Friedland and Robert S. Klein, "Transmission of the Human Immunodeficiency Virus," *NEJM* 317 (18 [29 October 1987]): 1128.

61. Curran et al., "Epidemiology of HIV," p. 612; CDC, "HIV Infection in the United States: A Review of Current Knowledge," *MMWR* 36 (S-6 [18 December 1987]): 24–27.

62. CDC, "HIV Infection in Transfusion Recipients and Their Family Members," *MMWR* 36 (20 March 1987): 137–40.

63. Curran et al., "Epidemiology of HIV Infection," p. 612; CDC, "HIV Infection in the United States," p. 27.

Chapter 4. The Risks of Heterosexual Intercourse

1. Personal communication, 3 February 1989.

2. Denise Grady et al., "Just How *Does* AIDS Spread?" *Time* 131 (12 [21 March 1988]): 61.

3. Personal communication.

4. See John Langone, *AIDS: The Facts* (Boston: Little, Brown, 1986), p. 98. See also Henry Gray, *Gray's Anatomy*, 13th ed., ed. Carmine D. Clemente (Philadelphia: Lea and Febiger, 1985), p. 1487.

5. William W. Darrow et al., "Risk Factors for Human Immunodeficiency Virus (HIV) Infections in Men," *AJPH* 77 (4 [April 1987]): 480.

6. Warren Winkelstein, Jr., "Sexual Practices and the Risk of Infection by the Human Immunodeficiency Virus: The San Francisco Men's Health Study," *JAMA* 257 (3 [16 January 1987]): 325.

7. Jay A. Nelson, et al., "Detection of the Human Immunodeficiency Virus in Bowel Epithelium from Patients with Gastrointestinal Symptoms," *Lancet*-I (8580 [6 February, 1988]), pp. 259–62.

8. Dennis Osmond et al., "Time of Exposure and Risk of HIV Infection in Homosexual Partners of Men with AIDS," *AJPH* 78 (8 August 1988]): 944–48, citing Michael Marmor et al., "Kaposi's Sarcoma in Homosexual Men," *Annals of Internal Medicine* 100 (6 [June 1984]): 809–15; Warren Winkelstein, Jr. et al., "Sexual Practices and Risk of Infection by the Human Immunodeficiency Virus: The San Francisco Men's Health Study," *JAMA* 257 (3 [16 January 1987]): 321–25; James J. Goedert et al., "Determinants of Retrovirus (HTLV-III) Antibody and Immunodeficiency Conditions in Homosexual Men," *Lancet*-II (8405 [29 September 1984]): 711–15; Janet K. A. Nicholson, et al., "Exposure to Human T-lymphotropic Virus Type III/Lymphadenopathy-Associated Virus and Immunologic Abnormalities in Asymptomatic Homosexual Men," *Annals of Internal Medicine* 103 (1 [July 1985]): 37–42; Eric Jeffries et al., "The Vancouver Lymphadenopathy-AIDS Study: 2. Seroepidemiology of HTLV-III Antibody," *Canadian Medical Association Journal* 132 (12 [15 June 1985]): 1373–77; Jerome E. Groopman et al., "Seroepidemiology of Human T-lymphotropic Virus Type III Among Homosexual Men with Acquired Immunodeficiency Syndrome or Generalized Lymphadenopathy and Among Asymptomatic Controls in Boston," *Annals of Internal Medicine* 102 (3 [March 1985]): 334–37; Cladd E. Stevens et al., "Human T-cell Lymphotropic Virus Type III Infection in a Cohort of Homosexual Men in New York City," *JAMA* 255 (16 [25 April 1986]): 2167–72.

9. Larry Thompson, "Safe Sex in the Era of AIDS," *Washington Post*, 31 March 1987, p. H12.

10. Darrow et al., "Risk Factors for HIV," p. 481.

11. L. A. Kingsley et al., "Risk Factors for Seroconversion to Human Immunodeficiency Virus Among Male Homosexuals," *Lancet*-I (8529 [14 February 1987]): 345–49.

12. Osmond et al., "Time of Exposure," pp. 944–48.

13. See Joan S. Chmiel et al., "Factors Associated with Prevalent Human Immunodeficiency Virus (HIV) Infection in the Multicenter AIDS Cohort Study," *AJE* 126 (4 [October 1987]): 574.

14. James I. Slaff and John K. Brubaker, *The AIDS Epidemic* (New York: Warner, 1985), p. 146: "Current estimates indicate infection in sexually active homosexual men in San

406 Notes

Francisco and New York to be 70–90 percent"; and Kathleen McAuliffe et al., "AIDS: At the Dawn of Fear," *U.S. News* 102 (2 [12 January 1987]): 62: "In New York City, it is estimated that . . . 70 percent of homosexuals and bisexuals carry the virus."

15. Nancy S. Padian et al., "Male-to-Female Transmission of Human Immunodeficiency Virus," *JAMA* 258 (6 [14 August 1987]): 789.

16. F. S. Sion, "The Importance of Anal Intercourse in Transmission of HIV in Women," IV International Conference on AIDS (Stockholm, Sweden) 12–16 June 1988, abstract 4007.

17. Neal H. Steigbigel et al., "Heterosexual Transmission of HIV Infection," IV Intl. Conf. on AIDS, abstract 4057.

18. See generally Padian et al., "Male-to-Female Transmission of HIV"; and James A. Wiley, Nancy Padian, and Warren Winkelstein, Jr., "Male-to-Female Transmission of Human Immunodeficiency Virus (HIV): Current Results and Infectivity Estimates" (henceforth "Current Results"), unpublished report (unnumbered).

19. Ann G. Fettner, "Playboy's AIDS Philosophy," *New York Native* 6 (26, iss. 164 [9 June 1986]): 21.

20. G. J. Stewart et al., "Transmission of Human T-cell Lymphotropic Virus Type III (HTLV-III) by Artificial Insemination by Donor," *Lancet*-II (8455 [14 September 1985]): 581–84.

21. Ann G. Fettner, "The Truth Hurts," *New York Native*, 14 September 1985, p. 21.

22. R. J. Pomerantz et al., "Human Immunodeficiency Virus (HIV) Infection of the Uterine Cervix," *Annals of Internal Medicine* 108 (3 [March 1988]): 321–27.

23. See Nancy S. Padian, "Heterosexual Transmission of Acquired Immunodeficiency Syndrome: International Perspectives and National Projections," *Review of Infectious Diseases* 9 (5 [September–October 1987]): 954.

24. Personal communication with Dr. Robert Redfield.

25. A. D. J. Robertson, letter to Rep. Dan Burton, 6 February 1986, p. 2.

26. Leo Bersani, "Is the Rectum a Grave?" *October* 43 (Winter 1987): 197.

27. Norman Podhoretz, "AIDS in Plain English," *New York Post*, September 24, 1985, p. 27. Patrick J. Buchanan, "AIDS Disease: It's Nature Fighting Back," *New York Post*, 24 May 1983, p. 31.

28. Padian et al., "Male-to-Female," p. 789.

29. Langone, *AIDS: The Facts*, pp. 95–96. See also Gray, *Gray's Anatomy*, 13th ed., p. 1579.

30. Langone, *AIDS: The Facts*, p. 91.

31. Denise Grady et al., "Just How *Does* AIDS Spread?" *Time* 131 (12 [21 March 1988]): 61.

32. Letter of Robertson to Burton, p. 2.

33. Langone, *AIDS: The Facts*, p. 2.

34. CDC, "HIV/AIDS Surveillance," *MMWR*, any 1989 issue.

35. New York City Department of Health, "AIDS Surveillance Update," 25 January 1989, p. 4.

36. Chmiel et al., "Factors Associated with Prevalent Human Immunodeficiency Virus (HIV)," p. 574.

37. Darrow et al., "Risk Factors for HIV," p. 480.

38. Ibid.

39. Calculated from Ibid.

40. Personal communication with Gayle Lloyd, public affairs specialist, CDC.

41. Personal communication with Dr. Padian, 14 February 1989.

42. Thomas A. Peterman et al., "Risk of Human Immunodeficiency Virus Transmission from Heterosexual Adults with Transfusion-Associated Infections," *JAMA* 259 (1 [1 January 1988]): 55–58.

43. H. Hunter Handsfield, "Heterosexual Transmission of Human Immunodeficiency Virus," *JAMA* 260 (13 [7 October 1988]): 1943, citing Richard Platt, Peter A. Rice and William McCormack, "Risk of Acquiring Gonorrhea and Prevalence of Abnormal Adnexal Findings Among Women Recently Exposed to Gonorrhea," *JAMA* 250 (23 [16 December 1983]): 3205–9.

44. Ibid., citing R. N. T. Thin, I. A. Williams, and C. F. Nicol, "Direct and Delayed Methods of Immunofluorescent Diagnosis of Gonorrhea in Women," *British Journal of*

Venereal Diseases 47 (1 [February 1971]): 27–30; and H. Hunter Handsfield et al., "Gonorrhea and Uncomplicated Gonococcal Infection," in King K. Holmes et al., eds., *Sexually Transmitted Diseases* (New York: McGraw-Hill, 1984), pp. 205–20.

45. Handsfield, "Heterosexual Transmission," p. 1943.

46. Langone, *AIDS: The Facts,* p. 94.

47. Jay A. Levy, "The Transmission of AIDS: The Case of the Infected Cell," *JAMA* 259 (20 [27 May 1988]): 3037.

48. Ibid., citing Constance B. Wofsy et al., "Isolation of AIDS-associated Retrovirus from Genital Secretions of Women with Antibodies to the Virus," *Lancet*-I (8480 [8 March 1986]): 527–29.

49. Levy, "Transmission of AIDS," p. 3037, citing M. W. Vogt et al., "Isolation Patterns of the Human Immunodeficiency Virus from Cervical Secretions During the Menstrual Cycle of Women at Risk for the Acquired Immunodeficiency Syndrome," *Annals of Internal Medicine* 106 (3 [1987]): 380–82.

50. Personal communication with Jay Levy, 9 May 1989.

51. Dr. Jonathan Mann, "AIDS in Africa," "Nightline," transcript of 20 October 1986, p. 5.

52. Kevin Hopkins and William Johnston, letter to *National Review,* 6 November 1988, p. 2 (on file at *National Review*).

53. For example, Peter Piot et al., "AIDS: An International Perspective," *Science* 239 (4840 [5 February 1988]): 573.

54. H. Hunter Handsfield et al., "Association of Anogenital Ulcer Disease with Human Immunodeficiency Virus Infection in Homosexual Men," III International Conference on AIDS (Washington, D.C.), 1–5 June 1987, abstract F.1.6; J. W. Curran et al., *Science* 239 (4840 [5 February 1988]): 610–16; J. Kreiss et al., *Genitourinary Medicine* 64 (1 [February 1988]): 1–2.

55. Levy, "Transmission of AIDS," p. 3037.

56. Piot et al., "AIDS: An International Perspective," pp. 574–75.

57. See J. Neil Simonsen, "Human Immunodeficiency Virus Among Men with Sexually Transmitted Diseases," *NEJM* 319 (5 [4 August 1988]): 275.

58. Piot et al., "AIDS: An International Perspective," pp. 574–75; see also Simonsen, "HIV Among Men," p. 275.

59. Panos Institute, *AIDS and the Third World,* p. 44, citing Francis Plummer et al., III Intl. Conf. on AIDS, abstract M.8.4. The abstract itself does not actually say this. Presumably the Panos Institute is referring to the whole paper or to the interview they conducted with Plummer, rather than simply the abstract.

60. David Katzenstein et al., "Risks for Heterosexual Transmission of HIV in Zimbabwe," III Intl. Conf. on AIDS, abstract M.8.3.

61. D. William Cameron et al., "Incidence and Risk Factors of Female to Male Transmission of HIV," IV Intl. Conf. on AIDS, abstract 4061.

62. Interview with Dr. Francis Plummer by Panos Institute as cited in Panos Institute, *AIDS in the Third World,* p. 185.

63. See Marcello Piazza et al., "Passionate Kissing and Microlesions of the Oral Mucosa: Possible Role in AIDS Transmission" (letter), *JAMA* 261 (2 [13 January 1989]): 244–45.

64. James W. Curran et al., "Epidemiology of HIV Infection and AIDS in the United States," *Science* 239 (4840 [5 February 1988]): 615.

65. Alan R. Lifson, "Do Alternate Modes for Transmission of HIV Exist?" *JAMA* 259 (9[4 March 1988]): 1353. But see also Stuart Logan et al., "Breast-Feeding and HIV Infection" (letter), *Lancet*-I (8598[11 June 1988]): 1346.

66. Personal communication with Chuck Fallis, public affairs specialist, CDC.

67. Kingsley et al., "Risk Factors for Seroconversion," pp. 345–48.

68. Darrow et al., "Risk Factors for HIV," p. 480.

69. William H. Masters, Virginia E. Johnson, and Robert C. Kolodny, *Crisis: Heterosexual Behavior in the Age of AIDS* (New York: Grove, 1988), pp. 119–20; Kevin R. Hopkins and William B. Johnston, "The Incidence of HIV Infection in the United States" (Indianapolis, Ind.: Hudson Institute, 19 August 1988), p. 3, citing Margaret Fischl et al., "Evaluation of Heterosexual Partners, Children, and Household Contacts of Adults with AIDS," *JAMA* 257 (5 [6 February 1987]): 643–44.

70. Fischl et al., "Evaluation of Heterosexual Partners," p. 644.

71. Ibid.

72. W. Rozenbaum et al., "HIV Transmission by Oral Sex," *Lancet*-I (8599 [18 June 1988]): 1395.

73. Lifson, "Alternate Modes," p. 1354.

74. David E. Dassey, R. Detels, and B. Visscher, "HIV and Orogenital Transmission" (letters), *Lancet*-II (8618 [29 October 1988]): 1023.

75. Personal communication.

76. Peter G. Spitzer and Neil J. Weiner, "Transmission of HIV Infection from a Woman to a Man by Oral Sex" (letter), *NEJM* 320 (9 [26 January 1989]): 251.

77. Ofelia T. Monzon and José M. B. Capellan, "Female-to-Female Transmission of HIV" (letter), *Lancet*-II (8549 [4 July 1987]): 40–41.

78. Personal communication, 10 February 1989.

79. Ibid.

80. Ibid.

81. Personal communication.

82. "AIDS and Heterosexuals: A Leading Expert Evaluates the Risks (Interview with Myron Essex)," *Washington Post*, 24 February 1987, p. H8.

Chapter 5. The "Perils" of Promiscuity

1. Linda Murray, "Straight Facts About Straight Sex," *Penthouse* 20 (1 [September 1988]): 206.

2. Robert E. Lee, *AIDS in America: Our Chances, Our Choices* (Troy, N.Y.: Whitston, 1987), p. 91.

3. Chris Norwood, *Advice for Life: A Woman's Guide to AIDS Risks and Prevention* (New York: Pantheon, 1987), citing Graham Hancock and Enver Carim et al., *AIDS: The Deadly Epidemic* (Gallancz: England, 1981).

4. Ann G. Fettner, "HTLV-III Disease, Not AIDS: An Interview with Major Robert Redfield," *New York Native* 5 (12, iss. 118 [17–30 June 1985]): 23.

5. U.S. Department of Health and Human Services, Public Health Service, "Surgeon General's Report on AIDS," 1986, p. 15.

6. See William H. Masters, Virginia E. Johnson, and Robert C. Kolodny, *Crisis: Heterosexual Behavior in the Age of AIDS* (New York: Grove, 1988), p. 5.

7. Office of the Surgeon General and CDC, "Understanding AIDS" (Rockville, Md.: U.S. Public Health Service, 1988), p. 3.

8. Joyce Price, "AIDS Risk for Women Rises with 'Casual' Sex," *Washington Times*, 17 April 1987, p. 6A.

9. "Modern Love," "Geraldo," transcript of 1 December 1987, p. 1.

10. Janice Hopkins Tanne, "The Last Word on Avoiding AIDS," *New York* 18 (39 [7 October 1985]): p. 29.

11. Marsha F. Goldsmith, "Sex in the Age of AIDS Calls for Common Sense and 'Condom Sense,'" *JAMA* 257 (17 [1 May 1987]): 2263.

12. C. Everett Koop, "Prepared Statement by C. Everett Koop, M.D., SC.D., Surgeon General, U.S. Public Health Service, Department of Health and Human Services," 1 March 1988, p. 5.

13. "A Consumer Guide," *U.S. News & World Report* 102 (15 [20 April 1987]): 61.

14. "At Risk," *USA Today*, 16 July 1988, p. 4D.

15. C. B. Broderick, "Adult Sexual Development," in Benjamin Wolman, ed., *Handbook of Developmental Psychology* (Englewood Cliffs, N.J.: Prentice-Hall, 1982), pp. 726–33.

16. Masters, Johnson, and Kolodny, *Crisis*, p. 55.

17. See, for example, College Press Service, "Collegians May Be Next at Risk in AIDS Epidemic," 8 October 1987.

18. Personal communication, 3 February 1989.

19. Editors of Heron House, *The Odds on Virtually Everything* (New York: G. P. Putnam, 1980), p. 194.

20. Ibid., p. 189.

21. Ibid., p. 119.

22. Warren Winkelstein Jr. et al., "The San Francisco Men's Health Study: III. Reduction in Human Immunodeficiency Virus Transmission among Homosexual/Bisexual Men, 1982–86," *AJPH* 76 (9 [June 1987]): 686, making references to the SFMHS results as well as those of a different cohort. Levels of seropositivity among homosexuals attending bathhouses would be higher than that in the general homosexual population in a given city, insofar as this group is by definition highly sexually active.

23. Diane D. Edwards, "Heterosexuals and AIDS: Mixed Messages," *Science News* 132(4 [25 July 1987]): 60.

24. Norman Hearst and Stephen B. Hulley, "Preventing the Heterosexual Spread of AIDS," *JAMA* 259 (16 [22–29 April 1988]): 2428–30.

25. Ibid., p. 2429.

26. Ibid., pp. 2428–29.

27. Ibid., pp. 2429–30.

28. Judy Ismach, "What Can We Believe?" *American Health* 7 (5 [June 1988]): 54.

29. Hearst and Hulley, "Preventing," p. 2431, citing CDC, "Occupant Restraint Usage in Fatal Crashes: Fatal Accident Reporting System," 1975–86, *MMWR* 38 (2 October 1987): 636–43.

30. Hearst and Hulley, "Preventing," p. 2432.

31. Ibid., p. 2431.

32. Personal communication.

33. See William A. Check, "Heterosexual AIDS Risk Studied," *Washington Post,* 17 April 1985, p. A7.

34. See Dave Carpenter, "Debate over Contacting AIDS Victims, Partners," UPI, 8 March 1987.

35. Nancy S. Padian et al., "Male-to-Female Transmission of Human Immunodeficiency Virus," *JAMA* 258 (6 [14 August 1987]): 789.

36. "Widespread Heterosexual Epidemic Not Foreseen by Secretary of HHS," *AIDS Policy and Law* 3 (1 [27 January 1988]): 2.

37. For example, Diane Salvatore, "AIDS and You," *Ladies Home Journal* 104 (10 [October 1987]): 121 (see page 183).

38. For example, Jo Coudert, "Nice Women *Can* Get AIDS," *Woman's Day* 50 (17 [27 October 1987]): 138.

39. Don C. Des Jarlais, "The Effectiveness of AIDS Educational Programs in Intravenous Drug Users," contractor document prepared for the Office of Technology Assessment, U.S. Congress, Washington, D.C., March 1988.

Chapter 6. "Russian Roulette," and Other Fearsome Fallacies

1. Susan Okie, "Heterosexual AIDS May Surge, Koop Says," *Washington Post,* 21 April 1987, p. A4.

2. Ibid.

3. Ellen Flax, "Koop Warns of an 'Explosion,' of AIDS Among Teen-Agers," *Education Week,* 24 June 1987, p. 10.

4. Susan Sontag, *Illness as Metaphor* (New York: Farrar, Straus & Giroux, 1978), p. 3.

5. Robert Bazell, "Surviving AIDS," *New Republic* 195 (21, iss. 3749 [24 November 1986]): 22.

6. Robert R. Redfield, testimony for Republican Leadership Task Force on Health Care, 10 June 1987 (Chairman Republican William Gradison, Ohio), transcript at 7.

7. See, for example, Kevin R. Hopkins and William B. Johnston, *The Incidence of HIV Infection in the United States* (Indianapolis, Ind.: Hudson Institute, 1988), p. 13.

8. See, for example, Gary L. Bauer and John P. Walters, "AIDS Hearing" (letter), *New Republic* 199 (10, iss. 3842 [5 September 1988]): 6.

9. Bengt Isaksson et al., "AIDS Two Months After Primary Human Immunodeficiency Virus Infection," *Journal of Infectious Diseases* 158 (4 [October 1988]): 866–68.

10. Personal communication, 15 May 1989.

11. Personal communication with Harold Jaffe, 16 May 1989.

12. See William Raspberry, "Will the 'Good' News Stop the Fight?" *Washington Post,* 28 October 1987, p. A19.

13. Laura Randolph, "Interview with U.S. Surgeon General C. Everett Koop, M.D.," *Ebony* 43 (11 [September 1988]): 156.

14. For example, Christian A. Nagle, "Cause for Alarm on AIDS Front," *Washington Times,* 19 December 1988, p. E5.

15. Anne Conover Heller, "Is There a Man in Your Man's Life?" *Mademoiselle,* 93 (July 1987): 134.

16. Jan Zita Grover, "AIDS: Keywords," *October* 43 (Winter 1987): 21.

17. Figures received from Chuck Fallis, public affairs specialist, CDC, 30 January 1989.

18. Ibid.

19. Figures calculated from Fallis and CDC, "AIDS Weekly Surveillance Report," 30 January 1989, p. 1.

20. Andrew R. Moss, "AIDS and Intravenous Drug Use: The Real Heterosexual Epidemic," *British Medical Journal* 294 (6569 [14 February 1987]): 1.

21. Mary E. Guinan and Ann Hardy, "Epidemiology of AIDS in Women in the United States," *JAMA* 257 (15 [17 April 1987]): 2040.

22. Chris Norwood, *Advice for Life: A Woman's Guide to AIDS Risks and Prevention* (New York: Pantheon, 1987), p. 9.

23. Kathryn Casey, "For Better, for Worse," *Ladies' Home Journal* 104 (5 [May 1987]): 151.

24. "AIDS May Dwarf the Plague," *New York Times,* 30 January 1987, p. A24.

25. See Allan M. Brandt, "AIDS and Metaphor," *Social Research* 55 (3 [Autumn 1988]): 430.

26. Ann Guidici Fettner, "Women and AIDS," *Health* 18 (11 [November 1986]): 62.

27. Caryl S. Avery, "The Love or Life Choice," *Self* 9 (8 [August 1987]): 124.

28. Brandt, "AIDS and Metaphor," pp. 430–31.

29. Bob Mondello, "Rewriting the Script: From Broadway to Hollywood," *Washington Post,* 29 December 1987, p. H11.

30. "Now That Sex Can Kill," "20/20," transcript of 12 February 1987, pp. 13–14.

31. Personal communication with Martin Bogner, New York Department of Health, Public Affairs, 1987.

32. Philip J. Hilts, "Data Shows AIDS Risk Widening," *Washington Post,* 21 October 1986, p. A1.

33. Ibid., p. A12.

34. Dianne Hales, "Are Women Like You Really at Risk for AIDS?" *Woman's Day* 50 (16 [1 October 1987]): 142.

35. "AIDS: Three-aspect Approach for Proper Education of Public," *Providence Journal* (Rhode Island), 24 August 1987, p. A10.

36. W. Shepherd Smith, "AIDS: A Threat to Heterosexuals Too" (letter), *Washington Post,* 30 January 1989, p. A8.

37. "MacNeil/Lehrer News Hour," rough draft 3232, transcript of 16 February 1987, pp. 8–9.

38. John Tierney, "Straight Talk," *Rolling Stone* (17 November 1988): 132.

39. John Allen Paulos, *Innumeracy: Mathematical Illiteracy and its Consequences* (New York: Hill & Wang, 1988), p. 8.

40. David Streitfeld, "The New Sexual Revolution," *Washington Post,* 11 April 1986, p. C5.

41. Henry Fairlie, "Fear of Living," *New Republic* 200 (4, iss. 3862 [23 January 1989]): 14.

42. For an excellent essay on the Great Suntan Scare see Michael Kinsley, "Fear of Frying" (editorial), *New Republic* 199 (10, iss. 3842 [5 September 1988]): 4.

43. Bauer and Walters, "AIDS Hearing," p. 6.

44. Tierney, "Straight Talk," p. 136.

45. Andrea Rock, "What You Don't Know About AIDS But Should," *Money* 16 (12 [November 1987]): 96.

46. Smith, "AIDS," p. A8.

47. Melvin J. Grayson and Thomas R. Shepard, *The Disaster Lobby* (Chicago: Follet, 1973).
48. Ibid., p. 99.
49. Rachel Carson, *Silent Spring* (New York: Houghton, Mifflin, 1962).
50. Grayson and Shepard, *Disaster Lobby*, p. 21.

Chapter 7. To Tell the Truth

1. Abraham Colles, as quoted in John Langone, *AIDS: The Facts* (Boston: Little, Brown, 1988), p. 66.
2. Personal communication with Allan Brandt, 12 May 1989.
3. John Tierney, "Straight Talk," *Rolling Stone* (17 November 1988): 124.
4. Ibid.
5. Ibid., pp. 124–26.
6. Ibid.
7. Ibid., p. 126.
8. Personal communication.
9. Ibid.
10. Katie Leishman, "Heterosexuals and AIDS," *Atlantic* 259 (2 [February 1987]): 46.
11. "Deadly Virus Blamed in Bishop's Death," *Washington Times*, 25 May 1987, p. 4A; "Bishop's Death Attributed to AIDS," *Washington Post*, 25 May 1987, p. A5.
12. See Hugh Aynsworth, "Houston's Gays Remember Late Bishop as One of Them," *Washington Times*, 5 June 1987, p. A1.
13. Personal communication, 3 February 1989.
14. Robert R. Redfield et al., "Heterosexually Acquired HTLV-III/LAV Disease (AIDS-Related Complex and AIDS)" (letter), *JAMA* 254 (15 [18 October 1985]): 2094.
15. Stephen Schultz et al., "Female-to-Male Transmission of HTLV-III" (letter), *JAMA* 255 (13 [4 April 1986]): 1704, citing M. A. Kock, "L'age-Stehr J: Der Heutigestand Unseres Wissens," *Deutsch Artzeblatt* 82 (1985): 2560.
16. John J. Potterat, L. Philips, and J. B. Muth, "Lying to Military Physicians About Risk Factors for AIDS" (letter), *JAMA* 257 (13 [3 April 1987]): 1727.
17. Personal communication, 2 February 1989.
18. Thomas C. Quinn et al., "Human Immunodeficiency Virus Infection Among Patients Attending Clinics for Sexually Transmitted Diseases," *NEJM* 318 (4 [28 January 1988]): 201.
19. Ibid., p. 198.
20. Michael Specter, "AIDS Survey Likely to Be Scaled Down," *Washington Post*, 20 October 1987, p. A4.
21. Personal communication with Rand Stoneburner; Alan R. Lifson et al., "HIV Infection in Sexually Active Heterosexual Adults Attending a New York City STD Clinic," III International Conference on AIDS (Washington, D.C.), 1–5 June 1987, abstract MP.83.
22. Thomas C. Quinn et al., "HIV Infection," citing J.W. Ward et al., "Epidemiological Characteristics of Blood Donors with Antibody to Human Immunodeficiency Virus," *Transfusion* 28 (4 [July–August]): 298.
23. "People Are Talking," WWOR, Secaucus, N.J., "The AIDS Lie," 3 March 1988.
24. Charles S. Rabkin et al., "Prevalence of Antibody to HTLV-III/LAV in a Population Attending a Sexually Transmitted Diseases Clinic," *Sexually Transmitted Diseases* 14 (1 [January–March 1987]): 48.
25. Personal communication.
26. William H. Masters, Virginia E. Johnson, and Robert C. Kolodny, *Crisis: Heterosexual Behavior in the Age of AIDS* (New York: Grove, 1988), p. 62.
27. Masters, Johnson, and Kolodny, *Crisis*, p. 9.
28. Ibid., p. 7.
29. Joyce I. Wallace, Jonathan Mann, and S. Beatrice, "HIV-I Exposure Among Clients of Prostitutes," IV International Conference on AIDS (Stockholm, Sweden), 12–16 June 1988, abstract 4055.
30. Robert E. Gould, "Reassuring News About AIDS," *Cosmopolitan* 204 (1 [January 1988]): 146.

31. Robert R. Redfield, "Frequent Transmission of HTLV-III Among Spouses of Patients with AIDS-Related Complex and AIDS," *JAMA* 253 (11 [15 March 1985]): 1571–73.

32. CDC, "HIV Infection in the United States: A Review of Current Knowledge," *MMWR* 36 (S-6 [18 December 1987]): 28.

33. Dennis Osmond et al., "Time of Exposure and Risk of HIV Infection in Homosexual Partners of Men with AIDS," *AJPH* 78 (8 [August 1988]): 946.

34. Redfield et al., "Frequent Transmission," p. 1572.

35. CDC, "HIV Infection in the United States," p. 37.

36. Kevin R. Hopkins and William B. Johnston, "The Incidence of HIV Infection in the United States" (Indianapolis, Ind.: Hudson Institute, 1988), p. 23.

37. Kirk Kidwell, "Heterosexuals and the AIDS Epidemic" *New American* 4 (10 [9 May 1988]): 11; See also Stanley K. Monteith, "Heterosexuals and AIDS" (letter), *Commentary* 85 (2 [February 1988]): 5.

38. Masters, Johnson, and Kolodny, *Crisis*, pp. 119–20; Hopkins and Johnston, "The Incidence of HIV Infection," p. 3, citing Margaret A. Fischl et al., "Evaluation of Heterosexual Partners, Children, and Household Contacts of Adults with AIDS," *JAMA* 257 (5 [6 February 1987]): 640–44.

39. "Generally, the News Is Not Good," *Newsweek* 111 (26 [27 June 1988]): 46–47, citing Margaret A. Fischl et al., "Seroprevalence of HIV in a Sexually Active Heterosexual Population," IV Intl. Conf. on AIDS, abstract 4067.

40. Monteith, "Heterosexuals and AIDS," p. 5; see also Chris Norwood, *Advice for Life: A Woman's Guide to AIDS Risks and Prevention* (New York: Pantheon, 1987), p. 18.

41. Norwood, *Advice for Life*, p. 100.

Chapter 8. Prostitutes: The "AIDS Assassins"

1. "Modern Love," "Geraldo," transcript of 1 December 1987, p. 16.

2. "Porn Stars and Their Families," "Geraldo," 9 January 1989.

3. "Modern Love," "Geraldo," pp. 2–3.

4. Judy Mann, "Laws Can't Stop AIDS," *Washington Post*, 13 May 1987, p. B3.

5. Joseph Carey et al., "AIDS: A Time of Testing," *U.S. News*, 102 (15 [20 April 1987]): 56.

6. "AIDS Conference," "The Health Show," transcript of 6 June 1987, p. 2.

7. Mark A. R. Kleiman, "Prostitution Isn't Victimless with AIDS Here," *Wall Street Journal*, 1 June 1987, p. 22.

8. For example, Courtland Milloy, "The Battle Against AIDS," *Washington Post*, 17 October 1985, p. DC1.

9. Joyce Price, "Media Blitz on AIDS Launched Today," *Washington Times*, 30 September 1987, p. A5.

10. Bruce Lambert, "AIDS Among Prostitutes Not as Prevalent as Believed, Studies Show," *New York Times*, 20 September 1988, p. B5.

11. "Newark to Require AIDS Tests for Prostitutes, Customers," *Washington Post*, 7 January 1988, p. A13.

12. Lambert, "AIDS Among Prostitutes," p. B5.

13. Ibid.

14. See Kleiman, "Prostitution Isn't Victimless," p. 22. The writer cites this as a possibility, without actually advocating it.

15. Ibid.

16. "Heterosexual AIDS: Horror or Hoax?" "Geraldo," transcript of 1 December 1987, p. 2.

17. Kleiman, "Prostitution Isn't Victimless," p. 22.

18. Steven Nahmias, "A Model of HIV Diffusion from a Single Source," *Journal of Sex Research* 26 (1 [February 1989]): 15.

19. Personal communication.

20. Personal communication with Ellen Castleberry, public affairs specialist, Office of the Surgeon General.

21. John F. Decker, *Prostitution: Regulation and Control* (Littleton, Colo.: Fred B. Rothman, 1979), pp. 11–15, 94.

22. Joyce I. Wallace et al., "HIV-I Exposure Among Clients of Prostitutes," IV International Conference on AIDS (Stockholm, Sweden), 12–16 June 1988, abstract 4055.
23. CDC, "Antibody to Human Immunodeficiency Virus in Female Prostitutes," *MMWR* 36 (11 [27 March 1987]): 157–61.
24. Ibid., p. 158.
25. Personal communication with Rand Stoneburner.
26. Eric Justice, "Prostitution 'Coverup' in Hetero AIDS," *Medical Tribune* 28 (25 [1 July 1987]): 8.
27. Department of Public Health, State of New Jersey, "AIDS Cases," 30 November 1988, p. 2.
28. CDC, "Antibody," p. 158.
29. Margaret A. Fischl et al., "Human Immunodeficiency Virus Among Female Prostitutes in South Florida," III International Conference on AIDS, (Washington, D.C.), 1–5 June 1987, abstract W.2.2.
30. U. Tirrelli, "HIV Infection Among Female and Male Prostitutes," III Intl. Conf. on AIDS, abstract WP. 95.
31. Personal communication with Mona Whittaker, public affairs specialist, National Institute of Drug Abuse.
32. Michael J. Rosenberg and Jodie M. Weiner, "Prostitutes and AIDS: A Health Department Priority?" *AJPH* 78 (4 [April 1987]): 421.
33. CDC, "Antibody to HIV," pp. 157–61.
34. Tirrelli, "HIV Infection."
35. G. L. Smith and K. F. Smith, "Lack of HIV Infection and Condom Use in Licensed Prostitutes" (letter), *Lancet*-II (8520 [13 December 1986]): 1392; S. E. Barton et al., "HTLV-III Antibody in Prostitutes" (letter), *Lancet*-II (8469–70 [21–28 December 1985]): 1424; Dominique Brenky-Faudeux and André Fribourg-Blanc, "HTLV-III Antibody in Prostitutes," *Lancet*-II (8469–70 [21–28 December 1985]): 1424.
36. Nancy Padian et al., "Human Immunodeficiency Virus (HIV) Infection in Nevada," III Intl. Conf. on AIDS, abstract WP.53.
37. Tirrelli, "HIV Infection."
38. "Heterosexual AIDS: Horror or Hoax?" p. 2.
39. William W. Darrow, "HIV-I Antibody in U.S. Prostitutes with No Evidence of IV-Drug Abuse," paper presented at III Intl. Conf. on AIDS, abstract 4054, p. 3.
40. Ibid., p. 5.
41. William W. Darrow et al., "HIV Antibody in 640 U.S. Prostitutes with No Evidence of Intravenous (IV) Drug Abuse," III Intl. Conf. on AIDS, abstract 4054.
42. Ibid.
43. Lambert, "AIDS Among Prostitutes," p. B5.
44. Personal communication with William W. Darrow.
45. M. Rosenberg, testimony presented at hearings on Prevention and Education, conducted by the Presidential Commission on the Human Immunodeficiency Virus Epidemic, Washington, D.C., 1 March 1988.
46. Justice, "Prostitution 'Coverup,' " p. 8.
47. Joyce I. Wallace et al., "Survey of Streetwalkers in New York City for Anti-HIV Antibodies," IV Intl. Conf. on AIDS, abstract 4046.
48. George Papaevangelou et al., "The Effectiveness of Education in Preventing HIV Infection in Greek Registered Prostitutes," IV Intl. Conf. on AIDS, abstract 4048.
49. Allan M. Brandt, *No Magic Bullet: A Social History of Venereal Disease in the United States since 1880* (New York and Oxford: Oxford University Press, 1985), p. 73.
50. Ibid., p. 72.
51. Ibid., p. 89.
52. Geoffrey Marks and William K. Beatty, *Epidemics* (New York: Charles Scribner's Sons, 1976), p. 90.
53. Richard Collier, *The Plague of the Spanish Lady* (New York: Atheneum, 1974), p. 83.
54. Brandt, *No Magic Bullet*, pp. 20–21.
55. Myram Borders, "Nevada's Legal Brothels Weather AIDS Scare," UPI, 26 April 1987.
56. Ibid.

57. Kenneth Charles Locking, "Prostitutes as AIDS Educators," III Intl. Conf. on AIDS, abstract 4047.

Chapter 9. But What About Africa?

1. *Newsweek* 108 (21 [24 November 1986]).
2. "AIDS in Africa," "Nightline," transcript of 20 October 1986, p. 2.
3. Ibid.
4. Larry J. Davis, "We Must All Work Together Against AIDS," *St. Petersburg Times,* 8 August 1987, p. 3D.
5. Kathleen McAuliffe et al., "AIDS: At the Dawn of Fear," *U.S. News & World Report,* 102 (2 [12 January 1987]): 62.
6. Senate Hearing Committee on Appropriations, Special Hearing, Health and Human Services, 99th Cong., 1st sess., 26 September 1985, p. 170.
7. "AIDS in Africa," "Nightline," transcript of 20 October 1986, p. 2.
8. "AIDS in Africa," "Nightline," transcript of 13 May 1988, p. 4.
9. Peter Younghusband, "AIDS Epidemic Threatens to Depopulate Much of Africa," *Washington Times,* 29 May 1987, p. 1A.
10. "AIDS in Africa," "60 Minutes," transcript of 8 November 1987, p. 10.
11. John Langone, *AIDS: The Facts* (Boston: Little, Brown, 1988), p. 111.
12. Blaine Harden, "AIDS Seen as Threat to Africa's Future," *Washington Post,* 31 May 1987, p. A18.
13. *Fodor's Kenya,* rev. ed. (New York: David McKay, 1987).
14. Michele Barry, "Ethical Considerations of Human Investigation in Developing Countries: The AIDS Dilemma," *NEJM* 319 (16 [20 October 1988]): 1084. See also Renée C. Sabatier, "Social, Cultural, and Demographic Aspects of AIDS," *Western Journal of Medicine* 147 (6 [December 1987]): 713.
15. Rod Nordland, Ray Wilkinson, and Ruth Marshall, "Africa in the Plague Years," *Newsweek* 108 (21 [24 November 1986]): 47.
16. Paul Raeburn, "Spread in Africa Provides Glimpse Into Future," AP, 30 December 1985.
17. John Pekkanen, "AIDS: The Plague that Knows No Boundaries," *Reader's Digest* 130 (782 [June 1987]): 53.
18. Lewis Thomas, "Science and Health—Possibilities, Probabilities, and Limitations," *Social Research* 55 (3 [Autumn 1988]): 381.
19. W. Shepherd Smith, "AIDS: A Threat to Heterosexuals Too," *Washington Post,* 30 January 1989, p. 8A.
20. "AIDS in Africa," "Nightline," transcript of 20 October 1986, p. 5.
21. Langone, *AIDS: The Facts,* pp. 109–10.
22. Larry Thompson, "What Are the Dangers for Heterosexuals?" *Washington Post,* 15 March 1988, p. 6.
23. "St. Louis Youth's Death in 1969 Linked to AIDS," *Washington Post,* 25 October 1987, p. A6; Christine Gorman et al., "Strange Trip Back to the Future," *Time* 130 (19 [9 November 1987]): 83.
24. "AIDS in Africa," "Nightline," p. 3.
25. Philip J. Hilts, "AIDS Takes Heavy Toll of African Children," *Washington Post,* 10 October 1987, p. A6.
26. Nordland et al., "Africa in the Plague Years," p. 46.
27. See A. R. Neequaye et al., "Preponderance of Females with AIDS in Ghana" (letter), *Lancet*-II (8513 [25 October 1986]): 978.
28. Jonathan M. Mann et al., "The International Epidemiology of AIDS," *Scientific American* 259 (4 [October 1988]): 85.
29. CDC, "Information/Education Plan to Prevent and Control AIDS in the United States (1987/1988)," 3 March 1987.
30. Hilts, "AIDS Takes Heavy Toll," p. A6.
31. S. F. Lyons, P. G. Jupp, and B. D. Schoub, "Survival of HIV in the Common Bedbug" (letter), *Lancet*-II (8497 [5 July 1986]): 45.

32. Panos Institute, *AIDS in the Third World*, 3d ed., (Philadelphia: New Society, 1989) p. 92.

33. Philippe Lepage and Philippe Van de Perre, "Nosocomial Transmission of HIV in Africa: What Tribute Is Paid to Contaminated Blood Transfusions and Medical Injections?" *Infection Control and Hospital Epidemiology* 9 (5 [May 1988]): 202.

34. "AIDS in Africa," "60 Minutes," p. 12.

35. Nordland et al., "Africa in the Plague Years," p. 46.

36. Karen Rafinski, "Africa: AIDS a Disaster of Unknown Proportions," Inter Press Service, 9 March 1987; Nordland et al., "Africa in the Plague Years," p. 47.

37. One comprehensive 1988 study found that "blood transfusions are recognized as an important risk factor of HIV infections . . . in Africa," and cited numerous individual studies showing seropositive Africans to have been far more likely to receive transfusions than seronegative ones. In two different Kinshasa studies, only 9 percent of seropositives had received transfusions in the previous few years, meaning that this was the maximum number that could have been infected this way. The other studies cited, however, showed much higher transfusion rates. Thirty-two percent of HIV-infected hospital workers in Kigali, Rwanda, had a history of blood transfusion in the previous three years (while only 6 percent of the seronegative ones had). Thirty-nine percent of pediatric Kigali AIDS or ARC cases with seronegative mothers (eliminating perinatal transmission as a possible mode of infection) interviewed were found to have a history of transfusion. Among hospitalized Kinshasa children under 24 months old whose mothers were seronegative, 31 percent of seropositive children had been transfused, as compared to 7 percent of seronegative children. For older children tested in Kinshasa, ages 2–14, 60 percent of all seropositives had a history of transfusion. Lepage and Van de Perre, "Nosocomial Transmission of HIV in Africa," pp. 201–2.

38. "AIDS in Africa," "60 Minutes," p. 12.

39. Viktor Belitsky, "Children Infect Mothers in AIDS Outbreak at a Soviet Hospital," *Nature* 337 (6207 [9 February 1989]): 493.

40. Jonathan M. Mann et al., "Surveillance for AIDS in a Central African City," *JAMA* 255 (23 [20 June 1986]): 3257.

41. Jonathan M. Mann et al., "HIV Seroprevalence Among Hospital Workers in Kinshasa, Zaire," *JAMA* 256 (22 [12 December 1986]): 3101.

42. Lepage and Van de Perre, "Nosocomial Transmission," p. 201.

43. Erich Schmutzhard, "AIDS and the African Traditional Healer" (letter), *Lancet*-II (8556 [22 August 1987]): 459.

44. Uli Linke, "AIDS in Africa" (letter), *Science* 231 (4735 [17 January 1986]): 203.

45. D. Vittecoq et al., "Acute HIV Infection After Acupuncture Treatments" (letter), *NEJM* 320 (4 [26 January 1989]): 250–51.

46. See Langone, *AIDS: The Facts*, pp. 111–12.

47. "AIDS in Africa," "Nightline," p. 4.

48. Blaine Harden, "AIDS Seen as Threat," p. A18.

49. "AIDS in Africa," "Nightline," p. 3.

50. Blaine Harden, "Uganda Battles AIDS Epidemic," *Washington Post*, 2 June 1986, p. A18.

51. Edgar Gregerson, *Sexual Practices* (New York: Franklin Watts, 1983), p. 183.

52. Ibid.; taken from *AIDS: The Facts*, p. 114.

53. Blaine Harden, "Tribal 'Cleansing' Customs Help Spread AIDS in Zambia," *Sunday News Journal* (Wilmington, Del.), 5 July 1987, p. A11.

54. Robert Bazell, "The Plague," *New Republic* 196 (22, iss. 3776 [1 June 1987]): 15.

55. Joan K. Kreiss et al., "AIDS Virus Infection in Nairobi Prostitutes," *NEJM* 314 (7 [13 February 1986]): 414–15.

56. Thomas C. Quinn, "Status on AIDS in Africa: Epidemiological Features," Testimony before the President's Commission on the Human Immunodeficiency Virus Epidemic, 11 April 1988, p. 3 (on file in the National Archives, Washington, D.C.).

57. F. I. D. Konotey-Ahulu, "AIDS: Origin, Transmission and Moral Dilemmas" (letter), *Journal of the Royal Society of Medicine* 80 (11 [November 1987]): 720.

58. Ibid.

59. Ann G. Fettner, "Flashpoint: A Safari Into the Origins of AIDS," *New York Native* 5 (7, iss. 113 [8–21 April 1985]): 29.

60. Cary Alan Johnson, "Inside Gay Africa," *New York Native* (13, iss. 150 [13 March 1986]): 29.

61. Alfred C. Kinsey, Wardell Pomeroy, and Clyde E. Martin, *Sexual Behavior in the Human Male* (New York: W. B. Saunders, 1948), p. 651.

62. D. Serwadda et al., "Slim Disease: A New Disease in Uganda and Its Association with HTLV-III Infection," *Lancet*-II (8460 [19 October 1985]): 849–52.

63. Robert E. Gould, "Reassuring News About AIDS," *Cosmopolitan* 204 (1 [1988]): 147.

64. Langone, *AIDS: The Facts*, p. 117.

65. Ibid., p. 118.

66. Johnson, "Inside Gay Africa," p. 29.

67. Ibid., p. 32.

68. Langone, *AIDS: The Facts*, p. 118.

69. Nancy Padian and John Pickering, "Female-to-Male Transmission of AIDS: A Reexamination of the African Sex Ratio of Cases" (letter), *JAMA* 256 (5 [1 August 1986]): 590.

70. O. P. Arya and F. J. Bennet, "Role of the Medical Auxiliary in the Control of Sexually Transmitted Disease in a Developing Country," *British Journal of Venereal Diseases* 52 (April 1976): 116–21.

71. Renée Sabatier, *Blaming Others* (Philadelphia: New Society, 1988), p. 71.

72. Panos Institute, *AIDS in the Third World*, p. 44.

73. A. O. Asoba, "Sexually Transmitted Diseases in Tropical Africa," *British Journal of Venereal Diseases* 57 (2 [April 1981]): 89.

74. Michael J. Rosenbert, Kenneth F. Schulz, and Nadine Burton, "Sexually Transmitted Diseases in Sub-Saharan Africa," *Lancet*-II (8499 [19 July 1986]): 152.

75. Lourdes J. D'Costa et al., "Prostitutes are a Major Reservoir of Sexually Transmitted Diseases in Nairobi, Kenya," *Sexually Transmitted Diseases* 12 (2 [April–June 1985]): 67.

76. Ibid., p. 66.

77. Don C. Des Jarlais et al., "Intravenous Drug Use and the Heterosexual Transmission of the Human Immunodeficiency Virus," *New York State Journal of Medicine* 87 (5 [May 1987]): 287.

78. Kreiss et al., "AIDS Virus Infection in Nairobi Prostitutes," p. 417.

79. Ibid., p. 414.

80. Ibid., p. 415.

81. Ibid.

82. Ibid., p. 414.

83. Ibid.

84. The Collaborative Study Group of AIDS in Haitian-Americans, "Risk Factors for AIDS Among Haitians Residing in the United States," *JAMA* 257 (5 [6 February 1987]): 637.

85. Kreiss et al., "AIDS Virus Infection in Nairobi Prostitutes," p. 416.

86. J. Neil Simonsen, "Human Immunodeficiency Virus Infection Among Men with Sexually Transmitted Diseases," *NEJM* 319 (5 [4 August 1988]): 275.

87. Aaron J. Fink, "A Possible Explanation for Heterosexual Male Infection with AIDS" (letter), *NEJM* 315 (18 [30 October 1986]): 1167.

88. Robert W. Enzenauer, "Circumcision and Heterosexual Transmission of HIV Infection to Men" (letter), *NEJM* 316 (24 [11 June 1987]): 1545.

89. "Circumcision Touted as Way to Reduce AIDS Risk," *Washington Times,* 17 June 1988, p. A7.

90. Simonsen, "Human Immunodeficiency Virus," pp. 275–6.

91. D. William Cameron, "Incidence and Risk Factor for Female to Male Transmission of HIV," IV International Conference on AIDS (Stockholm, Sweden), 6–12 June 1988, abstract 4061; personal communication with Cameron.

92. Aaron J. Fink, "Circumcision and Heterosexual Transmission of HIV Infection to Men (reply)," *NEJM* 316 (24 [11 June 1987]): 1546.

93. Ibid. See also Simonsen, "Human Immunodeficiency Virus," p. 276.

94. Thomas C. Quinn et al., "Serologic and Immunologic Studies in Patients with AIDS in North America and Africa," *JAMA* 257 (19 [15 May 1987]): 2620.

95. Ibid., p. 2621. See also Richard G. Marlink and Myron Essex, "Africa and

the Biology of Human Immunodeficiency Virus," *JAMA* 257 (19 [15 May 1987]): 2632–33.

96. Philip J. Hilts, "AIDS Seen Leveling Off in Africa," *Washington Post,* 21 March 1988, p. A1.

97. Ibid., p. A18.

98. Ibid.

99. Mann et al., "International Epidemiology of AIDS," p. 88.

100. John Maurice, "The Global Benefits of Spending Big," *New Scientist* 18 (1612 [12 May 1988]): 34.

101. Jim Hoagland, "Africa Faces the AIDS Threat," *Washington Post,* 17 January 1989, p. A23.

102. Felix I. D. Konotey-Ahulu, "AIDS in Africa: Misinformation and Disinformation" (letter), *Lancet*-II (8552 [(25 July 1987)]: 207.

103. William Greenfield, "Night of the Living Dead II: Slow Virus Encephalopathies and AIDS: Do Necromantic Zombiists Transmit HTLV-III/LAV During Voodooistic Rituals?" *JAMA* 256 (16 [24–31 October 1986]): 2199.

104. Ibid.

105. David Black, *The Plague Years* (New York: Simon & Schuster, 1986), p. 64.

106. Panos Institute, *AIDS in the Third World,* citing personal communication with Jean Pape in October 1987.

107. Black, *The Plague Years,* pp. 67–68.

108. AIDS Discrimination Unit of the New York City Commission on Human Rights, "AIDS and People of Color: The Discriminatory Impact," 7 August 1987, pp. 23–24.

109. Jean W. Pape et al., "Characteristics of the Acquired Immunodeficiency Syndrome (AIDS) in Haiti," *NEJM* 309 (16 [20 October 1983]): 949.

110. See Margaret A. Fischl and Gwendolyn B. Scott, "The Acquired Immunodeficiency Syndrome Among Haitian Adults and Infants: An Update," in *Advances in Host Defense Mechanisms* 5 (New York: Raven Press, 1985), p. 110.

111. Chris Norwood, *Advice for Life: A Woman's Guide to AIDS Risks and Prevention* (New York: Pantheon, 1987), p. 145.

112. Pape, "Characteristics . . . in Haiti," p. 948; Jean W. Pape, "The Acquired Immunodeficiency Syndrome in Haiti," *Annals of Internal Medicine* 103 (5 [November 1985]): 676.

113. Black, *Plague Years,* p. 63.

114. Pape, "Characteristics . . . in Haiti," p. 948; Collaborative Study Group of AIDS, "Risk Factors for AIDS Among Haitians," p. 637.

115. Ibid., "Risk Factors for AIDS Among Haitians," p. 637.

116. Janice Hopkins Tanne, "Fighting AIDS," *New York,* 20 (2 [12 January 1987]): 26.

117. Anne-Christine d'Adesky, "Haiti: The Great AIDS Cover-up," *New York Native* 6 (18, iss. 156 [14 April 1986]): 15.

118. Panos Institute, *AIDS in the Third World,* p. 37.

Chapter 10. The Agony of the Underclass

1. Martha Smilgis et al., "The Big Chill: Fear of AIDS," *Time* 129 (7 [16 February 1987]): 53.

2. Chris Norwood, *Advice for Life: A Woman's Guide to AIDS Risks and Prevention* (New York: Pantheon, 1987), p. 67; ODN Productions, *Sex Drugs and AIDS,* 1986, Franklin Getchall, director, Oralee Wachter and Lynne Smilow, producers.

3. *Atlantic* 260 (2 [February 1987]): cover.

4. Smilgis et al., "The Big Chill," cover.

5. *U.S. News & World Report* 102 (1 [12 January 1987]): cover.

6. *People* 29 (10 [14 March 1988]): cover.

7. "AIDS: A National Town Meeting," "Nightline," transcript of 5 October 1987, pp. 17–18.

8. See, for example, Kathryn Casey, "For Better, For Worse," *Ladies Home Journal,* 104 (5 [May 1987]): 89.

9. CDC, "AIDS Weekly Surveillance Report," 7 September 1987, p. 1.

10. CDC, "AIDS Weekly Surveillance Report," 4 January 1989, p. 1.

11. CDC, "AIDS Weekly Surveillance Report," 14 November 1988, p. 1.

12. CDC, "AIDS Weekly Surveillance Report," 4 January 1989, 1, with additional breakdown provided by CDC public affairs.

13. CDC, "AIDS Weekly Surveillance Report," 4 January 1988, p. 1, with additional breakdown provided by CDC public affairs.

14. CDC, "AIDS Weekly Surveillance Report," 14 November 1988, p. 1.

15. Richard M. Selik et al., "Racial/Ethnic Differences in the Risk of AIDS in the United States," *AJPH* 78 (12 [December 1988]): 1543.

16. Ibid., p. 1540.

17. Ibid.

18. CDC, "AIDS Weekly Surveillance Report," 4 January 1989, p. 1, with additional breakdown provided by CDC public affairs.

19. CDC, "AIDS Weekly Surveillance Report," 14 November 1988, p. 1.

20. CDC, "AIDS Weekly Surveillance Report," 4 January 1989, p. 1, with additional breakdown provided by CDC public affairs.

21. CDC, "Trends in Human Immunodeficiency Virus Infection among Civilian Applicants for Military Service—United States, October 1985–March 1988," *MMWR* 37 (44 [11 November 1988]): 678.

22. CDC, "Prevalence of Human Immunodeficiency Virus Antibody in U.S. Active-Duty Personnel, April 1988," *MMWR* 37 (30 [5 August 1988]): 462.

23. Tim Friend, "Children's AIDS Toll May Soar by 1991," *USA Today*, 20 July 1988, p. D1.

24. Judy Ismach, "What Can We Believe?" *American Health* 7 (5 [June 1988]): 54.

25. "Disturbing New AIDS Study," "Nightline," transcript of 13 January 1988.

26. "AIDS Is Reported as No. 9 Cause of Death Among Children 1 to 4," *New York Times*, 20 December 1988, p. A18.

27. Calculated from CDC, "AIDS Weekly Surveillance Report," 14 November 1988, p. 1.

28. CDC, "AIDS Weekly Surveillance Report," 14 November 1988, p. 1.

29. See John W. Ward et al., "Transmission of Human Immunodeficiency Virus (HIV) by Blood Transfusions Screened as Negative for HIV Antibody," *NEJM* 318 (8 [25 February 1988]): 473–77.

30. CDC, "AIDS Weekly Surveillance Report," 14 November 1988, p. 1.

31. Selik, "Racial/Ethnic Differences," p. 1542.

32. Calculated from figures provided by Chuck Fallis, public affairs specialist, CDC, and the Bureau of the Census.

33. L. Krueger, "Poverty and HIV Seropositivity: The Poor Are More Likely to Be Infected," IV International Conference on AIDS(Stockholm, Sweden), 12–16 June 1988, abstract 4119.

34. Lisa Levitt Ryckman, "AIDS and Minorities: Myths, Fear Shield Color-blind Killer" *News-Gazette* (Champaign-Urbana, Ill.), 31 July 1988, p. B1.

35. Carol Randolph, "AIDS Strikes Without Regard for Race," *Washington Times*, 26 August 1988, p. B1.

36. Wayne Greaves, "The Black Community," in *AIDS and the Law*, ed. Harlon L. Dalton, Scott Burris, and the Yale AIDS Law Project (New Haven, Conn.: Yale University Press, 1987), p. 283.

37. Sandra Boodman, "AIDS Message Misses Many Blacks, Hispanics," *Washington Post*, 31 May 1987, p. A18.

38. Greaves, "The Black Community," p. 282; and K. Castro, "Frequency of Opportunistic Diseases in AIDS Patients by Race/Ethnicity and HIV Transmission Categories," IV International Conference on AIDS (Stockholm, Sweden), 12–16 June 1988, abstract 4152.

39. Castro, "Frequency."

40. For example, Katherine Franke, "AIDS and Race," *Exchange* (publication of the National Lawyers' Guild), iss. 4, May 1987, p. 3; Joyce Price, " 'We Can't Ignore,' Problem of AIDS, Minorities," *Washington Times*, 10 August 1987, p. A1.

41. Greaves, "Black Community," p. 282.

42. Norwood, *Advice for Life*, pp. 27–28.

43. Susan Okie, "Genes May Play Role in Contracting AIDS," *Washington Post,* 12 May 1987, p. A3.

44. Personal communication with Harold Jaffe.

45. Lesley-Jane Eales, Keith E. Nye and Anthony J. Pinching, "Group-specific Component and AIDS: Erroneous Data," *Lancet*-I (8591 [23 April 1988]): 93.

46. CDC, "AIDS Weekly Surveillance Report," 14 November 1988, p. 1.

47. Personal communication with Mona Whittaker, National Institute of Drug Abuse, 11 May 1989.

48. Greaves, "Black Community," p. 282.

49. Beryl Koblin et al., "Racial Differences in HIV Infection in IVDUs," IV Intl. Conf. on AIDS, abstract 4537.

50. Don C. Des Jarlais et al., "HIV-I Infection Among Intravenous Drug Users in Manhattan, New York City, From 1977 Through 1987," *JAMA* 261 (7 [17 February 1989]): 1010.

51. Laurene Mascola et al., "HIV Seroprevalence in Intravenous Drug Users: Los Angeles, California, 1986," *AJPH* 79 (1 [January 1989]): 81.

52. W. Robert Lange, "Geographic Distribution of Human Immunodeficiency Virus Markers in Parenteral Drug Users," *AJPH* 78 (4 [April 1988]): 444, fig. 1.

53. Betsy Burkhard, "Rockford Hookers Dealing Deadly Virus," *Rockford Register Star,* 13 September 1987, p. A1.

54. Cathryn Donahoe, "Entering a Kingdom of Death Through a Needle," *Washington Times,* 13 December 1988, p. E12.

55. Perhrolov Pehrson et al., "HIV Infection Among IV Drug Abusers in Stockholm," IV Intl. Conf. on AIDS, abstract 4510.

56. Personal communication with Dr. Joyce Woods, Narcotic and Drug Research, Inc., New York, 2 August 1989. Dr. Woods notes that in Sweden, most IVDAs are amphetamine users and that, while most amphetamine injectors in the U.S. are also middle class, such usage in America is comparatively rare.

57. Richard E. Chaisson et al., "Human Immunodeficiency Virus Infection in Heterosexual Intravenous Drug Users in San Francisco," *AJPH* 77 (2 [February 1987]): 169–72.

58. See Jayne Garrison, "Saving San Francisco Addicts from AIDS," *San Francisco Examiner,* 13 March 1988, p. 1.

59. Ibid.

60. "Panacea in Needle Park," *U.S. News* 105 (20 [21 November 1988]): 18.

61. For interesting pieces of conversation with addicts concerning "safe injecting," see Samuel R. Friedman et al., "The Special Problems of Intravenous Drug Users as Persons at Risk for AIDS," *Medical Times* 115 (9 [September 1987]): 39–46.

62. Donahoe, "Entering a Kingdom of Death," p. E12.

63. Des Jarlais et al., "HIV Infection Among Intravenous Drug Users in Manhattan," p. 1010.

64. Ibid., p. 1011.

65. See Lawrence S. Brown et al., "Drug Treatment and Seropositivity" (letter), *New York State Journal of Medicine* 88 (3 [March 1988]): 156.

66. See Edward M. Brecher and the Editors of Consumer Reports, "Licit and Illicit Drugs" (Boston: Little, Brown, 1972), pp. 140–52, for a discussion of methadone maintenance success. According to Joyce Woods of Narcotic and Drug Research, Inc., New York, no follow-up studies have been done on drug-free programs. (Personal communication, 2 August 1989.)

67. "AIDS Prevention for Addicts," *Medical World News,* 11 January 1988, p. 11.

68. Ronald Sullivan, "Citing 'State of Emergency,' New York Starts Drug-Clinic Program to Fight AIDS," *New York Times,* 12 June 1987, p. B4.

69. Ibid.

70. Peter Kerr, "Drug Treatment Shortage Imperils AIDS Control," *New York Times,* 4 October 1987, p. A32.

71. See, for example, ibid.

72. Selik, "Racial/Ethnic Differences," p. 1543.

73. Ibid., p. 1541 (table 3).

74. Ibid.

75. Alan P. Bell and Martin S. Weinberg, *Homosexualities* (New York: Simon & Schuster, 1978), p. 55.

76. Ibid.

77. Sandra Boodman, "AIDS Spreading Faster Among D.C. Blacks," *Washington Post,* 8 August 1988, p. D1.

78. Ibid.

79. Ibid.

80. Sandra Boodman, "Hispanic Culture Redefines AIDS Fight," *Washington Post,* 28 December 1987, p. A15.

81. Joyce Price, "Though at Risk, Hispanics Shun Warnings About AIDS," *Washington Times,* p. A12 (story begins on p. A1).

82. Don C. Des Jarlais and Samuel R. Friedman, "Intravenous Cocaine, Crack, and HIV Infection" (letter), *JAMA* 259 (13 [1 April 1988]): 1945–46.

83. Ibid., p. 1946.

84. Peter Kerr, "Syphilis Surge and Crack Use Raising Fears on Spread of AIDS," *New York Times,* 29 June 1988, p. B5.

85. Ibid., p. B1.

86. Matt Clark, "AIDS," *Newsweek* 106 (7 [12 August 1985]): 20.

87. Kerr, "Syphilis Surge and Crack Use," p. B1.

88. Robert Rolfs et al., "Drug-Related Behavior and Syphilis in Philadelphia—Sex for Drugs," *AJE* 128 (4 [October 1988]): 898.

89. Kerr, "Syphilis Surge and Crack Use," p. B1.

90. Personal communication.

91. Testimony before U.S. Commission on Civil Rights, 18 May 1988, draft of hearings, 324–25 (on file with Office of General Counsel).

92. See generally, James H. Jones, *Bad Blood: The Tuskagee Syphilis Experiment* (New York: Free Press, 1981).

93. "Chicago Aide Apologizes for Religious Slurs," *Washington Post,* 3 May 1988, p. A12.

94. Allan M. Brandt, "The Syphilis Epidemic and its Relation to AIDS," *Science* 239 (4838 [22 January 1988]): 379.

95. CDC, "Syphilis and Congenital Syphilis—United States, 1985–1988," *MMWR* 37 (32 [19 August 1988]): 486.

96. CDC, "Continuing Increase in Infectious Syphilis—United States," *MMWR* 37 (3 [29 January 1988]): 36.

97. Joyce Price, "Funds Diversion to AIDS Pushes Other VD Rates Up," *Washington Times,* 17 August 1987, p. A5.

98. Testimony of Wendy Wertheimer before the Presidential Commission on the Human Immunodeficiency Virus Epidemic, 1 March 1988, p. 3.

99. Ibid., pp. 3–4.

100. Andrea Rock, "What You Don't Know About AIDS But Should," *Money* 16 (12 [November 1987]): 96.

101. These statistics appear on the last two pages of CDC, "Human Immunodeficiency Virus Infections in the United States, A Review of Current Knowledge and Plans for Expansion of HIV Surveillance Activities, A Report to the Domestic Policy Council," 30 November 1987.

102. Lisa Levitt Ryckman, "Educators Plot Strategy to Quell the Epidemic," AP, 31 July 1988.

103. Richard Goldstein, "AIDS and Race," *Village Voice* 32 (10 [10 March 1987]): 26.

104. Franke, "AIDS and Race," p. 1.

105. Linda S. Williams, "AIDS Risk Reduction: A Community Health Education Intervention for Minority High Risk Group Members," *Health Education Quarterly* 13 (4 [Winter 1986]): 416–17.

106. Lisa M. Krieger, "Blacks and Hispanics Missing Message on AIDS," *San Francisco Examiner,* 28 July 1987, p. B1.

107. Personal communication with Sunny Rumsey.

108. Goldstein, "AIDS and Race," p. 26.

109. Jeff Sklansky, "CDC Signals Sensitivity to Minorities," *Washington Post,* 16 August 1988, p. 1A.

110. Joyce Price, "District Officials' Concerns Scuttle Federal AIDS Survey," *Washington Times,* 16 August 1988, p. B3.

111. "Tony Brown's Journal," 13 January 1988.

112. Rick Wartzman, "AIDS Heaps Hardship on Washington Slum Called 'The Graveyard,' " *Wall Street Journal,* 4 November 1987, p. 1.

113. Personal communication with Randy Shilts, May 1987.

114. Office of Technology Assessment, U.S. Congress, *How Effective Is AIDS Education?* June 1988, p. 10.

Chapter 11. The Liberal Democratizers

1. "AIDS: Changing the Rules," AIDS Films, Inc., 1987, John Hoffman and Franklin Getchalt, producers.

2. George F. Will, "AIDS: The Real Danger," *Washington Post,* 7 June 1987, p. B7.

3. Chris Norwood, *Advice for Life: A Woman's Guide to AIDS Risks and Prevention* (New York: Pantheon, 1987), pp. 76–77.

4. Allan M. Brandt, *No Magic Bullet: A Social History of Venereal Disease in the United States Since 1880* (New York and Oxford: Oxford University Press, 1985), p. 21.

5. Ibid., p. 22.

6. "An 'Elegant' Disease: An Interview with Ann Guidici Fettner," *New York Native* (95 [30 July–12 August, 1984]): 27.

7. Ann G. Fettner, "Is the CDC Dying of AIDS?" *Village Voice* 31 (39 [30 September 1986]): p. 14.

8. Ann G. Fettner, "The Truth Hurts," *New York Native* 6 (20, iss. 158 [28 April 1986]): 26; Ann G. Fettner, "Belle Glade: Another Kind of Harvest," *New York Native* 5 (15, iss. 121 [29 July–11 August 1985]): 21–23; Ann G. Fettner, "A Place to Die and a Drink of Water," *New York Native* 16 (19, iss. 157 [21 April 1986]): 22–23.

9. For example, Ann G. Fettner, "Dropping the Other Shoe," *New York Native* 5 (13, iss. 119 [1–14 July 1985]): 25.

10. Ann G. Fettner, "The AIDS Scare: Answers to Frightening Questions," *Redbook,* April 1987, p. 30.

11. Ibid., p. 27.

12. Ann G. Fettner, "Playboy's AIDS Philosophy," *New York Native* 6 (26, iss. 164 [9 June 1986]): 21.

13. Fettner, "The AIDS Scare," p. 30.

14. Jeffrey Hart, " 'Safe Sex' and the Presence of Absence," *National Review* 39 (8 [May 1987]): 43.

15. Norwood, *Advice for Life,* p. 55.

16. "AIDS: What Is to Be Done?" *Harper's* 271 (1625 [October 1985]): 43.

17. Testimony of Elvira Arriola before the U.S. Commission on Civil Rights, 18 May 1988, draft at 336 (on file in the office of the General Counsel).

18. Kathleen McAuliffe et al., "AIDS: At the Dawn of Fear," *U.S. News* 102 (2 [12 January 1987]): 62.

19. *Everything You and Your Family Need to Know About AIDS,* HBO Productions, 1987 Gabby Monet, producer.

20. Dr. Walter Dowdle of CDC quoted in "Haitians Removed from AIDS Risk List," *New York Times,* 10 April 1985, p. A13.

21. Benjamin Schatz, "The AIDS Insurance Crisis: Underwriting or Overreaching?" *Harvard Law Review* 100 (7 [May 1987]): 1783.

22. Clif Cartland, *You Can Protect Yourself and Your Family from AIDS* (Tappan, N.J.: Flemming H. Revell, 1987), p. 81.

23. James I. Slaff and John Brubaker, *The AIDS Epidemic: How You Can Protect Your Family—Why You Must* (New York: Warner, 1985), p. 83.

24. Michael Ryan, "When No One Dared," *Parade* 5 June 1988, p. 18.

25. "AIDS Straight Talk," *New York Times,* 29 March 1989, p. C22.

26. Personal communication with Surveillance, Ep, and End Result Office of the National Cancer Institute, 21 June 1989.

27. "Coolfont Report: A PHS Plan for Prevention and Control of AIDS and the AIDS Virus," *Public Health Reports* 101 (4 [July-August 1986]): 342.

28. Susan Sontag, *AIDS and Its Metaphors* (New York: Farrar, Straus & Giroux, 1989), pp. 82–83.

29. See, for example, David Eisenman, "Sooner or Later We'll All Know an AIDS Victim," *News-Gazette* (Champaign-Urbana, Ill.), 5 April 1988, p. A5.

30. Cal Thomas, "AIDS and the Media," *Washington Times,* 18 February 1988, p. F4.

31. Ibid.

32. Joseph Cary, "And Now, a Worldwide War Against AIDS," *U.S. News* 102 (13 [6 April 1987)]: 13.

33. Ibid.

34. See *World Book Encyclopedia,* 1988 ed. (Chicago: World Book, 1987), p. 513.

35. Personal communication with Dr. Hans Lobell, Malaria Branch, CDC, 31 May 1989.

36. John Maurice, "The Global Benefits of Spending Big," *New Scientist* 118 (1612 [12 May 1988]): 34.

37. "MacNeil/Lehrer News Hour," Rough Draft 3232, 16 February 1987, p. 8.

38. *New York Times,* 24 December 1988, p. 33.

39. "Krim Takes a Bow for AIDS Work," *USA Today,* 3 November 1987, p. 2D.

40. George Johnson, "Dr. Krim's Crusade," *New York Times Magazine,* 14 February 1988, pp. 31–32.

41. Ibid., p. 34.

42. Lawrence K. Altman, "F.D.A. Approves First Drug for an AIDS-Related Cancer," *New York Times,* 22 November 1988, p. C3.

43. Johnson, "Dr. Krim's Crusade," p. 34.

44. Ibid., p. 32.

45. "Mixed Messages About AIDS," "Nightline," transcript of 22 January 1988, p. 6.

46. Barry Adkins, "The Human Response" (interview with Mathilde Krim), *New York Native* 6 (11, iss. 148 [17–23 February 1986]): 21.

47. Ibid., pp. 21–22.

48. Jennet Conant, "The Fashionable Charity," *Newsweek* 110 (26 [28 December 1987]): 54.

49. Conant, "Fashionable Charity," p. 54.

50. Ibid.

51. Lewis H. Lapham, "AIDS and the Political Right: Smugness, But Little Help," *New York Native* 57 (10, iss. 56 [20 May–2 June 1985]): 6. Lapham ironically identifies Krim as "right wing."

52. Sharon Churcher, "Intelligencer," *New York* 18 (21 [27 May 1985]): 14.

53. Charles Ortlieb, "Waltzing with Mathilde," *New York Native* 5 (11, iss. 117 [3–16 June 1985]): 6.

54. Ibid.

55. Ibid.

56. Lindsy Van Gelder, "Mathilde Krim," *Ms.,* 14 (7 [January 1986]): 37.

57. Copies of this ad are available from AmFAR, New York, New York.

58. See, for example, "AIDS: A Multi-Country Assessment," *Public Opinion* 11 (1 [May–June 1988]): 38, citing Gallup Organization figure that 25 percent of all Americans think that being coughed or sneezed on is a way to get AIDS.

59. Panos Institute, *AIDS and the Third World,* 3d ed. (Philadelphia: New Society, 1988), p. 93.

Chapter 12. Safe Sex and the Condom Wars

1. See Hans Zinsser, *Rats, Lice, and History* (Boston: Atlantic Monthly, 1934), p. 80.

2. "Surgeon General Gives Perspective on Condom Promoting, HIV Magnitude, Testing, His Near-term AIDS Emphasis," *AIDS Record* 1 (23 [15 November 1987]): 2–3.

3. See James Barron, "In Condom Ads, Focus is on Women," *New York Times,* 3 June 1987, p. C1.

4. See Terry E. Johnson, "An Unflinching AIDS Campaign," *Newsweek* 109 (21 [25 May 1987]): 24.

5. Sandra G. Boodman, "TV Networks Agree to Air AIDS Ads Mentioning Condoms," *Washington Post,* 4 October 1988, p. H9.

6. "California Valentine," *Dartmouth Review,* 2 March 1988, p. 4.

7. Carl Thitchener, "The Condom Conundrum," *Humanist* 47 (4 [July–August 1987]): 14.

8. "Morals, Assault File Turning Up to Haunt the 'Condom Pastor,'" *Washington Times,* 19 February 1987, p. D4.

9. "The Condom Preacher—And His Pantless Past," *Newsweek* 109 (9 [2 March 1987]): 69.

10. Kim Painter, "Safe-sex Solution: Condoms in Dorms," *USA Today,* 17 September 1987, p. B1.

11. "Campus Condoms" (editorial), *San Francisco Chronicle,* 19 August 1987, p. 50.

12. "U-Va. Dorm Machines to Sell Condoms, Not Cigarettes," *Washington Post,* 22 August 1988, p. A4.

13. Painter, "Safe-sex Solution," p. B1.

14. "College Paper to Include a Condom," *Philadelphia Inquirer,* 9 February 1988, p. 2B.

15. "Huge Cock in Oslo," *New York Native* 6 (52, iss. 190 [6 December 1986]): 13.

16. "Macabre Ads, Fairy Tales, UFOs, etc." (editorial), *Washington Times,* 22 January 1988, p. F2.

17. Debra W. Haffner, "AIDS and Adolescents" (Center for Population Options, Washington, D.C.), p. 17.

18. "Loose Lips," *City Paper* (Washington, D.C.), 15 April 1988, p. 4.

19. Ibid.

20. Chris McKenna, "Condom Classes Scrapped, for Now," *New York Post,* 25 July 1987, p. 5.

21. John Lofton, "Dipping into AIDS Research," *Washington Times,* 29 June 1988, p. F3.

22. "Modern Love," "Geraldo," transcript of 1 December 1987, p. 17.

23. See William K. Stevens, "Fear of AIDS Brings Explicit Advice to Campus, Caution to Singles Bar," *New York Times,* 17 February 1987, p. A21.

24. Haffner, "AIDS and Adolescents," p. 16.

25. See James W. Stout and Frederick P. Rivara, "Schools and Sex Education: Does it Work?" *Pediatrics* 83 (3 [March 1989]): 375.

26. "Killing All the Right People," "Designing Women," Linda Bloodworth-Thomason, executive producer, release date 5 October 1987.

27. Personal communication with Judy Margolin, publicist for "Designing Women," 18 May 1989.

28. Office of Technology Assessment, U.S. Congress, "How Effective Is AIDS Education?" June 1988, p. 56.

29. Leslie Cauley, "A New Life for an Old Industry," *Insight,* 16 March 1987, p. 50.

30. "Illinois Governor Kills 'Condom Rag' Jingle," *Washington Times,* 22 April 1987, p. A10.

31. Joyce Price, "Free Condom Triggers Boycott of Magazine," *Washington Times,* 3 November 1988, p. B2.

32. Madonna national tour, 1987.

33. "Tonight Show," 12 December 1988.

34. Art Ulene, *Safe Sex in a Dangerous World* (New York: Vintage, 1987), p. 31.

35. Robert R. Redfield and Wanda Kay Franz, *AIDS and Young People* (Washington, D.C.: Regnery-Gateway, 1987), p. 20.

36. See National Safety Council, *1988 Accident Facts* (Chicago, 1988), p. 52.

37. Ulene, *Safe Sex,* p. 35.

38. Ibid.

39. Allan M. Brandt, *No Magic Bullet: A Social History of Venereal Disease in the United States Since 1880* (New York: Oxford University Press, 1985), p. 37.

40. Ibid., p. 46.
41. Personal communication with Allan Brandt, 12 May 1989.
42. Brandt, *No Magic Bullet,* p. 46.
43. Ibid., p. 46.
44. William Styron, *In the Clap Shack* (New York: Random House, 1973), pp. 10–11.
45. Brandt, *No Magic Bullet,* p. 121.
46. Allan M. Brandt, "The Syphilis Epidemic and Its Relation to AIDS," *Science* 239 (4838 [22 January 1988]): 377.
47. David R. Hopkins, *Prince and Peasants: Smallpox in History* (Chicago: University of Chicago Press, 1983), p. 32.
48. Administrative Board of the U.S. Catholic Conference, "The Many Faces of AIDS," 1 December 1987.
49. "Bishops to Issue New AIDS Test," *HLI Reports* (Gaithersburg, Md.) 6 (8 [August 1988]): 4.
50. William F. Jasper, "A is for AIDS, and for Amorality," *New American* 3 (18 [31 August 1987]): 42.
51. "Good Morning America," 28 July 1987.
52. "Family Research," 2 (September–October 1987): 1.
53. "Did You Hear . . . ?," *New York Native* 7 (19, iss. 209 [20 April 1987]): 5.
54. Personal communication with James Warner.
55. Patrick L. Moore, " 'Safe Sex,' Claims and Liability," *Washington Times,* 13 May 1987, p. D2. For a similar statement by Theresa Crenshaw, see Caryl S. Avery, "The Love or Life Choice," *Self* 9 (8 [August 1987]): 125.
56. Edwin J. Haeberle, *The Sex Atlas* (New York: Continuum, 1983), p. 105.
57. Interestingly, according to Planned Parenthood representatives, there is no such study *per se,* in that Planned Parenthood conducts no surveys, although it does sometimes commission opinion polls through the Alan Guttmacher Institute. Planned Parenthood uses as its source for condom failure rates information provided by the Alan Guttmacher Institute. For the latest such data, see Elise F. Jones and Jacqueline Darroch Forrest, "Contraceptive Failure in the United States: Revised Estimates from the 1982 National Survey of Family Growth," *Family Planning Perspectives* 21 (3 [May–June 1989]): 105, table 2. The data show significant differences in failure depending on race, age, and marital status, all factors that would seem to have little to do with condom leakage.
58. U.S. Department of Education, "AIDS and the Education of Our Children," 6 October 1987, p. 16.
59. Margaret A. Fischl et al., "Evaluation of Heterosexual Partners, Children, and Household Contacts of Adults with AIDS," *JAMA* 257 (5 [6 February 1987]): 640–44.
60. Gary L. Bauer and John P. Walters, "AIDS Hearing" (letter), *New Republic* 842 (iss. 3 [5 September 1988]): 6.
61. From the HBO video, *Everything You and Your Family Need to Know About AIDS,* HBO Productions, 1987, Gabby Monet, producer.
62. Fischl et al., "Evaluation," p. 641.
63. David Seifman, "Flip-Flop Ed: Condoms are Russian Roulette," *New York Post,* 9 June 1987, p. 31.
64. Ibid.
65. "Can You Rely on Condoms?" *Consumer Reports* 54 (3 [March 1989]): 135; See also Marsha F. Goldsmith, "Sex in the Age of AIDS Calls for Common Sense and 'Condom Sense,' " *JAMA* 257 (17 [1 May 1987]): 2262–63, citing *Sexually Transmitted Diseases* 11 (1984): 94–95 and Marcus Conant et al., "Condoms Prevent Transmission of AIDS-Associated Retrovirus" (letter), *JAMA* 255 (13 [4 April 1986]): 1706.
66. "Can You Rely on Condoms?" p. 135.
67. E. N. Ngugi et al., "Prevention of Transmission of Human Immunodeficiency Virus in Africa: Effectiveness of Condom Promotion and Health Education Among Prostitutes," *Lancet*-II (8616 [15 October 1988]): 889.
68. Jonathan Mann et al., "Condom Use and HIV Infection Among Prostitutes in Zaire" (letter), *NEJM* 316 (6 [5 February 1987]): 345.
69. William W. Darrow, "Innovative Health Behavior: A Study of the Use, Acceptance, and Use-Effectiveness of the Condom as a Venereal Disease Prophylactic," Ph.D. diss., Emory University, Atlanta, Ga., 1973; C. W. Tucker, "Gonorrheal Recidivism in Richland

County, South Carolina," prepared for the U.S. Department of Health and Human Services, Centers for Disease Control, Atlanta, Ga., both as cited in Office of Technology Assessment, U.S. Congress, *How Effective is AIDS Education?*, June 1988, p. 7.

70. Lode Wigersma and Ron Ond, "Safety and Acceptability of Condoms for Use by Homosexual Men as a Prophylactic Against Transmission of HIV during Anogenital Sexual Intercourse," *British Medical Journal* 295 (6590 [11 July 1987]): 94.

71. Diane Richardson, *Women & AIDS* (New York: Methuen, 1988), p. 69.

72. Ibid., p. 78.

73. "An Interview with C. Everett Koop," *USA Today*, 18 September 1987, p. A13.

74. Michael W. Ross, "Problems Associated with Condom Use in Homosexual Men" (letter), *AJPH* 77 (7 [July 1987]): 877.

75. See, for example, advertisement of Whitman-Walker Clinic, *Washington Blade*, 15 July 1988, p. 31.

76. Brandt, "Syphilis Epidemic," p. 379.

77. Ronald Sullivan, "New York's AIDS Programs Shift Focus to Drug Abusers," *New York Times*, 23 Oct. 1987, p. B3.

78. Price, "Free Condom," p. B2.

79. "Condoms: Experts Fear False Sense of Security," *New York Times*, 18 August 1987, p. C9.

80. Hearing Before the Select Committee on Narcotics Abuse and Control, House of Representatives, 100th Cong., 1st sess., 27 July 1987, p. 112.

Chapter 13. The Conservative Alarmists

1. Elizabeth Mehren and Victor F. Zonana, "Krim's Crusade: In the Fight Against AIDS, She Is a Scientist, a Socialite, a Strategist, a Spokeswoman and Sometimes a Cheerleader in Sensible Shoes," *Los Angeles Times*, 27 November 1988.

2. Personal communication with Kathy Stone, medical epidemiologist, CDC.

3. Personal communication with Robert Rolfs, CDC, 3 August 1989. Exact data is lacking on this, but see Arnold L. Schroeter et al., "Therapy for Incubating Syphilis," *JAMA* 218 (5 [1 November 1971]): 711–13; Gavin Hart, "Epidemiologic Treatment of Syphilis," *Journal of the American Venereal Disease Association* 3 (2, pt. 2 [December 1986]): 177–80; and M. Brittain Moore, Jr. et al., "Epidemiologic Treatment of Contacts to Infectious Syphilis," *Public Health Reports* 78 (11 [November 1963]): 966–70.

4. "Where Candidates Stand on AIDS Policy," *Christian Science Monitor*, 12 June 1987, p. 7.

5. U.S. Congress, Senate, S. 1352, 100th Cong., 1st sess., sec. 5 (1987).

6. U.S. Congress, House, H.R. 2273, 100th Cong., 1st sess., sec. 1 (1987).

7. "Mandatory Testing Worked for Syphilis," *Human Events*, 27 June 1987, p. 1.

8. John D. Klenk, U.S. Department of Education, "Note to Bill Kristol," 18 June 1987.

9. Robert R. Redfield and Donald S. Burke, "Shadow on the Land: The Epidemiology of HIV Infection," *Viral Immunology* 1 (1 [Spring 1987]).

10. Allan M. Brandt, *No Magic Bullet: A Social History of Venereal Disease in the United States Since 1880* (New York: Oxford University Press, 1985), p. 136.

11. Ibid., p. 137.

12. Ibid., pp. 114–15.

13. Personal communication with Allan M. Brandt.

14. For a listing of the 22 states, see Nan Hunter, "AIDS Prevention and Civil Liberties: The False Security of Mandatory Testing," *SIECUS Report* (Sex Information and Education Council of the U.S.) 16 (1 [September–October 1987]): n. 20.

15. "Illinois May End Premarital AIDS Testing," *Washington Post*, 5 January 1989, p. B12.

16. Sandra Boodman, "Premarital AIDS Testing Annoying Many in Illinois," *Washington Post*, 30 July 1988, p. A9.

17. "Illinois May End," p. B12.

18. For broader discussions of the disadvantages of mandatory HIV testing, see generally Paul D. Cleary et al., "Compulsory Premarital Screening for the Human Im-

munodeficiency Virus," *JAMA* 258 (13 [2 October 1987]): 1757–62; and Michael A. Fumento, "Chicken Little with a Hypodermic," *Reason* 20 (6 [November 1988]): 30.

19. Testimony of Dr. John Seale before the California Senate Health and Human Services Committee, 29 September 1986, as reprinted in David Noebel, Wayne Lutton, and Paul Cameron, *AIDS: A Special Report* (Manitou Springs, Colo.: Summit Ministries, 1987), p. 174.

20. Report of Dr. John Seale to the British House of Commons, Social Services Committee, sec. 1986–87, vol. 3, p. 146.

21. Ibid., pp. 144–45.

22. Ibid., pp. 146–47.

23. "The AIDS Cover-up?" *Washington Inquirer,* 17 April 1987, p. 1.

24. Ibid., p. 3.

25. Wayne Lutton, "Hazardous to Your Health," *National Review* 39 (1 [30 January 1987]): 56.

26. "Robertson Has His Version of AIDS Facts," *Washington Post,* 20 December 1987, p. A12.

27. Gregory Fossedal, "Beyond Testing for AIDS," *Washington Times,* 23 June 1987, p. D2.

28. "AIDS," "Nightline," transcript of 30 June 1986, p. 3.

29. "AIDS: A National Town Meeting," "Nightline," transcript of 5 October 1987, p. 37.

30. Kenneth G. Castro et al., "Investigations of AIDS Patients with No Previously Identified Risk Factors," *JAMA* 259 (9 [4 March 1988]): 1339.

31. Family Research Institute, "ISIS Newsletter" 2 (July–August 1986): 1 (now called "Family Research").

32. Gene Antonio, *The AIDS Cover-up?* (San Francisco: Ignatius, 1986), p. 181.

33. Ibid., pp. 118–19.

34. John F. D. Shrewsbury, *A History of Bubonic Plague in the British Isles* (Cambridge, England: University Press, 1970), p. 6.

35. A. D. J. Robertson and James F. Grutcsh, Jr., "The Coming of AIDS," *The American Spectator* 19 (3 [March 1986]): 14.

36. Ibid., p. 13.

37. Ibid.

38. Ibid., p. 15.

39. Andrew Ferguson, "Count Me Out" (letter), *The American Spectator* 20 (1 [January 1987]): 9.

40. Personal communication with Wladyslaw Pleszczynski.

41. Mark Kleiman," Prostitution Isn't Victimless with AIDS Here," *Wall Street Journal,* June 1987, p. 22.

42. Katie Leishman, "The AIDS Debate That Isn't," *Wall Street Journal,* 27 February 1988, p. A14.

43. Katie Leishman, "Journalistic Uses of AIDS," *The New Republic* 199 (13, iss. 3,845 [26 September 1988]): 6.

44. Terry Krieger and Cesar Caceres, "The Unnoticed Link in AIDS Cases," *Wall Street Journal,* 24 October 1985, p. 32.

45. "AIDS Strategies," *Wall Street Journal,* 4 June 1987, p. 30.

46. Brandt, *No Magic Bullet,* p. 180.

47. "AIDS in Real Life," *AIDS Prevention* 1 (7 November 1987): 4.

48. H. Edward Rowe, letter to the author, 20 January 1988.

49. Brandt, *No Magic Bullet,* p. 65.

50. "Miss America and Sex," *AIDS Protection* 1 (10 [February 1988]): p. 6.

51. "Never Again!" *AIDS Protection* 1 (8 [December 1987]): 1.

52. Roger Ricklefs, "AIDS Videos for Schools," *Wall Street Journal,* 18 November 1987, p. 30.

53. Ibid.

54. David Black, *The Plague Years* (New York: Simon & Schuster, 1986), p. 103.

55. Brandt, *No Magic Bullet,* p. 27.

56. Lena Williams, "Teen-Age Sex: New Codes Amid the Old Anxiety," *New York Times,* 27 February 1989, p. A1.

57. Melvin Anchell, "A Psychoanalytic Look at Homosexuality," *Vital Speeches* 52 (9 [15 February 1986]): 286.

58. Paul Cameron, "Tattooing: A Reasonable Next Step," *Family Research* 2 (September–October 1987): p. 5.

59. "Compassion Grows Among Christian Groups Confronting Spread of AIDS," *Washington Post*, 29 October 1988, p. C11.

60. Ibid.

61. Larry Witham, "Misperception on AIDS is Noted," *Washington Times*, 9 September 1988, p. B5.

62. Calculated from CDC, "HIV/AIDS Surveillance," April 1989, p. 8.

63. John Crewdson, "U.S. AIDS Projection Down," *Chicago Tribune*, 22 November 1987, p. 22. Confirmed through personal communication with James Warner.

64. James W. Warner, "Estimating the Extent of HIV Infection," Draft Policy Memorandum, 23 October 1987, on file at White House.

65. Personal communication with James Warner.

66. Norman Podhoretz, "AIDS in Plain English," *New York Post*, 24 September 1985, p. 27.

67. Patrick J. Buchanan, "AIDS Disease: It's Nature Fighting Back," *New York Post*, 24 May 1983, p. 31.

68. See, generally, Randy Shilts, *And the Band Played On* (New York: St. Martin's Press, 1987).

69. "Masters and Johnson and Quackery" (editorial), *Washington Times*, 10 March 1988, p. F2.

70. George F. Will, "AIDS: The Real Danger," *Washington Post*, 7 June 1987, p. B7.

71. James J. Kilpatrick, "Aren't We Overreacting to AIDS?" *Washington Post*, 9 June 1988, p. A19.

72. Charles Krauthammer, "AIDS Hysteria," *New Republic* 197 (14, iss. 3,794 [5 October 1987]): 18.

73. Patrick Buchanan, "Turning on the Messenger," *Washington Times*, 9 November 1988, p. F1.

74. "Crossfire," CNN, 11 November 1987.

75. See, for example, "Who Gets the Fast Track?" *Wall Street Journal*, 30 January 1987, p. 22; "A New Era for Drugs," *Wall Street Journal*, 13 March 1987, p. 24; "First Do No Harm," *Wall Street Journal*, 21 December 1987, p. 20.

76. "Will the FDA Die of AIDS?" *National Review* 38 (5 [28 March 1986]): 23.

77. Ronald C. Docksi, "Department of Health and Human Services," in *Mandate for Leadership III: Policy Strategies for the 1990s*, ed. by Charles L. Heatherly and Burton Y. Pines (Washington, D.C.: Heritage Foundation, 1989), pp. 247–48.

78. Ferguson, "Count Me Out," p. 9.

Chapter 14. The Homosexual Lobby

1. Leviticus 18:22: "You shall not lie with a male as one lies with a female; it is an abomination." Leviticus 20:13 "If there is a man who lies with a male as those who lie with a woman, both of them have committed a detestable act; they shall surely be put to death."

2. Dennis Altman, *AIDS in the Mind of America* (Garden City, N.Y.: Anchor/Doubleday, 1986), p. 143.

3. Dennis Altman, *The Homosexualization of America* (New York: St. Martin's Press, 1982), p. 17.

4. Ibid., p. 79.

5. Altman, *AIDS in the Mind of America*, p. 144.

6. Randy Shilts, *And the Band Played On* (New York: St. Martin's Press, 1987), p. 40.

7. "St. Louis Youth's Death in 1969 Linked to AIDS," *Washington Post*, 25 October 1987, p. A6; Christine Gorman et al., "Strange Trip Back to the Future," *Time* 130 (19 [9 November 1987]): 83.

8. See Philip Ziegler, *The Black Death* (New York: John Day, 1969), p. 82.

9. See Susan Sontag, *Illness as Metaphor* (New York: Farrar, Straus & Giroux, 1978),

p. 14, and generally for a discussion of physical manifestations of disease and perceptions caused thereby.

10. Richard Goldstein, "State of Emergency," *Village Voice* 32 (26 [30 June 1987]): 21.

11. See Altman, *AIDS in the Mind of America,* p. 96.

12. Max Navarre, "PWA Coalition," *October* 43 (Winter 1987): 163.

13. See Jan Zita Grover, "AIDS: Keywords," *October* 43 (Winter 1987): 20.

14. See Ibid., p. 26.

15. National Association of People with AIDS, "Statement of Purpose," September 1986, on file at headquarters of NAPWA, Washington, D.C.

16. Navarre, "PWA Coalition," pp. 149–50.

17. Altman, *AIDS in the Mind of America,* pp. 118–19.

18. Ibid., p. 175.

19. Ibid., p. 176.

20. Ian Young, "Prescription for Suicide," *New York Native* 8 (40, iss. 282 [12 September 1988]): 18.

21. David Black, *The Plague Years* (New York: Simon & Schuster, 1986), p. 40.

22. Renée Sabatier, *Blaming Others* (Philadelphia: New Society, 1988), p. 47.

23. Larry Kramer, "1,112 and Counting," *New York Native* 3 (8, iss. 59 [14–27 March 1983]): 19.

24. "Kaposi's Sarcoma and Related Opportunistic Infection," hearings before House of Representatives Subcommittee on Health and the Environment, 13 April 1982, p. 2, as cited in Altman, *AIDS in the Mind of America,* p. 113.

25. See, generally, Shilts, *And the Band Played On.*

26. David A. Noebel et al., *AIDS,* 2d ed, p. 92 (Manitou Springs, Colo.: Summit Ministries, 1987), citing *Dallas Gay News,* 20 May 1983.

27. See Richard Cohen, "Falwell's Hate Mailing," *Washington Post,* 1 May 1987, p. A23.

28. Personal communication with Randy Shilts.

29. See Susan Sontag, "AIDS and its Metaphors," *New York Review of Books* 35 (16 [27 October 1988]): 89.

30. Robert S. Gottfried, *The Black Death* (New York: Free Press, 1983), p. 159.

31. Dorothy Nelkin and Sander L. Gilman, "Placing Blame for Devastating Disease," *Social Research* 55 (3 [Autumn 1988]): 365.

32. John Adams Wettergreen, "AIDS, Public Morality, and Public Health," *Claremont Review of Books* 4 (3 [Fall 1985]): 3.

33. Peter M. Nardi, "Attacks on 'AIDS, Public Morality, and Public Health' " (letter), *Claremont Review of Books* 4 (4 [Winter 1985]): 25, making reference to Harry Nelson and Robert Steinbrook, "Drug Users—Not Gays—Called First AIDS Victims," *Los Angeles Times,* 18 October 1985, p. 1.

34. Nelson and Steinbrook, "Drug Users—Not Gays," p. 35.

35. George E. Demetrakopoulos, "A Lesson from Greece," *New York Native* 3 (16, iss. 67 [4–17 July 1983]): 23.

36. For more on homosexuals blaming Haitians, see Robert Bazell, "The History of an Epidemic," *New Republic* 189 (5, iss. 3576 [1 August 1983]): 14.

37. Arthur F. Ide, *AIDS Hysteria* (Dallas: Monument Press, 1986), p. 52.

38. Arthur F. Ide, *Gomorrah and the Rise of Homophobia* (Las Colinas, Tex.: 1985).

39. Arthur F. Ide, *City of Sodom and Homosexuality in Western Religious Thought to 630 CE* (Dallas: Monument Press, 1988).

40. Altman, *AIDS in the Mind of America,* p. 174.

41. Lee Oliver, "AIDS and the Heterosexual Myth: The Scapegoating of the Gay Male Population," *New York Native* 5 (25, iss. 128 [30 September–6 October 1985]): 27.

42. Ibid., p. 28.

43. Robert E. Fay et al., "Prevalence and Patterns of Same-Gender Sexual Contact Among Men," *Science* 243 (4889 [20 January 1989]): 346.

44. Oliver, "AIDS and the Heterosexual Myth," p. 27.

45. George F. Will, "AIDS: The Real Danger," *Washington Post,* 7 June 1987, p. B7.

46. Neil Ravin, "AIDS: Mr. Will's Idle Speculations" (letter), *Washington Post,* 15 June 1987, p. A12.

47. "Kilpatrick on AIDS: 'Downright Meanness' " (letters), *Washington Post*, 18 June 1988, p. A21 (letters of Andrew D. Lautman, Garrett Lagnese, and Jeffrey S. Akman, in that order).

48. Testimony of Robert Kunst before United States Commission on Civil Rights (USCCR), 18 May 1988, draft at 916 (on file in the office of the General Counsel).

49. *The Weekly News* (Dade County, Fla.), advertisement, 27 January 1988, p. 18.

50. Cure AIDS Now, one-page promotional sheet.

51. Ibid.

52. Testimony before USCCR, p. 914.

53. U.S. Government Accounting Office, "AIDS: Information on Global Dimensions and Possible Impacts," October 1987, p. 10.

54. Cure AIDS Now, three-page promotional sheet, p. 1.

55. Ibid., p. 1.

56. Cure AIDS Now, one-page promotional sheet.

57. See, for example, Robert Kunst, "Testimony Before U.S. Commission on Civil Rights" (handout), 18 May 1988 (on file with the office of the General Counsel).

58. "Lottery Could Net $50 million for AIDS Study, Advocate Says," *Tampa Tribune*, 2 April 1988, p. 8B.

59. Bruce Lambert, "New York Called Unprepared on AIDS," *New York Times*, 14 July 1988, p. B1.

60. Ibid.

61. Ibid., p. B9.

62. Ibid.

63. Ibid.

64. Personal communication with Rand Stoneburner, and remarks by Mayor Edward I. Koch on Pediatric AIDS before the House Select Committee on Narcotics Abuse and Control, 27 July 1987, p. 8.

65. "Health Department Cuts in Half Estimate of HIV Infection in New York City," *The AIDS Record* 2 (14 [23 July, 1988]): 4.

66. Ibid.

67. Ibid.

68. Donna Minkowitz and John Soeder, "Police Probe ACT UP," *Village Voice* 33 (42 [18 October 1988]): 25.

69. See Rick Shur, "ACT-UP Demands Joseph's Removal," *New York Native* 9 (36, iss. 278 [15 August 1988]): 6.

70. *New York Native* 8 (37, iss. 279 [22 August 1988]): cover.

71. Bruce Lambert, "Halving of Estimate of AIDS is Raising Doubts in New York," *New York Times*, 20 July 1988, p. B4.

72. Alfred C. Kinsey, Wardell Pomeroy, and Clyde E. Martin, *Sexual Behavior in the Human Male* (Philadelphia: W. B. Saunders, 1948).

73. See, for example, testimony of Virginia M. Apuzzo, Subcommittee on Intergovernmental Relations and Human Resources, U.S. House of Representatives, 1 August 1983.

74. Julie Johnson, "Homosexual Groups and the Politics of AIDS," *New York Times*, 6 October 1988, p. B16.

75. Kinsey et al., *Sexual Behavior in the Human Male*, p. 651.

76. Ibid.

77. Fay et al., "Prevalence and Patterns," pp. 346–47.

78. Alfred C. Kinsey et al., *Sexual Behavior in the Human Female* (Philadelphia: W. B. Saunders, 1953), p. 474.

79. CDC, "HIV Infection in the United States: A Review of Current Knowledge," *MMWR* 36 (S-6 [18 December 1987]): 21 (table 1).

80. Patrick J. Buchanan, "Did Kinsey Cook His Figures?" *Washington Times*, 19 September 1988, p. F1.

81. New York City Department of Health, "Estimate of HIV-Infected New Yorkers" (working paper), July 1988, p. 7 (available from the Office of Public Affairs).

82. Ibid., pp. 7–8.

83. Ibid., p. 3.

84. Patrick J. Buchanan, "Turning on the Messenger," *Washington Times,* 9 November 1988, p. F4.

85. Bruce Lambert, "New Estimate Leaves Scars on AIDS Fight 'Partnership,' " *New York Times,* 21 July 1988, p. B2; see also Bruce Lambert, "Halving of Estimate on AIDS Is Raising Doubts in New York," *New York Times,* 20 July 1988, p. B4.

86. Heidi Evans, "State Won't Buy AIDS Cut," *New York Daily News,* 15 August 1988, p. 13.

87. Bruce Lambert, "Unabated Rise in AIDS Seen for New York," *New York Times,* 7 December 1988, p. B1.

88. Robert E. Gould, "Reassuring News About AIDS," *Cosmopolitan* 204 (1 [January 1988]): 146.

89. Donna Minkowitz, "Women Picket *Cosmopolitan* Magazine," *The Guardian* (New York) 4 (17 [27 January 1988]): 4.

90. Arthur S. Leonard, "On the Need for a Realistic View of the Epidemic," *New York Native,* 20 July 1987, p. 22.

91. Ibid., p. 23.

92. "Disturbing New AIDS Study," "Nightline," transcript of 13 January 1988, pp. 5–6.

93. Leo Bersani, "Is the Rectum a Grave?" *October* 43 (Winter 1987): 202–3.

94. Geoffrey Marks and William K. Beatty, *Epidemics* (New York: Charles Scribner's Sons, 1976), pp. 89–91.

95. National Gay and Lesbian Task Force, "Anti-Gay Violence, Victimization and Defamation in 1987," available from NGLTF, 1517 U Street, N.W., Washington, D.C. 20009.

96. Laurence Zuckerman, "Open Season on Gays," *Time* 131 (10 [7 March 1988]): 24.

97. House Committee on the Judiciary, Subcommittee on Criminal Justice, *Anti-gay Violence,* 99th Congress, 2nd sess., 9 October 1986, p. 43.

98. Ruben Rosario, "AIDS Spurs Gay Attacks," *New York Daily News,* 16 February 1986, p. 31.

99. Ibid.

100. Ibid.

101. Subcommittee on Criminal Justice, *Anti-gay Violence,* p. 43.

102. Ibid., pp. 7–8.

103. Ibid., p. 7.

104. D. Keith Mano, "Arresting Gays," *National Review* 40 (21 [28 October 1988]): 57.

105. James I. Slaff and John K. Brubaker, *The AIDS Epidemic* (New York: Warner, 1985), p. 146.

106. Kathleen McAuliffe et al., "AIDS: At the Dawn of Fear," *U.S. News* 102 (2 [12 January 1987]): 62.

Chapter 15. AIDS Goes to Hollywood

1. Allan M. Brandt, *No Magic Bullet: A Social History of Venereal Disease in the United States Since 1880* (Oxford and New York: Oxford University Press, 1985), p. 47.

2. "Mixed Messages About AIDS," clip shown on "Nightline," transcript of 21 January 1988, p. 2.

3. Ibid.

4. Universal Studios, *Casual Sex?* Genevieve Robert, director, 1988.

5. Peter Biskind, "The Big Chill," *Premiere* 2 (1 [September 1988]): 60.

6. Ibid.

7. Ibid., p. 62.

8. Radio bite, 1 November 1988.

9. Biskind, "The Big Chill," p. 62.

10. John M. Wilson, "Cinema's New Rules About Sex," *Washington Post,* 30 August 1987, p. G1.

11. Biskind, "The Big Chill," p. 62.

12. Wilson, "Cinema's New Rules," p. G1.

13. Bob Mondello, "Rewriting the Script: From Broadway to Hollywood," *Washington Post,* 29 December 1987, p. H11.

14. "Killing All the Right People," "Designing Women," 5 October 1987, Harry Thomason, director, Linda Bloodworth-Thomason, producer.

15. "Women and AIDS," "Geraldo," transcript of 27 June 1988, p. 2.

16. "Killing All the Right People," "Designing Women."

17. Matt Roush, "A Tiptop Topical 'Women,' " *USA Today,* 27 June 1988, p. D3.

18. Ibid.

19. "Three Series' Episodes to Deal with AIDS," AP, 22 January 1986.

20. C. Wallace, "Charmin' Harmon," *People* 25 (4 [27 January 1986]): 46–48.

21. "Family Feud," "St. Elsewhere," 29 January 1986, Mark Tinker, director, Bruce Paltrow, executive producer.

22. Sandy Rovner, "Can AIDS Travel from Women to Men?" *Washington Post,* 8 January 1986, p. H11.

23. "After It Happened," "Midnight Caller," 13 December 1988, Robert Singer, producer.

24. Matt Roush, "A Tense AIDS Drama," *USA Today,* 13 December 1988, p. 3D.

25. John M. Wilson, "Cinema's New Rules," p. G1.

26. Ibid.

27. "AIDS and Hollywood," "Nightline," transcript of 19 September 1985, p. 4.

28. Ibid., p. 5.

29. "AIDS Scare Rocks Rambo," *Globe* 35 (28 [12 July 1988]): 9.

30. "New AIDS Terror Hits Stars," *Globe* 35 (41 [11 October 1988]): 8.

31. Personal communication with Tony Miles, *Globe.*

32. Mary Murphy, "The AIDS Scare," *TV Guide* 36 (43, iss. 1856 [22 October 1988]): 5.

33. Ibid., p. 9.

34. Eloise Salholz with Peter McAlevey, "AIDS: Hollywood Jitters," *Newsweek* 106 (9 [26 August 1985]): 73.

35. Jared Rutter, "John Holmes: The Man Behind the Myth," *High Society,* September 1988, p. 42.

36. Ibid., p. 43.

37. Robert W. Stewart, "Holmes Told Author He Never Knew Killers' Identities," *Los Angeles Times,* 15 March 1988, pt. 2, p. 3.

38. Chuck Conconi, "Personalities," *Washington Post,* 17 March 1988, p. D3.

39. "Porn Star Holmes Died of AIDS," *USA Today,* 8 March 1988, p. 5A.

40. Jim Zarroli, "Porn After AIDS," *Seven Days* 2 (9 [8 March 1989]): 17. Zarroli notes that one of the men Holmes had sex with on film died of AIDS.

41. Charlie Airwaves, "Porn Star Spotlight: Kascha," *High Society,* September 1988, p. 27.

42. "Porn Star Spotlight: Barbara Dare," *High Society,* June 1987, p. 33.

43. John Paone, "Porn Star Spotlight: Angela Baron," *High Society,* December 1987, p. 26.

44. Charlie Airwaves, "Porn Star Spotlight: Angel Kelly," *High Society,* July 1988, p. 35.

45. John Paone, "Porn Star Spotlight: Sheri St. Clair," *High Society,* November 1987, p. 35.

46. "Porn Star Spotlight: Krista Lane," *High Society,* July 1987, p. 33.

47. "Meet Missy, Republican Porn Star!" *Playboy* 34 (1 [January 1987]): 178.

48. Ibid.

49. Katie Leishman, "Heterosexuals and AIDS," *Atlantic* 259 (2 [February 1987]): 58.

50. Ibid.

51. *AIDS: Changing the Rules,* AIDS Film Productions, 1987, John Hoffman and Franklin Getchalt, producers.

52. Ibid.

53. Mickey Kaus et al., "The 'Small Health Problem' of AIDS," *Newsweek* 110 (2 [13 July 1987]): 46.

54. "AIDS: Changing the Rules," *Washington Post,* 12 November 1987, p. A22.
55. Edward M. Levine, "How the Gay Lobby Has Changed Television," *TV Guide* 29 (22 [30 May 1981]): 3.
56. Ibid., p. 6.

Chapter 16. The Death of the Sexual Revolution (Again)

1. David Gelman et al., "The Social Fallout from an Epidemic," *Newsweek* 106 (7 [12 August 1985]): 29.
2. Edward Cornish, "Farewell, Sexual Revolution. Hello, New Victorianism," *Futurist* 20 (1 [January–February 1986]): 48.
3. "Modern Love," "Geraldo," transcript of 1 December 1987, p. 2.
4. Martha Smilgis et al., "The Big Chill: Fear of AIDS," *Time* 129 (7 [16 February 1987]): 50.
5. Ibid., p. 51.
6. "A Current Affair," Fox TV, transcript of 9 January 1989.
7. "Scared Sexless," NBC, transcript of 30 December 1987, p. 1.
8. Ibid., p. 13.
9. Edwin Diamond and Alan Mahoney, "Once it was 'Harvest of Shame'—Now We Get 'Scared Sexless,' " *TV Guide* 36 (35 [27 August 1988]): 6.
10. "Spread of AIDS May Send Sex Mores Back to the '50s," *Washington Times,* 21 April 1986, p. A4.
11. Tom Kelly, "For Many Singles, the Party Is Over," *Washington Times,* 7 October 1987, p. E1.
12. Ed Foster-Simeon, "Looking for Love in the Era of AIDS," *Washington Times,* 7 October 1987, p. E1.
13. Lucy Schulte, "The New Dating Game," *New York* 19 (9 [3 March 1986]): 94.
14. William K. Stevens, "Fear of AIDS Brings Explicit Advice to Campus, Caution to Singles Bar," *New York Times,* 17 February 1987, p. A21.
15. "Dating in the '80s; Do Services Work?" *USA Today,* 16 November 1988, p. 4D.
16. Karen S. Peterson and Christopher Farley, "But Singles Like Their Freedom," *USA Today,* November 16, 1988, p. 1D.
17. William H. Masters, Virginia E. Johnson, and Robert C. Kolodny, *Crisis: Heterosexual Behavior in the Age of AIDS* (New York: Grove, 1988), p. 50.
18. Ibid., p. 133.
19. CDC, "Number of Sex Partners and Potential Risk of Sexual Exposure to Human Immunodeficiency Virus," *MMWR* 37 (37 [23 September 1988]): 565–68.
20. Roy M. Anderson and Robert M. May, "Epidemiological Parameters of HIV Transmission," *Nature* 333 (6173 [9 June 1988]): 516, citing AIDS Advertising Campaign, Report on Four Surveys During the First Year of Advertising 1986–87 (British Market Research Bureau, London).
21. Morton Hunt, *Sexual Behavior in the 1970s* (Chicago: Playboy, 1974), p. 152.
22. Ibid., p. 154.
23. Ibid., pp. 154–55.
24. Marilyn Elias, "Safe Sex and the Heterosexual," *USA Today,* 3 November 1987, p. 2D, quoting the psychologist Jerome Sherman, a regular on ABC's "Good Morning Houston."
25. Foster-Simeon, "Looking for Love," p. E1.
26. "AIDS: A National Town Meeting," "Nightline," transcript of 5 October 1987, p. 17.
27. Cal Thomas, "AIDS Week and the Politics of AIDS," *Washington Times,* 11 June 1987, p. D3.
28. Harold W. Jaffe et al., "National Case Control Study of Kaposi's Sarcoma and *Pneumocystis Carinii* Pneumonia in Homosexual Men: Part 1, Epidemiological Results," *Annals of Internal Medicine* 99 (2 [August 1983]): 146.

29. David Black, *The Plague Years* (New York: Simon & Schuster, 1986), p. 183.

30. See Randy Shilts, *And the Band Played On* (New York: St. Martin's Press, 1987), p. 19.

31. See, generally, Shilts, *And the Band Played On.*

32. Dennis Altman, *The Homosexualization of America* (New York: St. Martin's Press, 1982), p. 79.

33. Leo Bersani, "Is the Rectum a Grave?" *October* 43 (Winter 1987): 206.

34. John L. Martin, Marc A. Garcia, and Sara T. Beatrice, "Sexual Behavior Changes and HIV Antibody in a Cohort of New York City Gay Men," *AJPH* 79 (4 [April 1989]): 502. Twenty percent of the group continued to engage in anal receptive intercourse without a condom.

35. Linda Murray, "Straight Facts About Straight Sex" *Penthouse* 20 (1 [September 1988]): 206.

36. John Leo and Maureen Dowd, "The New Scarlet Letter," *Time* 120 (5 [2 August 1982]): 66.

Chapter 17. Lies, Damned Lies, and Statistics

1. Marlene Cimons, "Heterosexual AIDS Warning Issued," *Los Angeles Times,* 15 December 1987, p. 20.

2. Jean Seligmann et al., "The AIDS Epidemic," *Newsweek* 101 (16 [18 April 1983]): 74.

3. *Life* 8 (8 [July 1985]): cover.

4. Matt Clark et al., "AIDS," *Newsweek* 106 (7 [12 August 1985]): 20.

5. Claudia Wallis et al., "AIDS: A Growing Threat," *Time* 126 (6 [12 August 1985]): 40.

6. Tom Morgenthau et al., "The AIDS Epidemic: Future Shock," *Newsweek* 108 (21 [24 November 1986]): 31.

7. Kathleen McAuliffe et al., "AIDS: At the Dawn of Fear," *U.S. News & World Report* 102 (2 [12 January 1987]): 60.

8. Martha Smilgis et al., "The Big Chill: Fear of AIDS," *Time* 129 (7 [16 February 1987]): 50.

9. Joseph Carey et al., "AIDS: A Time of Testing," *U.S. News* 102 (15 [20 April 1987]): 56.

10. Michael Kramer, "Facing Life in the AIDies," *U.S. News* 102 (23 [15 June 1987]): 13.

11. Some examples from William Check: "Beyond the Political Model of Reporting: Nonspecific Symptoms in Media Communication About AIDS," *Reviews of Infectious Diseases* 9 (5 [September–October 1987]): 989; J. E. Bishop, "Lethal New Ailment Claims Another Group of Victims: Children," *Wall Street Journal,* 10 December 1982, p. 1; "First it killed gay men. Then drug addicts. Now children are dying, and some medical investigators fear the disease could spread through the nation's blood banks." S. West, "One Step Behind a Killer," *Science* 83, March 1983, p. 36. "AIDS began as the 'Gay Plague.' Now it has spread beyond that community and become America's deadliest epidemic." B. D. Colen, "Is There Death After Sex?" *Rolling Stone,* 3 February 1983, p. 17; C. Wallis, "Battling a Deadly New Epidemic: Some Experts Feel AIDS Will Strike Beyond the Gay Community," *Time* 121 (13 [28 March 1983]): 53.

12. For an at-length discussion of the furor over the Fauci statement, see Randy Shilts, *And the Band Played On* (New York: St. Martin's Press, 1987), pp. 299–301.

13. William Check, "Beyond the Political Model," p. 990.

14. David Black, *The Plague Years* (New York: Simon & Schuster, 1986), p. 191.

15. Marlise Simons, "For Haiti's Tourism, the Stigma of AIDS is Fatal," *New York Times,* 29 November 1983, p. A2. See also Joseph B. Treaster, "Haiti's Hotels Hit Hard as Tourists Shun Island," *New York Times,* 11 October 1984, p. 14.

16. Simons, "Haiti's Tourism," p. 62.

17. Quoted in Black, *Plague Years,* p. 62.

18. See Joe Dolce, "The Politics of Fear: Haitians and AIDS," *New York Native* 3 (8, iss. 16 [1–27 August 1983]): 16.

19. See Dennis Altman, *AIDS in the Mind of America* (New York: Anchor/Doubleday, 1986), p. 72.

20. "Haitians Removed from AIDS Risk List," *New York Times,* 10 April 1985, p. A13.

21. W. Meade Morgan and James W. Curran, "Acquired Immunodeficiency Syndrome: Current and Future Trends," *Public Health Reports* 101 (5 [September–October 1986]): 462.

22. Ibid.

23. Ibid., p. 464.

24. "Coolfont Report: A PHS Plan for Prevention and Control of AIDS and the AIDS Virus," *Public Health Reports* 101 (4 [July–August 1986]): 343.

25. Personal communication with W. Meade Morgan.

26. Ibid.

27. Helen Singer Kaplan, *The Real Truth About Women and AIDS* (New York: Fireside, 1987), p. 27.

28. Chris Norwood, *Advice for Life: A Woman's Guide to AIDS Risks and Prevention* (New York: Pantheon, 1987), p. 145.

29. "Infection Will Spread Outside High-Risk Groups," *USA Today,* 16 July 1988, p. 4D.

30. "AIDS: Deadly but Hard to Catch," *Consumer Reports* 51 (11 [November 1985]): 726.

31. Margaret Engel, "Newslines from Washington," *Glamour* 86 (1 [January 1987]): 110.

32. "AIDS Goes from Bad to Worse," *U.S. News* 100 (24 [23 June 1986]): 8.

33. Kathleen McAuliffe, "AIDS and 'Straights': Unsettling Questions?" *U.S. News* 103 (7 [17 August 1987]): 34.

34. "Cases Rising Fastest Among Heterosexuals," *USA Today,* 1 June 1987, p. 6D.

35. Lucille Beachy, "In the Shadow of AIDS," *Savvy* (June 1987): 58.

36. Philip J. Hilts, "Data Shows AIDS Risk is Widening; Increase in Cases Among Heterosexuals Is Causing Concern," *Washington Post,* 21 October 1986, p. A1.

37. Andrea Rock, "What You Don't Know About AIDS But Should," *Money* 16 (12 [November 1987]): 96.

38. Lee Siegel, "Fear of AIDS Spreads among Heterosexuals," AP, 6 April 1987.

39. Niki Cervantes, "Women Stampeding AIDS-testing Clinics," UPI, 13 March 1987. The reporter used the same figures four days later in "County Agrees to Open Two More AIDS Testing Centers," UPI, 17 March 1987.

40. Tom Morgenthau et al., "Future Shock," p. 31.

41. Mickey Kaus et al., "The 'Small Health Problem' of AIDS," *Newsweek* 110 (2 [13 July 1987]): 46.

42. Dave Carpenter, "Debate over Contacting AIDS Victims' Partners," AP, 8 March 1987.

43. Myron Brenton, "What Every Woman *Must* Know About Condoms," *Cosmopolitan* 202 (5 [May 1987]): 108.

44. Michael A. Fumento, "AIDS: Are Heterosexuals at Risk?" *Commentary* 84 (5 [November 1987]): 21.

45. Jennet Conant, "The Fashionable Charity," *Newsweek* 110 (26 [28 December 1987]): 54–55.

46. "The Facts About Straight Sex and AIDS" (interview with Randy Shilts), *Village Voice* 33 (8 [23 February 1988]): 21.

47. Judy Ismach, "What Can We Believe?" *American Health* 7 (5 [June 1988]): 53.

48. Susan J. Blumenthal, "Women's Health: A Medical Update," *McCall's* 115 (6 [March 1988]): 88.

49. Katie Leishman, reply in *Atlantic* 260 (4 [October 1987]): 10.

50. Katie Leishman, "Heterosexuals and AIDS," *Atlantic* 259 (2 [February 1987]): 40.

51. Ed Sikov, "Media Watch," *New York Native* 7 (13, iss. 203 [9 March 1987]): 24.

52. "Heterosexual AIDS: Horror or Hoax?" "Geraldo," transcript of 1 December 1987, p. 5.

53. Ibid., p. 6.

54. "Surgeon General C. Everett Koop Forecasts the Death Toll from AIDS: 170,000 Americans in Just Four Years," *People Weekly* 27 (11 [16 March 1987]): 44. For virtually identical wording, see speech before the NAACP in New York City on 8 July 1987,

transcript p. 7; Kathy Sawyer, "No AIDS Vaccine Seen Before 2000," *Washington Post*, 30 March 1987, p. A5 (quoting from CBS News's "Face the Nation." The "ninefold, twentyfold" language was also repeated in "America's Number One Health Threat" (interview with C. Everett Koop), *American Legion Magazine* 123 (2 [August 1987]): 40.

55. "Surgeon General C. Everett Koop Forecasts," p. 44.

56. Otis R. Bowen, "The War Against AIDS," *Journal of Medical Education* 62 (7 [July 1987]): 544.

57. See transcript of debate in *New York Times*, 14 October 1988, p. A15.

58. "This Week with David Brinkley," transcript of 15 February 1987, p. 2. How much of the confusion over the alleged rise in the heterosexual percentage due to Fauci is unknown. Among references to it is: Kaplan, *Real Truth About Women and AIDS*, p. 27 (Dr. Anthony Fauci . . . commenting on the rapidly rising rate of heterosexual transmission, estimated that "we expect 10 percent of U.S. AIDS cases to be heterosexually transmitted by 1991"), citing *Scientific References, Group I: The Epidemiology of AIDS*.

59. Ann V. Bollinger, "N.Y. Women Face Greatest AIDS Risk," *New York Post*, 3 June 1987, p. 14.

60. Lawrence K. Altman, "AIDS Expert Sees No Sign of Heterosexual Outbreak," *New York Times*, 5 June 1987, p. A17.

61. William A. Check, "Public Education on AIDS: Not Only the Media's Responsibility," *Hasting Center Report* (special supplement) 15 (4 [August 1985]): 31.

62. Smilgis et al., "Big Chill," p. 51.

63. McAuliffe, "AIDS and 'Straights,'" p. 34.

64. U.S. Department of Health and Human Services, PHS, "Surgeon General's Report on AIDS," 1986, p. 15.

65. See, "Changing Patterns of Groups at High Risk for Hepatitis B in the United States" (leads from the *MMWR*), *JAMA* 260 (6 [12 August 1988]): 761.

66. Ibid., p. 765.

67. See Fred Hiatt, "Japan Seeks to Slow Spread of AIDS," *Washington Post*, 14 January 1989, p. A17.

68. See New York City Department of Public Health AIDS Surveillance Unit, "AIDS Surveillance Update," any 1989 issue.

69. CDC, "AIDS Weekly Surveillance Report—United States AIDS Program," 4 January 1989, p. 3.

70. Joseph F. Sullivan, "Jersey and SUNY Centers to Study the AIDS Virus in Heterosexuals," *New York Times*, 16 December 1988, p. A26.

Chapter 18. The Media and the Doctors of Doom

1. New York City Department of Health, AIDS Surveillance Unit, "AIDS Surveillance Update," 25 January 1989, p. 7.

2. Tim Friend, "Children's AIDS Toll May Soar by 1991," *USA Today*, 20 July 1988, p. D1.

3. William A. Check, "Beyond the Political Model of Reporting: Nonspecific Symptoms in Media Communication About AIDS," *Review of Infectious Diseases* 9 (5 [September–October 1987]): 993.

4. John Langone, "AIDS: Special Report," *Discover* 6 (12 [December 1985]): 42.

5. Philip M. Boffey, "Top Health Official and Expert Seek Greater Rise in AIDS Money," *New York Times*, 27 September 1985, p. A16.

6. Ibid.

7. Morton Hunt, "Teaming Up Against AIDS," *New York Times Magazine*, 2 March 1986, p. 42.

8. Helen Mathews Smith, "AIDS: Lessons from History," *MD* 30 (9 [September 1986]): 47.

9. Senate Hearing Committee on Appropriations, *Special Hearing, Health and Human Services*, 99th Cong., 1st sess., 26 September 1985, p. 170.

10. Ibid., p. 172.

11. Ibid., p. 170.

12. Ibid., p. 180.

13. Ibid., p. 181.

14. Ibid., p. 204.

15. Ibid., p. 214.

16. Ibid.

17. Ibid.

18. Joyce Price, "Researchers Suggest 'Manhattan Project' to Fight the AIDS Virus," *Washington Times,* 2 September 1987, p. B8.

19. Margaret Engel, "Prostitutes Transmitting AIDS to U.S. Soldiers," *Washington Post,* 27 September 1985, p. A20.

20. See, for example, William A. Check, "Heterosexual AIDS Risk Studied," *Washington Post,* p. A7. For other criticism of Haseltine's assertion on this point, and Haseltine's reply, see James M. James, Michael A. Morgenstern, and John A. Hatten, "HTLV-III/LAV-Antibody-Positive Soldiers in Berlin" (letter), *NEJM* 314 (1 [2 January 1986]): 55–56.

21. Check, "Beyond the Political Model," 993.

22. Ibid., citing personal communication.

23. Robert Redfield et al., "Frequent Transmission of HTLV-III Among Spouses of Patients with AIDS-Related Complex and AIDS," *JAMA* 253 (11 [15 March 1986]): 1571–73.

24. Check, "Heterosexual AIDS Risk Studied," p. A7.

25. T. Morgenthau et al., "The AIDS Epidemic: Future Shock," *Newsweek* 108 (21 [24 November 1986]): 31.

26. Ibid., pp. 30–39.

27. Robert R. Redfield, Testimony for Republican Leadership Task Force on Health Care, 10 June 1987 (chairman Representative William Gradison, R-Ohio), transcript, p. 17.

28. Philip J. Hilts, "The Advocate for AIDS Testing," *Washington Post,* 27 December 1986, p. C3.

29. Susan Okie, "AIDS Virus Rate Stable for U.S. Recruits," *Washington Post,* 15 May 1987, p. A1.

30. Ibid.

31. William A. Check, "Public Education on AIDS: Not Only the Media's Responsibility," *Hastings Center Report* (special supplement) 15 (4 [August 1985]): 31.

32. Personal communication with William Check.

33. Ann Guidici Fettner, "The Truth Hurts: *Playboy*'s AIDS Philosophy," *New York Native* 6 (6, iss. 164 [9 June 1986]): 20–21.

34. Ann Guidici Fettner, "The Facts About Straight Sex and AIDS," *Village Voice,* 33 (8 [23 February 1988]): 21.

35. For a breakdown on how often and why needlesticks occur, see Janine Jagger et al., "Rates of Needle-Stick Injury Caused by Various Devices in a University Hospital," *NEJM* 319 (5 [4 August 1988]): 284–88.

36. L.B. Seeff et al., "Type B Hepatitis after Needle-Stick Exposure: Prevention with Hepatitis B Immune Globulin," *Annals of Internal Medicine* 88 (3 [March 1978]): 290; Barbara G. Werner and George F. Grady, "Accidental Hepatitis B Surface-Antigen-Positive Inoculations," *Annals of Internal Medicine* 97 (3 [September 1982]): 368.

37. Paul Raeburn, "AIDS Shows Signs of Spreading to General Population, Researchers Say," AP, 17 April 1985.

38. Robert Byrd, "AIDS Researchers Say 'High-Risk' Designation Becoming Obsolete," AP, 20 February 1987.

39. See, for example, Charles S. Taylor, "AIDS Spread Among Heterosexuals," UPI, 20 February 1987.

40. See William H. Foege, "Plagues: Perceptions of Risk and Social Responses," *Social Research* 55 (3 [Autumn 1988]): 339.

41. "AIDS and Heterosexuals: A Leading Expert Evaluates the Risks" (interview with Max Essex), *Washington Post,* 24 February 1987, p. H9.

42. Richard Stengel et al., "Testing Dilemma," *Time* 129 (23 [8 June 1987]): 21.

43. William H. Masters, Virginia E. Johnson, and Robert C. Kolodny, *Crisis: Heterosexual Behavior in the Age of AIDS* (New York: Grove, 1988), p. 7.

44. Michael Specter, "Heterosexual AIDS Study Denounced," *Washington Post,* 8 March 1988, p. A3.

45. Linda Murray, "Straight Facts About Straight Sex," *Penthouse* 20 (1 [September 1988]): 96.
46. Michael Specter, "Sex Researchers Warning About Heterosexual AIDS," *Washington Post*, 6 March 1988, p. A3.
47. Murray, "Straight Facts," p. 94.
48. Kim Painter, "Masters and Johnson Join AIDS Fray," *USA Today*, 7 March 1988, p. D2.
49. John Lofton, "Up to Our Ears in Scientific Peers," *Washington Times*, 16 March 1988, p. F3.
50. "Masters and Johnson and Quackery," *Washington Times*, 10 March 1988, p. F2.
51. Thomas Sowell, "Years to Tell Who's Right," *Washington Times*, 18 March 1988, p. F3.
52. Kevin R. Hopkins and William B. Johnston, *The Incidence of HIV Infection in the United States* (Indianapolis, Ind.: Hudson Institute, 1988).
53. Masters, Johnson, and Kolodny, *Crisis*, p. 56.
54. Ibid., p. 50.
55. Ibid., pp. 162–63.
56. "Questionable New AIDS Book," "Nightline," transcript of 7 March 1988, p. 3.
57. Painter, "Masters and Johnson Join AIDS Fray," p. D2.
58. Masters, Johnson, and Kolodny, *Crisis*, p. 88.
59. Ibid., p. 89.
60. Bernie Zilbergeld and Michael Evans, "The Inadequacy of Masters and Johnson," *Psychology Today* 14 (3 [August 1980]): 29–30.
61. Cynthia Crossen, "Masters Developing AIDS Product for Problem He Warns of in Book," *Wall Street Journal*, 14 March 1988, p. 32.
62. William H. Masters, Virginia E. Johnson, and Robert C. Kolodny, "Sex in the Age of AIDS" (excerpt from *Crisis: Heterosexual Behavior in the Age of AIDS*), *Newsweek* 111 (11 [14 March 1988]): 45.
63. "Firing Line," national release, 22 April 1988.
64. Terence Monmaney, "The AIDS Threat: Who's at Risk?" *Newsweek* 111 (11 [14 March 1988]): 42–44.
65. Alan E. Nourse, "A Doctor Comments on *Crisis,*" *Good Housekeeping* 206 (5 [May 1988]): 266, 274–75.
66. Introduction to William H. Masters, Virginia E. Johnson, and Robert C. Kolodny, "Our Nation's Blood Supply is Not Safe," *Redbook* 171 (2 [June 1988]): 99.
67. Christine Gorman et al., "An Outbreak of Sensationalism?" *Time* 131 (12 [21 March 1988]): 59.
68. Steven Findlay and Joanne Silberner, "What the Press Release Left Out," *U.S. News* 104 (11 [21 March 1988]): 59–60.
69. Steve Findlay, "AIDS is Rising Among Heterosexuals," *USA Today*, 3 June 1987, p. D6.
70. Murray, "Straight Facts," p. 96.

Chapter 19. An Epidemic of Media Hype

1. David Kline, "A Crisis of Mounting AIDS Hysteria," *MacLean's* 96 (31 [1 August 1983]): 8.
2. Kim Painter, "Women's Risk on Upswing," *USA Today*, 7 November 1988, p. D1.
3. "AIDS: The Danger to Heterosexuals," "Nightline," transcript of 22 April 1985, p. 2.
4. "AIDS," "Nightline," transcript of 30 June 1986, p. 2.
5. Address Given by C. Everett Koop, M.D., Surgeon General, U.S. Public Health Service, Department of Health and Human Services, to the NAACP, New York City, 8 July 1987, p. 7.
6. Ibid.
7. Ellen Hale and Kim Painter, "High AIDS Level Found on Campus," *USA Today*, 2 November 1988, p. A1.
8. Ibid.

9. Connie Leslie et al., "Amid the Ivy, Cases of AIDS," *Newsweek* 62 (20 [14 November 1988]): 65.

10. Maggie Mahar, "Pitiless Scourge," *Barron's* 69 (11 [13 March 1989]): 16.

11. "A Scary Little Survey of AIDS on Campus," *U.S. News* 105 (19 [14 November 1988]): 12.

12. See Alfred C. Kinsey, Wardell B. Pomeroy, and Clyde E. Martin, *Sexual Behavior in the Human Male* (Philadelphia: W. B. Saunders, 1948), p. 651.

13. "Could This Be Your Daughter?" "20/20," 17 May 1989.

14. Personal communication with Chuck Fallis, public affairs specialist, CDC, 23 May 1989.

15. Warren E. Leary, "Campus AIDS Survey Finds Threat Is Real but Not Rampant," *New York Times,* 23 May 1989, p. 24.

16. "AIDS Rate on Campus Causes Concern," *Washington Times,* 23 May 1989, p. A6.

17. "Generally, the News Is Not Good," *Newsweek* 111 (26 [27 June 1988]): 46.

18. *World Almanac* (New York: Ballantine, 1986), p. 1377.

19. Paul Raeburn, "Expert Estimates One in 30 Men Middle-Aged and Younger Infected with AIDS," AP, 2 June 1987.

20. Maureen Orth, "Talking to . . . Mathilde Krim," *Vogue* 177 (10 [October 1987]): 246.

21. CDC, "HIV Infection in the United States: A Review of Current Knowledge," *MMWR* 36 (S-6 [18 December 1987]): 40.

22. See Edward M. Brecher, "Straight Sex, AIDS, and the Mixed-up Press," *Columbia Journalism Review* 25 (3 [March–April 1988]): 50.

23. For example, Ann Guidici Fettner, "Women and AIDS," *Health* 18 (11 [November 1986]): 62.

24. Lucille Beachy, "In the Shadow of AIDS," *Savvy,* June 1987, p. 58.

25. Personal communication with Randolph Lockwood, Humane Society of the United States.

26. Personal communication with Arch Stanaland, president of the American Pit Bull Owners Association.

27. "Nightline," transcript of 20 July 1987, show 1607.

28. "Reagan's Program Is Urgently Needed," *USA Today,* 27 April 1984, p. A10.

29. Jay T. Harris, "Lost: 100 Children Every Day," *USA Today,* 27 April 1984, p. A10.

30. *USA Today,* 1 June 1983, p. A10.

31. *USA Today,* 1 May 1985, p. A10.

32. Jeff Riggenbach, "Missing Kids Hysteria Is Terrorizing Families," *USA Today,* 19 July 1985, p. A10.

33. "Missing Need Help; Problem Is No Myth," *USA Today,* 1 May 1985, p. A10.

34. "It's Not Hysteria to Aid Missing Kids," *USA Today,* 19 July 1985, p. A10.

35. Ibid.

36. One wag, connecting the pit bull and AIDS scares, began selling bumper stickers reading "This Car Protected By a Pit Bull with AIDS."

37. Interview with Ruth Savolaine, National Safety Council, Chicago, Illinois.

38. Carol S. Avery "The Love or Life Choice," *Self* 9 (8 [August 1987]): 123, quoting Martha Gross.

39. "The AIDS Story," "Media Monitor" (Center for Media and Public Affairs) 1 (9 [December 1987]): 2.

40. Ibid., p. 3.

41. Ibid., p. 5.

42. Ron Dorfman, "AIDS Coverage: A Mirror of Society," *The Quill* 75 (10 [November 1987]): 16.

43. Gerald Clarke et al., "AIDS: A Growing Threat," *Time* 126 (6 [12 August 1985]): 40.

44. Peter Carlson and Carole Patton, "Fatal, Incurable, and Spreading," *People* 23 (24 [17 June 1985]): 42.

45. David A. Noebel, Paul Cameron, and Wayne C. Lutton, "AIDS Warning," *New American* 3 (2 [19 January 1987]): 11.

46. "The Burks Have AIDS," "60 Minutes," 6 October 1985.

47. "People Are Talking," WWOR Secaucus, N.J., "The AIDS Lie," 3 March 1988.

48. Bruce Lambert, "Unlikely AIDS Sufferer's Message: Even You Can Get It," *New York Times,* 11 March 1989, p. L29.

49. "Could This Be Your Daughter?" "20/20," 17 May 1989.

50. Personal communication with Chuck Fallis, public affairs specialist, CDC, 9 May 1989.

51. Personal communication with public affairs spokeswoman at Ogilvy & Mather, November 1987.

52. "Now That Sex Can Kill You," "20/20," transcript of 12 February 1987, p. 13.

53. Jude Wanniski, *The 1988 Media Guide* (Morristown, N.J.: Polyconomics, 1988), p. 20.

54. Katie Leishman, "Heterosexuals and AIDS," *Atlantic* 259 (2 [February 1987]): 40.

55. See Ann M. Hardy et al., "Review of Death Certificates to Assess Completeness of AIDS Case Reporting," *Public Health Reports* 102 (4 [July–August 1987]): 386–91.

56. Letters to the Editor, *Atlantic* 259 (5 [May 1987]): 12.

57. Leishman, "Heterosexuals and AIDS," pp. 42–43.

58. Ibid., p. 39.

59. Charles Trueheart, "Picks of the Periodical Profession," *Washington Post,* 5 April 1988, p. D7.

60. Hal Quinley, "The New Facts of Life: Heterosexuals and AIDS," *Public Opinion* 11 (1 [May–June 1988]): 53.

61. Charles Truehart, "Of Ignorance & Bliss," *Washington Post,* 20 June 1987, p. E7.

62. "Vivre avec le SIDA," and accompanying short pieces, *Ca M'Interesse* 97 (March 1989): 6. The word "homosexual" did appear once, but only as a means of identifying an AIDS victim in the piece.

63. Holly G. Miller, "Elizabeth Taylor's Crusade Against AIDS," *Saturday Evening Post* 259 (6 [September 1987]): 102.

64. See generally, Peter Braestup, *Big Story* (New York: Anchor/Doubleday, 1978).

65. Timothy Johnson, "AIDS: A New Perspective," "The Health Show," transcript of 13 June 1987, p. 4.

66. Ibid.

67. Betsy Burkhard, "Rockford Hookers Dealing Deadly Virus," *Rockford Register Star,* 13 September 1987, p. A1.

68. "Women Living with AIDS," "Oprah Winfrey Show," transcript of 18 February 1987, p. 2.

69. Ibid., p. 7.

70. Janet Cooke, "Jimmy's World," *Washington Post,* 28 September 1980, p. A1. For more about the Cooke affair, see Thomas Griffith, "The Pulitzer Hoax—Who Can Be Believed?" *Time* 117 (18 [4 May 1981]): 50.

71. Quoted from interviews with reporters in Jay. A. Winsten, "Science and the Media: The Boundaries of Truth," *Health Affairs* (Spring 1985): 5–23, as cited in William A. Check, "Public Education on AIDS: Not Only the Media's Responsibility," *Hastings Center Report* (Special Supplement) 15 (4 [August 1985]): 29.

72. William A. Check, "Beyond the Political Model of Reporting: Nonspecific Symptoms in Media Communication About AIDS," *Reviews of Infectious Diseases* 9 (5 [September–October 1987]): 997.

73. Jonathan Alter, "Skipping Through the News," *Newsweek* 107 (23 [9 June 1986]): p. 85.

74. John Langone, "How to Block a Killer's Path," *Time* 133 (5 [30 January 1989]): 60.

75. Harry W. Haverkos and Robert Edelman, "The Epidemiology of Acquired Immunodeficiency Among Heterosexuals," *JAMA* 260 (13 [7 October 1988]): 1926.

76. Joyce Price, "Blacks Hit Hardest with Heterosexual AIDS Cases," *Washington Times,* 7 October 1988, p. A1.

77. See "Backlash Against Gays Appears to Be Levelling Off," *Gallup Report* 258 (March 1987): 13, indicating 55 percent polled don't favor legalization of consensual homosexual relations.

78. S. Robert Lichter and Stanley Rothman, "Media and Business Elites," *Public Opinion* 4 (5 [October–November 1981]): 44.

79. Linda Murray, "Straight Facts About Straight Sex," *Penthouse* 20 (1 [September 1988]): 96.

80. Helen Singer Kaplan, *The Real Truth About Women and AIDS* (New York: Simon & Schuster, 1987), p. 11.

81. Ibid., p. 12.

82. Ibid., p. 13.

83. "People are Talking," WWOR, Secaucus, N.J., "The AIDS Lie," 3 March 1988.

84. "Modern Love," "Geraldo," transcript of 1 December 1987, pp. 4–5, 12.

85. John Langone, *AIDS: The Facts* (Boston: Little, Brown, 1988), pp. 85–86.

86. John Langone, "AIDS Update: Still No Reason for Hysteria," *Discover* 7 (9 [September 1986]): 30.

87. *Citizen Kane*, RKO Pictures, 1941, Orson Welles director and producer.

Chapter 20. The Terror, Revisited

1. Paula Treichler, "AIDS, Homophobia, and Biomedical Discourse: An Epidemic of Signification," *October* 43 (Winter 1987): 34.

2. John Tierney, "Straight Talk," *Rolling Stone*, iss. 539 (17 November 1988): 125.

3. Ibid., p. 130.

4. Ibid., p. 135.

5. Ibid., p. 137.

6. Michael Crichton, "Panic in the Sheets," *Playboy* 35 (1 [January 1988]): 184.

7. David Black, *The Plague Years* (New York: Simon & Schuster, 1986), pp. 16–17.

8. Walker Percy, *Lost in the Cosmos* (New York: Farrar, Straus & Giroux, 1983), p. 58.

9. John Bartlett, *Bartlett's Familiar Quotations*, ed. Emily Morrison Beck (Boston: Little, Brown, 1980), p. 743 (from *The Malakand Field Force* [1898]).

10. Testimony of Becky Adler, Teen AIDS Hotline, Montgomery County, Md., before the Select Committee on Children, Youth, and Families, House of Representatives, 100th Cong., 1st sess., 18 June 1987, p. 132. A page earlier in the transcript 17-year-old Adler states, "Saving lives gives a feeling of complete satisfaction and is something each of us do with each phone call."

11. Susan Sontag, "AIDS as Metaphor," *New York Review of Books* 35 (16 [27 October 1988]): 98.

12. Caryl S. Avery, "The Love or Life Choice," *Self* 9 (8 [August 1987]): 123.

13. Joseph Hooper, "The Straight Dope," *Seven Days* 1 (6 [4 May 1988]): 8.

14. Rae Corelli et al., "AIDS and Sex," *MacLean's* 100 (35 [31 August 1987]): 33.

15. Chris Norwood, *Advice for Life: A Woman's Guide to AIDS Risks and Prevention* (New York: Pantheon, 1987), p. 151.

16. See Wendell W. Hoffman, "A Campaign of Disinformation," *Christianity Today* 31 (12 [4 September 1987]): 36 (photograph).

17. Hal Quinley, "The New Facts of Life: Heterosexuals and AIDS," *Public Opinion* 11 (1 [May–June 1988]): 54.

18. See CDC, "Number of Sex Partners and Potential Risk of Sexual Exposure to Human Immunodeficiency Virus," *MMWR* 37 (37 [23 September 1988]): 565–68.

19. Quinley, "New Facts of Life," p. 54.

20. William H. Masters, Virginia E. Johnson, and Robert C. Kolodny, *Crisis: Heterosexual Behavior in the Age of AIDS* (New York: Grove, 1988), p. 133.

21. Warren Winkelstein Jr., et al., "Selected Sexual Practices of San Francisco Heterosexual Men and Risk of Infection by the Human Immunodeficiency Virus," *JAMA* 257 (11 [20 March 1987]): 1470–71.

22. Quinley, "New Facts of Life," p. 54.

23. Masters, Johnson, and Kolodny, *Crisis*, p. 133.

24. CDC, "Comparison of Observed and Self-Reported Seat Belt Use Rates—United States," *MMWR* 37 (36 [16 September 1988]): 549–51.

25. Office of Technology Assessment, U.S. Congress, *How Effective Is AIDS Education?* June 1988, p. 62.

26. Joyce Price, "Single Women Don't Say No to Sex Despite AIDS Scare, Report Shows," *Washington Times*, 28 July 1988, p. A1.

Chapter 21. The Incredible Shrinking Epidemic

1. Lawrence K. Altman, "Global Program Aims to Combat AIDS 'Disaster,' " *New York Times*, 21 November 1986, p. A1.

2. Matt Clark et al., "AIDS," *Newsweek* 106 (7 [12 August 1985]): 20.

3. Stephen Jay Gould, "The Terrifying Normalcy of AIDS," *New York Times Magazine*, 19 April 1987, p. 33.

4. Theresa L. Crenshaw, "Survival or Extinction: The Choice is Ours," paper presented to House Subcommittee on Health and the Environment, 10 February 1987.

5. For example, Tom Morgenthau et al., "The AIDS Epidemic: Future Shock," *Newsweek* 108 (21 [24 November 1986]): 31.

6. Senate Hearing Committee on Appropriations, *Special Hearing, Health and Human Services*, 99th Cong., 1st sess., 26 September 1985, p. 204.

7. Susan Okie, "Heterosexual AIDS May Surge, Koop Says," *Washington Post*, 21 April 1987, p. A4.

8. Michael Kramer, "Facing Life in the AIDies," *U.S. News* 102 (23 [15 June 1987]): 13.

9. "Cases Rising Fastest Among Heterosexuals," *USA Today*, 1 June 1987, p. 6D.

10. For example, Diane Richardson, *Women & AIDS* (New York: Methuen, 1988), p. 13. I have been unable to locate the origin of that figure.

11. See, for example, James W. Curran, "The Epidemiology and Prevention of the Acquired Immunodeficiency Syndrome," *Annals of International Medicine* 103 (5 [November 1985]): 657.

12. See Marilyn Chase, "AIDS Is Causing Far More Illness Than the Official Figures Convey," *Wall Street Journal*, 30 May 1986, p. 23.

13. Stanley K. Monteith, "Seriousness of the AIDS Situation," *AIDS Protection* 1 (9 [January 1988]): 5.

14. Curran, "Epidemiology and Prevention," p. 657.

15. William H. Masters, Virginia E. Johnson, and Robert C. Kolodny, *Crisis: Heterosexual Behavior in the Age of AIDS* (New York: Grove, 1988).

16. Ibid., p. 206.

17. David Chilton, *Power in the Blood* (Brentwood, Tenn.: Wolgeman & Hyatt, 1987), p. 6.

18. Wayne Lutton, "Sickness Unto Death," *National Review* 40 (10 [27 May 1988]): 49.

19. See Helen Singer Kaplan, *The Real Truth About Women and AIDS* (New York: Simon & Schuster, 1987), p. 30.

20. Personal communication with Harold Jaffe.

21. A. D. J. Robertson, "The Virulence of AIDS" (letter), *Wall Street Journal*, 31 October 1985, p. 33.

22. W. J. Hamerman et al., "Why is Atlanta CDC Covering Up the AIDS Story?" *Executive Intelligence Review* 12 (38 [27 September 1985]): 52–53, as cited in T. R. Mader, ed., *The Death Sentence of AIDS* (Gillette, Wyo.: Ram Foundation, 1987), p. 104.

23. Mader, *Death Sentence of AIDS*, p. 102. The group was Americans Against AIDS, affiliated with The Conservative Caucus, Inc., based in Vienna, Va. The actual quote was, "AIDS cases are doubling every six months. That's so fast the *Indianapolis Star* said AIDS could kill 262,000,000 Americans by the year 2000. That's more than every single American alive today!"

24. David Black, *The Plague Years* (New York: Simon & Schuster, 1986), p. 16.

25. Allan Parachini and Lynn Simross, "Who Will Pay the Bill for AIDS Treatment?" *Los Angeles Times*, 4 June 1987, sec. V, pp. 8–9.

26. Kevin R. Hopkins and William B. Johnston, *The Incidence of HIV Infection in the United States* (Indianapolis; Ind.: Hudson Institute, 1988). For a full critical review, see Michael Fumento, "The AIDS Numbers Racket: Chapter 37," *National Review* 40 (20 [14 October 1988]): 45.

27. For a critique of Masters, Johnson, and Kolodny's *Crisis: Heterosexual Behavior in the Age of AIDS*, see Michael Fumento, "The AIDS Cookbook," *New Republic* 198 (14, iss. 3820 [4 April 1988]): 19.

28. Robert E. Lee, *AIDS in America: Our Chances, Our Choices* (Troy, Mich.: Whitsit, 1987), p. 99.

29. Gene Antonio, *The AIDS Cover-up?* (San Francisco: Ignatius, 1986), pp. 133–34.

30. Hopkins and Johnston, *Incidence of HIV Infection,* p. 57.

31. Alfred Kinsey, Wardell Pomeroy, and Clyde E. Martin, *Sexual Behavior in the Human Male* (Philadelphia: W. B. Saunders, 1948).

32. Masters, Johnson, and Kolodny, *Crisis,* pp. 3–4.

33. Helen Singer Kaplan, *The Real Truth About Women and AIDS* (New York: Simon & Schuster, 1987), p. 27.

34. See, for example, William L. Heyward and James W. Curran, "The Epidemiology of AIDS in the U.S.," *Scientific American* 259 (4 [October 1988]): 72.

35. CDC, "HIV Infection in the United States: A Review of Current Knowledge," *MMWR* 36 (S–6 [18 December 1987]): 38.

36. Laurene Mascola et al., "HIV Seroprevalence in Intravenous Drug Users: Los Angeles, California, 1986," *AJPH* 79 (1 [January 1987]): 81–82.

37. Marilyn Chase, "As Many as 380,000 in U.S. are Expected to Have AIDS by 1992, Researcher Says," *Wall Street Journal,* 14 June 1988, p. 8.

38. Calculated from CDC, "HIV Infection in the United States," p. 15.

39. Ibid., p. 41.

40. See Joel W. Hay, Dennis H. Osmond, and Mark A. Jacobson, "Projecting the Medical Costs of AIDS and ARC in the United States," *Journal of Acquired Immune Deficiency Syndromes* 1 (5 [October 1988]): 469.

41. Personal communication with Joel Hay, 10 August 1988.

42. U.S. Department of Health and Human Services, Public Health Service, "Coolfont Report: A PHS Plan for Prevention and Control of AIDS and the AIDS Virus," *Public Health Reports* 101 (4 [July–August 1986]): 341–48.

43. CDC, "Update: Acquired Immunodeficiency Syndrome—United States, 1981–1988," *MMWR* 38 (14 [14 April 1989]): 229; George W. Rutherford, Susan F. Payne, and George F. Lemp, "Impact of the Revised AIDS Case Definition on AIDS Reporting in San Francisco" (letter), *JAMA* 259 (15 [15 April 1988]): 2235.

44. Personal communication with Joel Hay, 10 August 1988.

45. Kim Painter, "450,000 AIDS Cases by 1993, Experts Say," *USA Today,* 6 June 1988, p. 1A.

46. Personal communication with James W. Curran.

47. CDC, "Quarterly Report to the Domestic Policy Counsel on the Prevalence and Rate of Spread of HIV and AIDS," *MMWR* 37 (36 [16 September 1988]): 552.

48. Abigail Trafford, "The AIDS Numbers Game," *Washington Post,* 26 July 1988, p. H6.

49. John Pickering et al., "Modeling the Incidence of Acquired Immunodeficiency Syndrome (AIDS) in San Francisco, Los Angeles, and New York," *Mathematical Modelling* 7 (5–8 [1986]): 661.

50. Ibid.

51. Personal communication with Harold Jaffe.

52. Personal communication with W. Meade Morgan, chief statistician, CDC. The numbers are roughly shown in CDC, "Quarterly Report," p. 552.

53. Personal communication with James W. Curran.

54. Diane Johnson and John F. Murray, M.D., "AIDS Without End," *New York Review of Books* 35 (13 [18 August 1988]): 57.

55. "Questionable New AIDS Book," "Nightline," transcript of 7 March 1988, p. 4.

56. For a thoroughly enjoyable discussion of the comings and goings of epidemics, see generally Hans Zinsser, *Rats, Lice and History* (Boston: Atlantic Monthly, 1963).

57. Nancy Hessol et al., "Seroconversion to HIV Among Homosexual and Bisexual Men Who Participated in Hepatitis B Vaccine Trials," IV International Conference on AIDS (Stockholm, Sweden), 12–16 June 1988, abstract 4614.

58. See Michael Specter, "AIDS Virus Likely Fatal to All Infected," *Washington Post,* 3 June 1988, p. A1, referencing Kung-Jong Lui, William W. Darrow, and George W. Rutherford III, "A Model-Based Estimate of the Mean Incubation Period for AIDS in Homosexual Men," *Science* 240 (1857 [3 June 1988]): 1333–35. But see also John Laurit-

sen, "The Epidemiology of Fear," *New York Native* 8 (4, iss. 276 [1 August 1988]): 13, where Specter's interpretation is challenged.

59. Personal communication with Mary Ellen Pesa, CDC (for AIDS cases through 1988); and CDC, "HIV/AIDS Surveillance," June 1989, p. 8 (for total cases).

60. Personal communication with Mary Ellen Pesa.

61. Department of Health (U.K.) Press Office.

62. See Duncan Campbell, "AIDS: The Race Against Time," *New Society and the New Statesman* 2 (31 [6 January 1989]): 14.

63. Steve Connor and Sharon Kingman, "AIDS Cases 'Set to Grow Fifteenfold,'" *New Scientist* 120 (1641 [3 December 1988]): 23.

64. Personal communication.

65. "Enter the AIDS Pandemic," *Time* 128 (22 [1 December 1986]): 45.

66. Personal communication, 22 July 1988.

67. Ibid.

68. Ibid.

69. Jonathan M. Mann et al., "The International Epidemiology of AIDS," *Scientific American* 259 (4 [October 1988]): 88.

70. Julie Johnson, "Bush Is Urged to Be a Leader in the Fight on AIDS," *New York Times*, 2 December 1988, p. B6.

71. "Reported AIDS Cases Almost Doubled in '88," *Washington Post* (Reuter), 5 January 1988, p. A5.

72. Ibid.

73. "The Dilemma of Resources," *WorldAIDS* 1 (1 [January 1989]): 8.

74. Daniel Q. Haney, "Report Warns of Massive AIDS Epidemic in Western Hemisphere," AP, 13 April 1989.

75. Panos Institute, *AIDS and the Third World*, 3d ed. (Philadelphia: New Society, 1988), p. 93.

76. Larry Kramer, "1,112 and Counting," *New York Native*, 14–27 March 1983, p. 18.

77. Anthony Pascal, "The Costs of Treating AIDS Under Medicaid: 1986–1991" (Santa Monica, Calif.: Rand Corporation, 1986).

78. Lewis J. Lord et al., "The Staggering Price of AIDS," *U.S. News*, 102 (23 [15 June 1987]): 16.

79. Ann M. Hardy et al., "The Economic Impact of the First 10,000 Cases of Acquired Immunodeficiency Syndrome in the United States," *JAMA* 255 (2 [10 January 1986]): 209–11.

80. Hay, Osmond, and Jacobson, "Projecting the Medical Costs of AIDS and ARC," p. 474.

81. Ibid., p. 481.

82. "AIDS," "Nightline," transcript of 9 January 1987, p. 2.

83. Personal communication with Joel Hay, 7 February 1989.

84. Dennis Altman, *AIDS in the Mind of America* (New York: Anchor/Doubleday, 1986), p. 134.

85. See Gary Bauer and John P. Walters, "AIDS Hearing" (letter), *New Republic* 199 (10, iss. 3842 [5 September 1988]): 6, for an example of an alarmist laying the groundwork for claiming that anti-alarmists were just lucky guessers.

86. "Widespread Heterosexual Epidemic Not Foreseen by Secretary of HHS," *AIDS Policy & Law* 3 (1 [27 January 1988]): 1.

87. Personal communication with Chuck Fallis, public affairs specialist, CDC AIDS program.

88. James D. Watkins et al., *Report of the Presidential Commission on the Human Immunodeficiency Virus Epidemic*, 24 June 1988.

89. National Academy of Sciences/Institute of Medicine, *Confronting AIDS: Update 1988* (Washington, D.C.: National Academy Press, 1989).

90. William A. Blattner, Book Review of Shilts, *And the Band Played On, Scientific American* 259 (4 [October 1988]): 148.

91. Theresa L. Crenshaw, "Speaking Out on AIDS: A Humanist Symposium," *The Humanist* 47 (4 [July–August 1987]): 22.

92. "AIDS May Dwarf the Plague," *New York Times,* 30 January 1987, p. A24.
93. Richard Goldstein, "Heartsick: Fear and Loving in the Gay Community," *Village Voice* 28 (26 [28 June 1983]), as cited in Simon Watney, *Policing Desire* (Minneapolis: University of Minnesota Press, 1987), p. 13.

Chapter 22. The AIDS Lobby: Are We Giving It Too Much Money?

1. Susan Okie, "Assessing the War on Cancer," *Washington Post,* 22 August 1988, p. A13.
2. Spending figures are for fiscal year 1989, were allocated in the Labor, Health and Human Services and Education Appropriations Act of 1989, and were relayed to me by the Health and Human Services and Education Subcommittee. Cancer and heart disease death rates are from the Bureau of the Census.
3. Susan Okie, "Cutbacks, AIDS Emphasis Seen Slowing Cancer Fight," *Washington Post,* 28 December 1988, p. A9.
4. Stephen Dilsaver and Jeffrey Coffman, "Are We Spending Too Much Money on AIDS?" *The Scientist* 2 (11 July 1988): 11.
5. Okie, "Cutbacks," p. A9.
6. William Booth, "No Longer Ignored, AIDS Funds Just Keep Growing," *Science* 242 (4880 [11 November 1988]): 859.
7. Figures for federal patient costs are from a personal communication with Hay.
8. "Major AIDS Study on Drug-free Heterosexuals," AP, 16 December 1988.
9. Daniel Perry and Robert N. Butler, "Aim Not Just for Longer Life, But Extended 'Health Span,'" *Washington Post,* 20 December 1988, p. H20.
10. "Kaposi's Sarcoma and Related Opportunistic Infection," hearings before House of Representatives Subcommittee on Health and the Environment, 13 April 1982, p. 2, as cited in Dennis Altman, *AIDS in the Mind of America* (New York: Anchor/Doubleday, 1986), p. 113.
11. Altman, *AIDS in the Mind of America,* p. 190.

Chapter 24. The 1989 Montreal Conference on Aids

1. Marilyn Chase, "Activists Steal Show at AIDS Conference," *Wall Street Journal,* 12 June 1989, p. B4.
2. Ibid.
3. Ibid.
4. Randy Shilts, "Invisible Ink," *Seven Days* 2 (22 [7 June 1989]): 7.
5. Robert Wood et al., "Predicting HIV Risk Behaviors Among Gay Men," V International Conference on AIDS (Montreal, Canada), 5–9 June 1989, abstract M.D.P.35, p. 716.
6. Marilyn Chase, "U.S. Weighs New Program to Fight AIDS," *Wall Street Journal,* 1 June 1989, p. B4.
7. This figure obtained from the Surveillance, Epidemiology, and End Result Office of the National Cancer Institute.
8. See American Cancer Society, *Cancer Facts and Figures* (Atlanta: American Cancer Society, 1989), p. 10.
9. This is the same argument I have used against mandatory testing. There is no reason to assume that persons forced to learn their test results will act as altruistically as those who voluntarily receive their results. See Michael Fumento, "Chicken Little with a Hypodermic," *Reason* 20 (6 [November 1988]): 30.
10. Chase, "U.S. Weighs New Program," p. B4.
11. Timothy J. Dondero et al., "Evaluation of the Estimated Number of HIV Infections Using a Spreadsheet Model and Empirical Data," V Intl. Conf. on AIDS, abstract M.A.O.4, p. 45.
12. Kim Painter, "Best Guess at AIDS in USA: 1.5M," *USA Today,* 6 June 1989, p. 1A.
13. Personal communication with Joel Hay, 20 June 1989.
14. Joel W. Hay, "AIDS Infection Data Difficult to Refute" (letter), *Wall Street Journal,* 28 May 1989, p. A15, referencing W. Meade Morgan, "Comments for the Forecast-

Appendix A

1. Charles Perrow & Mauro F. Guillén, *The AIDS Disaster* (New Haven and London, Yale University Press, 1990), pp. 181–183.

2. CDC, "HIV/AIDS Surveillance," February 1993, p. 9, table 3.

3. John Pekkanen, "Are We Closing in on AIDS?" *Reader's Digest* 135 (12[December 1989]): 80.

4. World Health Organization, "WHO Revises Global Estimates of HIV Infection" (press release), 31 July 1990, p. 1.

5. Marlene Cimons, "'Alarming' Increase in AIDS Reported," *Los Angeles Times*, 13 June 1990, p. A1.

6. CDC, "Estimates of HIV Prevalence and Projected AIDS Cases: Summary of a Workshop, October 31—November 1, 1989, *MMWR* 39 (110 [23 February 1990]): 110.

7. "Fifth of World May Have AIDS in Next Century Expert Says," *Reuters*, 14 December 1992.

8. Gene Antonio, *AIDS: Rage and Reality* (Arlington, Tex.: Anchor, 1993).

9. Geoffrey Cowley, Mary Hager, and Ruth Marshall, "AIDS: The Next Ten Years," *Newsweek* 115 (26 [25 June 1990]): 21.

10. (London) *Daily Mail*, 10 January 1985.

11. *Doctor*, 1 August 1985.

12. (London) *Daily Telegraph*, 5 December 1986.

13. Department of Health (United Kingdom), Quarterly AIDS Figures, 21 January 1991, ref. no. H-91/22.

14. Christine Doyle, "AIDS: A Timely Warning—or Crying Wolf?" *Daily Telegraph*, 16 February 1990, p. 17.

15. Victoria Macdonald, "Cuts Hit Fight Against AIDS,"(London)*Sunday Telegraph*, 22 November 1992; for a perspective on the British AIDS hoax, *see*, Robert Whelan, "The AIDS Scandal," *Economic Affairs* 11 (4 June 1991, p. 16) or Susil Gupta, "The AIDS Hoax," *Analysis*, 1 (1 [January 1992]): 22.

16. Steve Connor, "Spreading the Notion that Lifestyle, not a Virus, is to Blame," *The Independent*, 21 May 1993, p. 6.

17. Liz Hunt, "AIDS Cases 'Could be Fewer than Predicted,'" *The Independent*, 8 June 1993, p. 2.

18. Dunstan McNichol, "Shalala Tells Congress America Will Perish if AIDS Crisis is Ignored," States News Service, 3 February 1993.

19. Robert Steinbrook, "Slower Spread of AIDS in Gays Seen Nationally," *Los Angeles Times* 5 January 1990, p. 1; Philip J. Hilts, "Forecast of AIDS Cases is Cut by 10 Percent," *New York Times*, 4 January 1990, p. D20.

20. CDC, "Estimates of HIV Prevalence and Projected AIDS Cases: Summary of a Workshop, October 31—November 1, 1989," *MMWR* 39 (110 [23 February 1990]): 110.

21. Kevin R. Hopkins, "Business May Harm the Real AIDS Fight," *USA Today*, 28 March 1990, p. 8A.

22. CDC, "Projections of the Number of Persons Diagnosed with AIDS and the Number of Immunosuppressed HIV-Infected Persons—United States, 1992–94," *MMWR* 41 (RR-18 [25 December 1992]): 8; *see also*, "U.S. Says Spread of AIDS to Slow," *New York Times*, 15 January 1993, p. A8.

23. CDC, "Projections," p. 5.

24. Joseph Palca, "Is the AIDS Epidemic Slowing?" *Science*, 246 (4937 [22 December 1989]): 1560.

25. Calculated from CDC case data.

26. Ibid.

27. Michael Fumento, "AIDS So Far," *Commentary* 92(6[December 1991]): 46.

28. Elizabeth M. Whelan, "Fringe of Science" (letter), *Policy Review* 54(Fall 1990): 70.

29. Jean Pierre Aboulker and Ann Marie Swart, "Preliminary Analysis of the Concorde Trial," (letter) *Lancet* 341 (8849 [3 April 1993]): 889; *see also*, Lawrence K. Altman, "New Study Questions Use of AZT in Early Treatment of AIDS Virus," *New York Times*, 2 April

1993, p. A1, and David Brown, "Popular U.S. Treatment for HIV is Challenged by European Study," *Washington Post*, 9 June 1993, p. A4.

30. *See*, CDC, *MMWR* 36 (S-6 [18 December 1987]): table 12, p. 38, and figure 13, p. 48.

31. CNN's "Late Night with Dennis Wholley," 17 February 1990.

32. Gregg Easterbrook, "Antonia Novella," *Los Angeles Times*, 12 January 1992, p. M3.

33. Steinbrook, p. 1.

34. Maurice Chittenden, "AIDS Author Claims British Blacklist," *Sunday Times* (London), 11 February 1990.

35. Roy M. Anderson *et al.*, "The Significance of Sexual Partner Contact Networks for the Transmission Dynamics of HIV," *Journal of Acquired Immune Deficiency Syndromes*, 3 (4 [April 1990]): 418.

36. CDC, "HIV/AIDS Surveillance," February 1993, p. 6, table one and other pages.

37. Ibid., January 1992, p. 6, table one, and other pages.

38. NBC's "The Today Show," 23 January 1993.

39. Easterbrook, p. M3.

40. CBS Evening News, 11 June 1993.

41. CDC, "HIV/AIDS Surveillance," February 1993, p. 9, table 3.

42. Ibid., p. 9, table 3.

43. Ibid., February 1993, p. 9, table 3.

44. CDC, "HIV/AIDS Surveillance Report," January 1992, page 9, table 3.

45. Calculated from the National Opinion Research Center (Chicago) polls of 1988–1992 (2.5 percent of all men claim to have had homosexual relations in the past year), the "National Household Survey on Drug Abuse" (1991) of the National Institute of Drug Abuse (1.9 percent of Americans claim to have injected illegal drugs), and CDC, "HIV/AIDS Surveillance Report," February 1993, p. 9, table 3.

46. Calculating from National Cancer Institute data on cancer deaths (approximately 500,000 a year) and the National Opinion Research Center polls on sexual preference (97.5 percent of the population heterosexual), equals 1,335 heterosexual cancer deaths a day.

47. About 43,000 women will die of breast cancer this year, according to the National Cancer Institute.

48. National Commission on AIDS, p. 154.

49. Gina Kolata, "Targeting Urged in Attack on AIDS," *New York Times*, 7 March 1993, p. 16.

50. CDC, "HIV/AIDS Surveillance," January 1990, January 1991, January 1992, February 1993, p. 8, table 2.

51. CDC, *National HIV Serosurveillance Summary: Results Through 1990*, (Atlanta: Centers for Disease Control, June 1992), pp. 2–3.

52. Ibid., p. 8.

53. Ibid., p. 18, figure 6.

54. CDC, "HIV/AIDS Surveillance," February 1993, p. 4, figures 2 and 3.

55. Ibid., p. 3.

56. Ibid., p. 23, figure 14.

57. Ibid., p. 21, figure 11.

58. Ibid., p. 4.

59. Nancy Padian, S. Shiboski, and N. Jewell, "Female-to-Male Transmission of the Human Immunodeficiency Virus," *JAMA* 266 (12 [25 September 1991]): 1664.

60. Okey C. Nwanyanwu *et al.*, "Increasing Frequency of Heterosexually Transmitted AIDS in Southern Florida: Artifact or Reality?" *American Journal of Public Health* 83 (4 [April 1993]): 571.

61. Personal communication with Carol A. Ciesielski. Ciesielski was a co-author.

62. Nwanyanwu *et al.*, p. 572.

63. CDC, "HIV/AIDS Surveillance," February 1993, p. 11, table 5.

64. CNN News Night, 28 November 1991.

65. Pico Iyer, "It Can Happen to Anybody. Even Magic Johnson," *Time* 138 (20 [18 November 1991]): 26.

66. Laurie Garrett, *Newsday*, 10 November 1991, p. 3.

67. CDC, "HIV/Surveillance," January 1992, p. 9, table three.

68. Charles Leerhsen *et al.*, "Magic's Message," p. 61.

69. Jerry Adler *et al.*, "Living with the Virus," *Newsweek* 21 (118 [18 November 1991]): 84.

70. Marilyn Chase, "Johnson Disclosure Underscores Facts of AIDS in Heterosexual Population," *Wall Street Journal*, November 11, 1991, p. B.

71. Charles Leerhsen *et al.*, "Magic's Message," p. 60.

72. "A Critical Need for Magic" (editorial), *Chicago Tribune*, 18 November 1991, p. 18.

73. *Newsweek* began its article about the Johnson's revelation, "It was an event that evoked the old Kennedy assassination question, 'Where were you when you heard the news'?" *See*, Charles Leerhsen *et al.*, "Magic's Message," 58.

74. Earvin Johnson, as told to Roy S. Johnson, "I'll Deal with It," *Sports Illustrated* 75 (22 [18 November 1991]): 25.

75. As quoted in "Magic Raises AIDS Consciousness," *The Outlook* (Santa Monica, California), p. 1.

76. William A. Henry III, "A Synonym for Glorious Excess," *Time* 129 (7 [16 February 1987]): 82.

77. Thomas Bonk, "Magic Answers the Rumors Again," *Los Angeles Times*, 24 October 1991, p. C8.

78. Bruce Horovitz, "Sidelined; Sponsors Reconsider Magic Johnson Ads," *Los Angeles Times*, 28 December 1991, p. D1.

79. David Streitfeld, "Magic's Story: $4 Million and Counting," *Washington Post*, 26 November 1991, p. B1.

80. Mark Heisler, "Magic Johnson's Career Ended by HIV-Positive Test," *Los Angeles Times*, 8 November 1991, p. 1.

81. "Navratilova Slams Magic for Promiscuity, Sees Double Standard," *Reuters*, 20 November 1991.

82. *See*, Michael Specter and Richard Pearson, "Rep. Stewart B. McKinney Dies of AIDS Complications," *Washington Post*, 8 May 1987, p. A1.

83. Clifford D. May, "Friends say McKinney had Homosexual Sex," *New York Times*, 8 May 1987, Sec. 2, p. 33.

84. Howard Kurtz, "You Can't Date City Hall; Chicago Reporter is Out of a Job," *Washington Post*, 16 November 1991, p. D1.

85. Paul Pringle, "Abstinence Best Policy, Quayle Says," *Outlook* (Santa Monica), 9 November 1991, p. A10.

86. Magic Johnson and Roy S. Johnson, p. 21.

87. Charles Leerhsen *et al*, "Magic's Message," p. 58.

88. Tom Callahan, "Stunned by Magic," *US News & World Report* 3 (21 [18 November 1991]):83.

89. Gene Herd, "Magic Johnson Confronts AIDS," *Los Angeles Times*, November 13, 1991, p. B6.

90. Michael Fumento, "Do You Believe in Magic," *American Spectator*, 25 (2 [February 1992]: 16.

91. Dave Kindred, "Magic Should Face Reality," *Sporting News*, October 12, 1992, p. 7.

92. *See*, David Aldridge, "Nothing Magic about Gossiping," *Washington Post*, 27 October 1992, p. E7.

93. Fred Kerber, "Magic Slam Dunks Rumors," *New York Post*, 22 October 1992.

94. Peter Vecsey, "Magic Has Better Things to Do," *USA Today*, 27 October 1992, p. 5C.

95. Elliot Almond, "There are No Simple Explanations," *Los Angeles Times*, 3 November 1992, p. C1.

96. Alex S. Jones, "Reports of Ashe's Illness Raise Old Issue for Newspaper Editors," *New York Times*, April 10, 1992, p. A15.

97. "Why Arthur Ashe Kept it Secret" (editorial), *New York Times*, 10 April 1992, p. A36.

98. Victor F. Zonana, "Ashe Case Raises Fame vs. Privacy Debate," *New York Times*, April 10, 1992, p. A20.

99. "Why Arthur Ashe Kept it Secret," p. A36.

100. Haynes W. Sheppard *et al.*, "Effect of New AIDS Case Definition on Numbers of

Cases Among Homosexual and Bisexual Men in San Francisco" (letter) *JAMA* 266 (16 [23–30 October 1991]): 2221.

101. Ibid., p. 8.

102. CDC, "HIV/AIDS Surveillance," January 1992; April 1992; February 1993; May 1993, tables 8.

103. CDC, "1993 Revised Classification System for HIV Infection and Expanded Surveillance Case Definition for AIDS Among Adolescents and Adults," p. 4.

104. Lauran Neergaard, "CDC Bows to Activists, Adds New Diseases to Proposed AIDS Definition," *Associated Press*, October 27, 1992.

105. George M. Carter, "ACT-UP, the AIDS War & Activism" (Westfield, New Jersey: Open Magazine Pamphlet Series, January 1992), p. 5.

106. Easterbrook, p. M3.

107. CBS Evening News, 20 April 1992.

108. CDC, "HIV/AIDS Surveillance," January 1992, p. 9, table 3.

109. Ibid., p. 9, table 3.

110. CDC, "HIV/AIDS Surveillance," February 1993, p. 9, table 3.

111. Antonia C. Novella, "A Woman-to-Woman Call to Arms," *Los Angeles Times*, 29 June 1993, p. B7.

112. Boyce Rensberger, "AIDS Spreads Among Young Women," *Washington Post*, 29 July 1993, p. A1.

113. "Women and AIDS," *USA Today*, 27 November 1991, p. D1.

114. Ed Parsons, "Women Become Top U.S. AIDS Risk Group" (letter), *New York Times*, 18 November 1991, p. A14.

115. "AIDS Test," *New York Times*, 16 August 1992, sec. 9 (Styles), p. 1 and chart, p. 10.

116. CDC, "HIV/AIDS Surveillance," February 1993, p. 11, table 5.

117. "The Top Ten Health Trends," *U.S. News & World Report* 112 (17 [4 May 1992]): 95.

118. Dolores Kong, "AIDS Runs Wild Among Teenagers," *Honolulu Star-Bulletin*, 14 April 1992, p. 1.

119. Barbara Kantrowitz *et al.*, "Teenagers and AIDS," *Newsweek*, 120 (5 [3 August 1992]): cover and p. 45.

120. News Conference, 26 March 1992, transcript available from Federal Information Systems Corporation, Federal News Service, Washington, D.C.

121. Select Committee on Children, Youth and Families, "A Decade of Denial: Teens and AIDS in America" (Washington, D.C.: Government Printing Office, May 1992), (GPO 55–439): 2; *see also*, "House Panel Says U.S. Ignores the AIDS Risk Faced by Teen-Agers," *New York Times*, 13 April 1992, p. A9.

122. Select Committee on Children, Youth and Families, p. 1.

123. Ibid., p. 5.

124. Scott Williams, "Show About AIDS Among Teens Very Scary," *Associated Press*, 18 September 1991.

125. Marlene Cimons, "Aim AIDS Prevention at Youth, National Panel Advises," *Los Angeles Times*, 3 June 1993, p. A9.

126. CDC, "HIV/AIDS Surveillance," January 1992, op. cit. (The table actually states 160 cases for 1991 but this was revised downward by one case in the next annual report.)

127. Ibid.

128. Ibid.

129. CDC, "HIV/AIDS Surveillance," February 1993, p. 12, table 6.

130. Personal communication, National Center for Health Statistics.

131. National Safety Council, *Accident Facts* (Itasca, Ill.: National Safety Council, 1992), p. 52.

132. Nancy Gibbs, "Teens: The Rising Risk of AIDS," *Time* 138 (9 [2 September 1991]): 60.

133. CDC, "HIV/AIDS Surveillance," Jan. 1990 and Feb. 1993, p. 12, table 6.

134. Ibid., February 1993, p. 12, table 6 and p. 9, table 3. Teen cases were 0.33 percent of all AIDS cases in 1992 compared to 0.35 percent in 1991. Cases in those age 20 to 24 were 3.2 percent of the total in 1991 and 3.0 percent in 1992.

135. CDC, "HIV/AIDS Surveillance," February 1993, p. 13, table 7.

136. Ibid., p. 12, table 6.

137. Ibid., February 1993, p. 14, table 8.

138. Donald S. Burke *et al.*, "Human Immunodeficiency Virus Infections in Teenagers," *JAMA* 263 (15 [18 April 1990]): 2077, table 6. (April 1988-March 1989).

139. Ibid., p. 2075, table 2.

140. CDC, "National HIV Serosurveillance Summary," p. 3.

141. CNN News Night, 28 November 1990.

142. Helene D. Gayle *et al.*, "Prevalence of the Human Immunodeficiency Virus among University Students," *New England Journal of Medicine* 323 (22 [29 November 1990]): 1538.

143. WGBH-TV Boston, "AIDS in the Shadow of Love: A Teen AIDS Story," Judith Stoia, executive producer, original air date on PBS 18 September 1991.

144. Williams, "Show About AIDS Among Teens Very Scary."

145. Scott Williams, "'In the Shadow of Love: A Teen AIDS Story' on PBS, ABC," *Associated Press*, 18 September 1991.

146. John Koch, "Enlightening 'In the Shadow of Love' Packs a Powerful Punch," *Boston Globe*, 18 September 1991, p. 78.

147. Lynne Hefley, "TV Review: An AIDS Resource for Teens," *Los Angeles Times*, 18 September 1991, p. F10.

148. John H. O'Connor, "Making AIDS a Reality with a Teen-Age Drama," *New York Times*, p. C18.

149. Joan Hanauer, untitled, United Press International distribution to New York and New York Metro area, 18 September 1991.

150. Sandy Rovner, "TV Drama Tells Teens Harsh Facts of AIDS," *Washington Post*, 17 September 1991, p. ZB.

151. Dennis McDougal, "The Young & the Randy," *Los Angeles Times*, 18 September 1991, p. F10.

152. A.M. Rosenthal, "The Price of Vendetta," *New York Times*, March 19, 1990, Sec. 4, p. 19.

153. Jonathan Mann, Daniel J.M. Tarantola, and Thomas W. Netter, eds. *AIDS in the World* (Cambridge, Mass.: Harvard University Press, 1992) unnumbered page, towards beginning.

154. "Harvard-based AIDS Study Sets Stage for Advanced Global Mobilization," *U.S. Newswire*, 30 November 1992.

155. "AIDS—Ein Kontinent vor dem Abgrund," ("AIDS-A Continent Before the Abyss"), *Der Spiegel*, 18 (47 [3 May 1993]): 1993, cover and p. 172.

156. Jonathan Mann, Daniel J.M. Tarantola, and Thomas W. Netter, eds., p. 886, tables 2.3A and 2.3B.

157. Ibid., p. 874.

158. Chris Mihill, "Spread of AIDS May Now Be Beyond Control," *Manchester (England) Guardian Weekly*, 7 February 1993, p. 11.

159. "Leading Authority Says Fight Against AIDS has Stalled," *Reuters*, 11 December 1992.

160. Jacqueline Frank, "World AIDS Experts Fear Disease Out of Control," *Reuters*, 30 November 1992.

161. Daniel Tarantola and Jonathan Mann, "Coming to Terms with the AIDS Pandemic," *Issues in Science and Technology*, Spring 1993, p. 43.

162. CDC, "Premarital Sexual Experience Among Adolescent Women—United States, 1970–1988," *Morbidity and Mortality Weekly Report*, 39 (51 & 52 [4 January 1991]): 929.

163. Barbara A. DeBueno, Stephen H. Zinner, and Maxim Daamen, *et al.*, "Sexual Behavior of College Women in 1975, 1986, and 1989," *New England Journal of Medicine* 322 (12 [22 March 1990]): 824; *see also*, Freya L. Sonenstein, Joseph H. Pleck, and Leighton C. Ku, "Sexual Activity, Condom Use and AIDS Awareness Among Adolescent Males," *Family Planning Perspectives* 21 (4 [July-August 1989]): 152.

164. Noni E. MacDonald, *et al.*, "High-Risk STD/HIV Behavior among College Students," *JAMA* 263 (23 [20 June 1990]): 3155.

165. "Driving the Message Home" (editorial), *Los Angeles Times*, 9 June 1993, p. B6.

166. Ron Stall, *et al.*, "Relapse from Safer Sex: The AIDS Behavioral Research Project," VI International Conference on AIDS, abstract Th.C. 108, p. 160.

167. CDC, "Trends in Gonorrhea in Homosexual Active Men—King County, Washington, 1989," *Morbidity and Mortality Weekly Report* 38 (44 [10 November 1989]): 763.

168. "Study Finds Significant Number of Young Gay Men Practicing Unsafe Sex," *Business Wire*, 9 June 1993. For further information, contact Ruthann Richter, University of California, San Francisco, 415–476–3804.

169. David Gelman, *et al.*, "The Young and the Reckless," *Newsweek* 121 (3 [11 January 1993]): 60.

170. Allan M. Brandt, *No Magic Bullet* (New York: Oxford University Press, 1985), p. 129.

171. CDC, "Sexually Transmitted Disease Surveillance 1991," June 1991, p. 152, Table 5B.

172. CDC, "HIV/AIDS Surveillance," February 1993, p. 10, table 4, and page 11, table 5.

173. Ibid.

174. CDC, "HIV/AIDS Surveillance," February 1993, p. 11, table 5.

175. John G. McNeil, *et al.*, "Trends of HIV Seroconversion Among Young Adults in the U.S. Army, 1985 to 1989," *JAMA* 265 (13 [3 April]): 1711. Note especially figures 2 and 3.

176. CDC, "HIV/AIDS Surveillance," February 1993, p. 10, table 4.

177. *See* Arthur Hu, "How Much AIDS?" *Asian Week* 12 (36 [19 April 1991]): 10.

178. CDC, "HIV/AIDS Surveillance," February 1993, p. 10, table 4.

179. Jeff Fast, "Shanti to Quit Housing PWAs," *Bay Area Reporter*, 20 May 1993, p. 1. *See also*, Jeff Fast, "Shanti 'On Probation' Says City AIDS Office," *Bay Area Reporter*, 27 May 1993, p. 1.

180. James Gliden, "Yeah, a Gay Disease. So What?" *Washington Blade* 24 (15 [9 April 1993]): 45.

181. "Ad Group to Fight AIDS," *Wall Street Journal*, 9 May 1991, p. 35.

182. Kevin Goldman, "TV Starts to 'Just Say No' to Antidrug Ads," *Wall Street Journal*, 30 April 1993, p. B3.

183. Scott Harris, "Johnson Brings New Stature to AIDS Funding," *Los Angeles Times*, 13 November 1991, p. A1.

184. *For example*, Shari Roan, "Long Hard Fight Still Seen Before Cancer is Conquered," *Los Angeles Times*, 13 November 1991, p. A1; Shari Roan, "Bold New Approaches Explored in Hunt for Clues to Prevention," *Los Angeles Times*, 13 November 1991, p. A14. *See especially*, box on page A16 "Advances in Treatment."

185. Marlene Cimons, "Advisory Panel Bemoans Lack of Funding for Cancer Research," *Los Angeles Times*, 13 November 1991, p. A15.

186. Marlene Cimons, " 'We Can Do Better,' AIDS Commission Pleads in its Final Report," *Los Angeles Times*, 29 June 1993, p. A13.

187. James Risen, "Clinton's Budget Seeks $1.5 Trillion," *Los Angeles Times*, 9 April 1993, p. A20.

188. Wendy Melillo, "Whatever Happened to AIDS?; The National Commission Prepares a Status Report of the Epidemic," *Washington Post*, 24 September 1991, p. Z10.

189. Warren King, "AIDS Battle Loses Focus, Expert Says—Health Workers Called Unfair Targets," *Seattle Times*, 5 October 1991, p. A8.

Appendix B

1. Craig Wilson and Kim Painter, "Counting the AIDS Losses after Nine Years," *USA Today*, 19 June 1990, p. 1D.

2. CDC, "HIV/AIDS Surveillance," February 1993, p. 9, table 3.

3. Ibid., p. 14, table 8.

4. "Women and AIDS," *USA Today*, 27 November 1991, p. D1.

5. Ed Parsons, "Women Become Top U.S. AIDS Risk Group" (letter), *New York Times*, 18 November 1991, p. A14.

6. Robert Steinbrook, "Slower Spread of AIDS in Gays Seen Nationally," *Los Angeles Times*, 5 January 1990, p. 1.

7. Roy M. Anderson *et al.*, "The Significance of Sexual Partner Contact Networks for

the Transmission Dynamics of HIV," *Journal of Acquired Immune Deficiency Syndromes*, 3 (4 [April 1990]): 418.

8. "The Top Ten Health Trends," *U.S. News & World Report* 112 (17 [4 May 1992]): 95.

9. Dolores Kong, "AIDS Runs Wild Among Teenagers," *Honolulu Star-Bulletin*, 14 April 1992, p. 1.

10. Barbara Kantrowitz *et al.*, "Teenagers and AIDS," *Newsweek*, 120 (5 [3 August 1992]): cover and p. 45.

11. Select Committee on Children, Youth and Families, p. 1.

12. Ibid., p. 5.

13. CDC, "HIV/AIDS Surveillance Report," January 1992, p. 12, table 6; CDC, "HIV/AIDS Surveillance Report," February 1993, p. 12, table 6.

14. Donald S. Burke, *et al.*, "Human Immunodeficiency Virus Infections in Teenagers," *JAMA* 263 (15 [18 April 1990]): 2077, table 6.

15. NBC's "The Today Show," 23 January 1993.

16. Gregg Easterbrook, "Antonia Novella," *Los Angeles Times*, 12 January 1992, p. M3.

17. CDC, "HIV/AIDS Surveillance Report," February 1993, p. 6, table 1, and other pages.

18. Ibid., January 1992, p. 6, table 1, and other pages.

19. Easterbrook, p. M3.

20. CBS Evening News, 20 April 1992.

21. CDC, annual reports going by various names, currently "HIV/AIDS Surveillance."

22. CDC, "HIV/AIDS Surveillance," February 1993, p. 9, table 3.

23. CDC, "HIV/AIDS Surveillance," February 1993, p. 10, table 4.

24. Ibid., p. 10, table 4.

Grateful acknowledgement is made to the following for permission to reprint:

Figure 4.1 on p. 53, from H. Hunter Handsfield, "Heterosexual Transmission of the Human Immunodeficiency Virus," *JAMA* 260 (13 [7 October 1988]): 1944. Copyright © 1988. Reprinted with permission of the American Medical Association.

Table 5.1 on p. 64, adapted from Harvey V. Fineberg, "Education to Prevent AIDS: Prospects and Obstacles," *Science* 239 (4850 [5 February 1988]): 593. Copyright © 1988, by the AAAS.

Table 5.2 on p. 68, from Susan Okie, "Heterosexuals Told to Avoid Risky Partners," *Washington Post*, 22 April 1988. Copyright © *The Washington Post*.

Figure 21.1 on p. 315, adapted from Michael A. Fumento, "The Incredible Shrinking AIDS Epidemic," *The American Spectator* 22 (5 [May 1989]): 24. Used by permission of *The American Spectator*.

Figure 21.2A on p. 316, from Eduardo Cortes et al., "HIV-I, HIV-II, and HTLV-I Infection in High-Risk Groups in Brazil," *NEJM* 320 (15 [13 April 1989]): 1006. Reprinted by permission of the *New England Journal of Medicine*.

Figure 21.2B on p. 316, from the Panos Institute, *AIDS in the Third World*, 3d ed. (Philadelphia: New Society, 1988), p. 128. Used by permission of the Panos Institute.

INDEX
